Clinical Medicine and Healthcare

Clinical Medicine and Healthcare

Editor: Maxim Clement

AMERICAN
MEDICAL PUBLISHERS
www.americanmedicalpublishers.com

AMERICAN
MEDICAL PUBLISHERS
www.americanmedicalpublishers.com

Cataloging-in-Publication Data

Clinical medicine and healthcare / edited by Maxim Clement.
p. cm.
Includes bibliographical references and index.
ISBN 978-1-63927-637-0
1. Clinical medicine. 2. Medical care. 3. Medicine. 4. Public health. I. Clement, Maxim.
RC48 .C55 2023
616--dc23

American Medical Publishers,
41 Flatbush Avenue,
1st Floor, New York,
NY 11217, USA

ISBN 978-1-63927-637-0 (Hardback)

Contents

Preface

Over the recent decade, advancements and applications have progressed exponentially. This has led to the increased interest in this field and projects are being conducted to enhance knowledge. The main objective of this book is to present some of the critical challenges and provide insights into possible solutions. This book will answer the varied questions that arise in the field and also provide an increased scope for furthering studies.

Clinical medicine is a field of medicine that deals primarily with the practice and study of medicine based on the direct examination of the patient. This field is concerned with the assessment of patients that includes diagnosis, treatment and prevention of a disease. There are a range of diagnostic devices such as stethoscope, thermometer, tongue depressor, etc. used for the physical examination of a patient. In the field of clinical medicine, a number of medical diagnostic techniques and examinations such as blood tests, biopsy, ultrasound, CT scan, MRI, X-ray, etc. are performed to assess the type and severity of a disease. The data collected from tests and physical examination is used to prescribe appropriate treatments such as medications, therapies and surgeries. This book is compiled in such a manner, that it will provide in-depth knowledge about clinical medicine and healthcare. A number of latest researches have been included to keep the readers up-to-date with the global concepts in this area of medicine. The book will serve as a valuable source of reference for graduate and post graduate students.

I hope that this book, with its visionary approach, will be a valuable addition and will promote interest among readers. Each of the authors has provided their extraordinary competence in their specific fields by providing different perspectives as they come from diverse nations and regions. I thank them for their contributions.

Editor

1

Three Drug Combinations in the Treatment of Fit Elderly Multiple Myeloma Patients

Hélène Gardeney [1], Arthur Bobin [1], Cécile Gruchet [1], Florence Sabirou [1], Anthony Lévy [1], Laly Nsiala [1], Laura Cailly [1], Cécile Tomowiak [1], Jose Torregrosa [1], Niels Moya [1], Cyrille Hulin [2], Xavier Leleu [1,3,*] and Stéphanie Guidez [1]

1 Service d'Hematologie et Therapie Cellulaire, and Inserm CIC U1402, 86000 Poitiers, France; helene.gardeney@gmail.com (H.G.); arthur.bobin@gmail.com (A.B.); cecile.gruchet@gmail.com (C.G.); sabirou.florence@hotmail.fr (F.S.); anthonyfoot90@hotmail.fr (A.L.); Lalynsiala@hotmail.fr (L.N.); Laura.cailly20@gmail.com (L.C.); Cecile.TOMOWIAK@chu-poitiers.fr (C.T.); Jose-Miguel.TORREGROSA-DIAZ@chu-poitiers.fr (J.T.); niels.moya@gmail.com (N.M.); Stephanie.GUIDEZ@chu-poitiers.fr (S.G.)

2 Service d'Hématologie et de Thérapie Cellulaire, CHU de Bordeaux, 33000 Bordeaux, France; Cyrille.hulin@chu-bordeaux.fr

3 Service d'Hématologie et Thérapie Cellulaire, Universite de Medecine et Pharmacie, 33000 Poitiers, France

* Correspondence: xavier.leleu@chu-poitiers.fr

Abstract: The multiple myeloma (MM) non transplant eligible (NTE) population is growing in line with the aging of the population in Western countries. Historically, this population has been known for having a greater risk of treatment related toxicity, and therefore drug development was slow and rather oriented towards the improvement of safety profile than the optimization of disease control. However, NTE MM patients, at least for the fit/non frail patients in recent years, seemed to have benefited more from a less palliative care to improve the depth of response and then prolong survival. NTE MM being a quite heterogeneous population, there are still a number of groups of patients that are in need of more efficient therapy, avoiding unnecessary toxicity, particularly for the frail patients. The use of triplet regimen with a melphalan-prednisone (MP) backbone has long been the standard of care for NTE MM, often dedicated to non-frail patients. New standards of care, triplet, and even quadruplet combinations, are emerging on the basis of the MP backbone but also on the more recently approved lenalidomide-dexamethasone (Rd) backbone. These developments were largely possible in line with the development of antibody-based immunotherapies (IT) in MM. The objective to improve outcomes with an acceptable safety profile will see other key therapeutic developments such as the dropping of dexamethasone early in the disease course or various attempts to allow permanent treatment discontinuation with a prolonged disease control. In that context, it is possible that immunomonitoring, minimal residual disease (MRD), and genomic risk-adaptation will become key elements of the treatment decisions on triplet-based regimens.

Keywords: elderly; multiple myeloma; treatment; frailty; survival

---

1. Introduction

Multiple myeloma (MM) typically develops among elderly patients with a median age at diagnosis of 70 years old, with an increased incidence with age. At the time of diagnosis 26% of MM patients are between 65 and 74 years old, increasing to 37% above 75 years old [1]. The prevalence of MM is expected to rise in the foreseeable future because of an aging population in Western countries and new therapeutic options have led to a longer survival of elderly MM patients [2]. Therefore, the percentage of elderly and very elderly patients with MM is expected to rise significantly.

MM, a hematologic cancer characterized by malignant proliferation of plasma cells in the bone marrow is an incurable neoplasm, and as such the main goal for MM patients is to improve survival without a negative impact of treatments on the quality of life (QoL). Although the overall survival (OS) of elderly MM has improved with the advent of proteasome inhibitors (PI) and immunomodulatory drugs (IMIDs), advanced age / frailty remains a poor prognostic factor [3]. There is no evidence to support a different biology causing a worse prognostic in elderly MM. Indeed, looking at "high risk" MM (HRMM) defined by cytogenetic abnormalities, the incidence rate of t(4;14) is less frequent with aging (14% in ≤65, 10.9% between 66 and 74 and 8.3% in ≥75 years old), and the rate of del17p similar across age categories, around 6% [4].

The inferior outcome of elderly patients seems rather to be related to the frequency of frailty factors due to aging (comorbidities and polymedication, decreased physiological reserve, cognitive impairment) [5], all leading to an increased risk of treatment related toxicity. It is therefore impossible for most elderly newly diagnosed multiple myeloma (NDMM) patients to undergo an intensive treatment like triplet induction regimen followed by autologous stem cell transplant (ASCT), the current standard of care for younger MM transplant eligible patients. These patients are thus called non transplant eligible (NTE) rather than elderly MM.

Nevertheless, NTE is quite a diverse group of patients, with very heterogenous characteristics and various degrees of impaired function and numbers of coexisting comorbidities. Consequently, the biggest challenges in the care of NTE MM are to identify and characterize the degree of frailty, in order to determine the optimal treatment approach, a balance between safety profile and disease control. Further drug development is needed to ultimately reach an optimal safety/efficacity balance allowing no dose reduction across NTE MM patients whatever their frailty score. The development of immunotherapy has led to this path.

2. Frailty Scores for NTE MM

The assessment of the patients' fitness or frailty associated with advanced aging is key to the treatment selection for NTE MM. Historically, treatment selection was based upon chronological age with the traditional cut-off of 65 years old and performance status quoted with the Karnofsky or ECOG indexes for instance. However, the multiplication of treatment options for NTE NDMM and the variety of frailty characteristics in that population led us to stratify this population in several subgroups taking into account the heterogeneity of their overall physical condition and their treatment objectives. Thus, in recent years, the frailty assessment has become a major challenge.

In this context, the concept of personalized medicine based on patients' fitness or frailty profile emerged since the report of the European Myeloma Network in 2011 [1]. Besides clinical judgment, in order to help the physician to perform this careful geriatric evaluation, some scores specifically adapted to elderly MM have developed such as the International Myeloma Working Group Frailty Score (IMWG) [6] or the Revised Myeloma Comorbidity Index (R-MCI) [7].

The IMWG frailty score has first proposed a scoring system with a range from 0 to 5, based on age, comorbidities (quoted with Charlson comorbidity index) and the evaluation of dependence for the (instrumental) activities of daily living (ADL and IADL scores). The IMWG score has been validated in the FIRST trial [8] and fit patients had an awaited superior outcome compared to frail with a median progression free survival (PFS) of 24.0 versus 19.4 months (HR 1.36 95% CI 1.21–1.53, $p < 0.0001$) and a median OS of 70.1 versus 42.1 months (HR 1.86 95% CI 1.63–2.12, $p < 0.0001$), respectively.

On the other hand, the R-MCI takes into account age, the glomerular filtration rate (eGFR) estimated with MDRD formula, the presence of a pulmonary comorbidity and its severity, Karnofsky index, and cytogenetics.

Combining the 2 scores, it is possible to identify 3 prognostic groups in terms of risk of severe adverse events (AEs), risk of premature treatment withdrawal, progression free survival (PFS) and overall survival (OS): fit patients (IMWG score = 0, R-MCI ≤ 3), intermediate-fit (IMWG score = 1, R-MCI 4–6), or frail (IMWG score ≥ 2, R-MCI > 6). Other scores are under validation such as the

UK Myeloma Research Alliance Risk Profile (MRP) [9] or the Hematology Oncology Frailty (HOF) scores [10].

The combination of the scores indicates if a patient is able to tolerate a full dose treatment or whether dose adaptation is preferable to limit treatment related toxicity. The 2014 consensus of the IMWG [11] has proposed upfront full dose conventional triplet based chemotherapy for fit NDMM aged between 70 and 75 years old and suggested reduced-dose therapy, regardless of their age, for patients older than 75 years old (or even 80 years old) or frail patients.

However, in the studies detailed below, patients are often only divided in frail/non frail groups so data on survival are rarely available for the intermediate fit group individualized by the frailty score mentioned above.

3. Objectives to Improve Survival in NTE MM

It has been shown that reaching the best response achievable, whenever possible a complete response (CR), was associated with improved survival, including for the eldest patients (≥75 years old) [12]. One step further, the ALCYONE trial [13] confirmed the value of deepening the response in the NTE population by showing that MRD negativity is associated with a diminution of the risk of progression or death, regardless of the treatment combination. These results call for a less palliative and a more active treatment approach for fit/non frail NTE MM to improve depth of response and prolong outcomes.

Transplant ineligibility has historically been above the cut-off of 65 years old, and more recently moved closer to 70 in real-world clinical practice [14–16]. However, non-frail/fit elderly MM patients, regardless of age, might be considered for upfront triplet-based induction and even possibly followed by ASCT, similarly to younger MM patients, while being cautious with drug management to avoid dose reductions that could impact the response. Indeed, there has never been any consensual age cut-off for transplant eligibility, since biological age and overall physical condition of elderly patients can differ from chronological age. ASCT has been evaluated in a retrospective fashion in the older MM population and it was concluded that ASCT can be safely performed in selected ≥65- and even >70-year-old MM patients. It has been shown that with adequate supportive care and control of complications, namely transfusions, antibiotics, and pain killers for mucositis, toxicity is similar with no excess in transplant-related mortality as compared to a younger cohort and with non-inferior outcomes (EFS, OS) or response [14,16–18].

The exact role of ASCT in the therapeutic arsenal in the care of elderly MM patients is not clearly defined, and only "selected" MM are considered transplant eligible beyond 65, and even more so beyond 70 years of age in real life. That clearly speaks to the need to develop better therapeutic options for NTE MM, including for non-frail/fit patients. Hope lies in the recent development of triplet-based combinations of proteasome inhibitors (PI) or anti CD38 immunotherapy (IT) plus IMIDs with induction and prolonged consolidation/maintenance to achieve a deep response, ultimately MRD negativity, hopefully associated to better outcomes.

4. Triplet-Based Combinations in NTE NDMM

All the data of trials in the NTE NDMM setting is summarized in Table 1.

4.1. Historical Melphalan Prednisone-Based Strategy

MPT (melphalan-prednisone-thalidomide) [19] has historically been the first triplet regimen to be approved for NDMM NTE in first line. However, the development of **VMP** (bortezomib-melphalan-prednisone, phase III VISTA study (VMP versus MP) [20]) has slowly replaced MPT. The addition of twice weekly IV bortezomib to MP has improved OS by 13 months and increased CR to 30% versus 4% with MP alone. The development of the sub-cutaneous (SC) bortezomib version has immediately improved the safety profile, particularly the neurotoxicity, but bortezomib can still not be given for a very prolonged time, although the continuous approach of most treatments has proved to improve survival.

Table 1. Results of trials upfront in non transplant eligible newly diagnosed multiple myeloma (NTE NDMM).

Studies	Regimen	RC (%)	MRD^{-5} (%)	PFS (Median, Months)	OS (Median, Months)	SAEs (%)	Discont (%)	High-Risk HR (95% IC)
VISTA	VMP (1)	30	/	24	56.4	91	15	/
CLARION	KMP (2)	25.9	/	22.3				/
FIRST	Rd (3)	22	/	26	59.1	/	/	1.27 (0.81–2.01)
SWOG-S0777	VRD-Rd (4)	15.7	/	43	75	/	/	/
Rd Lite	VRD-VR (5)	32	/	35.1	nr	/	4	/
IRd Kumar	IRD-I (6)	32	/	35.4	nr	52	14	/
ALCYONE	DaraVMP-D (7)	42.6	22.3	nr	nr	41.6	4.9	0.78 (0.43–1.43)
MAIA	DRd (8)	47.6	24.2	nr	nr	62.9	7.1	0.85 (0.44–1.65)

(1) VMP = Bortezomib, melphalan, prednisone. (2) KMP = Carfilzomib, melphalan, prednisone. (3) Rd = Lenalidomide, dexamethasone until progression. (4) VRD -Rd = Bortezomib, lenalidomide, dexamethasone triplet induction followed by maintenance by lenalidomide-dexamethasone until progression. (5) VRD -Rd = Bortezomib, lenalidomide, dexamethasone triplet induction followed by bortezomib-lenalidomide. (6) IRD -I = Ixazomib-lenalidomide-dexamethasone triplet induction followed by maintenance by ixazomib alone until progression. (7) DaraVMP-DaraD = Daratumumab-bortezomib-melphalan-prednisone quadruplet induction followed by maintenance by daratumumab-dexamethasone until progression. (8) DRd = Daratumumab-lenalidomide-dexamethasone until progression. CR = complete response. MRD-5 = MRD negativity at 10^{-5}. PFS = progression free survival. OS = overall survival. SAEs = serious adverse events. HR = high risk. 95%CI: confidence interval with an alpha risk of 5%. Discont. = discontinuation. Nr = not reached. Regimen = induction-maintenance.

Several attempts sought to improve the PI+ MP-based triplet combinations, starting with the CLARION study (**KMP** versus VMP) [21], evaluating the addition of carfilzomib (K), a second generation proteasome inhibitor of epoxyketone type in NTE NDMM. KMP failed to show a gain in PFS, the median PFS at 22.4 and 22.1 months respectively, $p = 0.159$. Several adjustments were proposed to improve the KMP regimen, including a greater carfilzomib dose concentration at either 20/56 or 20/70 mg/m^2 as published in the Relapsed/Refractory MM setting (RRMM) [22–24], but to date only VMP remains the approved standard of care for the NTE MM.

4.2. Lenalidomide-Dexamethasone (Rd), a More Convenient Backbone for Triplet Combinations and Continuous Approach

The final analysis of the FIRST trial [25] confirmed the superior outcome with doublet oral therapy Rd until progression over triplet oral therapy MPT with a median OS of 60 months and a median PFS of 25.5 months with a gain of 4.3 months over MPT. In addition, the safety profile of Rd was appealing with grade ≥ 3 AEs appreciably less frequent with continuous Rd than with alkylating agent based MPT (70% versus 78%) and lower rates of hematologic events and peripheral neuropathy (NP). Thus, Rd has become a standard of care since 2017, widely popular due to being entirely oral, and MPT is no longer a standard of care in NTE NDMM.

Unlike for MPT, there was no head to head randomized trial comparing Rd to VMP. A 2017 meta-analysis [26] compared Rd to different melphalan-based combinations (VMP, MPT, and MP) and was in favor of a superior activity of Rd doublet therapy until progression, with an improved OS and PFS over melphalan-containing triplet therapy. However, the Larocca et al. study [27] focusing on NTE NDMM with high-risk cytogenetics (e.g., t(4;14), t(14;16), and del17p), induction therapy including bortezomib, and thus VMP combination, has shown prolonged survival over Rd with a median OS of 62.4 versus 43.2 months, respectively (HR 0.68; 95% CI 0.47–0.96).

Thus, Rd and VMP remain the two standards of care for NTE NDMM but need to be improved. The former might become the new backbone for future triplet-based combinations gaining in convenience and ability to be given continuously but has demonstrated the lack of survival improvement for high-risk NTE NDMM, and the latter hardly can be given continuously. In that context, two options emerged: improving Rd on a triplet basis benefiting from all the convenience of this backbone or trying to further improve VMP towards a quadruplet-based regimen, but then the quadruplet agent must have a remarkable safety profile.

4.3. The Addition of a Proteasome Inhibitor (PI) to the Rd Backbone

The first Rd based triplet regimen proposed was **VRd** (bortezomib-lenalidomide-dexamethasone) based on the SWOG-S0777 trial (VRd versus Rd) [28]. It was a 2017 US phase III randomized, open label study that evaluated the VRd induction regimen administered in 21 days cycles with bortezomib twice-weekly intravenously (IV), lenalidomide 25 mg from day 1 to 14 plus 20 mg dexamethasone in NDMM without immediate ASCT planned, for 8 cycles followed by continuous Rd until progression. The median PFS was 43 months in the VRd group with a gain of 13 months compared to Rd ($p = 0.0018$) and the median OS was improved by 11 months. Among HRMM, the gain of PFS was not statistically significant even though the median PFS was 38 months with VRd versus 16 months for Rd alone. Noticeably, the median age of the study's population was 63 years old, patients being characterized as NTE for different reasons compared to "rest of the world" definition, with a greater proportion ≥ 65 in the Rd group (48% versus 38%). Finally, the improved PFS for ≥ 65 years of age in the VRd group was not statistically significant. The safety profile of this VRd regimen scheme was considered significant with 82% of AEs grade ≥ 3 for the VRd group (versus 75% in the Rd group) and around one fifth of patients (16%) had to stop treatment due to toxicity; but the increased toxicity profile is mainly due to the intravenous administration of bortezomib.

This increased toxicity led to elaborate dose adjustment with the "VRd lite" [29]. VRd induction regimen was given on 35 day cycles with bortezomib weekly SC, lenalidomide at a reduced dose of 15 mg from day 1 to day 21, and dexamethasone 20 mg. The induction regimen included 9 cycles and then patients were given consolidation with bortezomib and lenalidomide for 6 cycles; no maintenance therapy was mandatory. In this phase II study for NTE NDMM, the median age was 73 years old (range: 65–91). The primary endpoint was the overall response rate (ORR) after cycle 4 VRd and was 86%, with 66% ≥ very good partial response (VGPR), the median PFS was 35.1 months and OS was not reached. This modified bortezomib and lenalidomide schedule did not seem to negatively balance VRd's survival benefit over Rd, with excellent tolerability in a frailer population. Indeed, only 4% of patients discontinued treatment due to toxicity and 74% completed induction. With regard to neurotoxicity, NP of any grade occurred in 62% of patients but only 1 patient experienced a grade 3 NP.

Although VRd has been established as a new standard of care, improving Rd with an acceptable safety profile, it still does not appear to be the best solution when it comes to improving outcomes for patients with high-risk disease [28], including with the dose and schedule modification [30] brought by the VRd lite schema.

In order to improve the PI + Rd regimen, increase the QoL and allow more continuous approach, another triplet attempt was developed with the use of ixazomib, **IRd** (ixazomib, a boronate acid oral-based PI lenalidomide-dexamethasone). Kumar et al.'s phase I/II study [31] evaluated IRd with ixazomib given at a flat dose of 4 mg on days 1, 8, and 15 of 28 day cycles for 12 cycles followed by ixazomib alone maintenance. The ORR was 80% including 32% ≥ CR. The median PFS was 35.4 (95% CI 17.84–44.12) and in ≥65 years old, 21.4 (95% CI 12.9–46) months. Although 86% of patients experienced ≥ grade 3 AEs, dose reductions due to AEs primarily impacted R (45%) and d (38%), mainly due to fatigue, NP, and diarrhea. The dose intensity of ixazomib was preserved with 96.3% of the planned dose administered. NP of any grade was reported in 45% but with only 2 patients reporting grade 3. Treatment withdrawal due to treatment toxicity was reported in only 14% of patients. The twice-weekly 3mg ixazomib schedule studied in Richardson's phase I/II study [32] in younger patients with a median age of 63.5 years old, and not specifically NTE, demonstrated similar results overall. Sadly, the phase III, randomized, double blind, multicenter study TOURMALINE-MM2 trial (NCT01850524) evaluating IRd versus Rd in 700 NTE NDMM, did not meet its primary endpoint and failed to show a statistically significant improvement in PFS (HR, 0.83; $p = 0.073$, Takeda's recent update [33]).

In an effort to continue to improve the PI + Rd regimen, carfilzomib was also studied in association to Rd. The previous encouraging results and outcomes in RRMM based on the ASPIRE study [34], and in first line for NDMM eligible for ASCT based on the FORTE trial [35], positioned **KRd** (carfilzomib-lenalidomide-dexamethasone) as a serious option in the race to the best Rd-based triplet combination in NTE NDMM. However, the results of the ongoing phase III ENDURANCE trial [36] (E1A11, NCT01863550) comparing VRD versus KRd as induction therapy in standard risk NDMM with a median age of 65 years, appeared disappointing in that regard. Indeed, the median PFS was superimposable across the two arms with 34.4 and 34.6 months respectively (HR 1.04; 95% CI 0.8–1.3: $p = 0.74$), with no differences seen based on age, presence or absence of t(4;14), or disease stage. Three-year OS was also similar in both arms, with 84% in the VRd arm (95% CI 80–88) and 86% in the KRd arm (95% CI 82–89). Regarding the toxicity profile, only 42% of patients completed the induction protocol in the VRd arm with 299 patients over 527 who discontinued the treatment early. On the other hand, fewer patients stopped treatment in the KRd arm with 202 discontinuations but it is unknown if the difference is statistically significant. The main reasons for treatment discontinuation in the VRd arm are AEs and in first place peripheral neuropathy, which is well known to be related to the use of bortezomib and even more likely to happen knowing that bortezomib was administrated either via IV or SC. NP rates are higher with VRd with 8% compared to < 1% in KRd. However, the KRd arm experienced a significantly higher rate of cardio-pulmonary and renal toxicities (16% compared to 5% in the VRd arm) and overall grade 3–5 AEs were more frequent in the KRd arm with 44% versus 22% with VRd ($p < 0.001$). So, it is likely that the higher rate of early treatment discontinuation in the VRd arm is due to NP which has a great impact on quality of life and despite a lower rate of severe AEs compared to KRd.

As a conclusion, triplet-based Rd regimens have proved a great benefit to NTE NDMM patients, although the data were mainly available for fit/non frail patients. VRd will likely remain the main standard of care across the PI + Rd options.

5. The New Area of Immunotherapy in NTE NDMM

Monoclonal therapeutic antibodies (mAb) have been developed for years in MM, essentially based on antibody dependent cell mediated cytotoxicity (ADCC), antibody dependent cellular phagocitosis (ADPC), and specific target monoclonal antibodies (MOAs). They have always failed in MM, until the recent development of antiSLAMF7 and CD38 targeting. The first fully humanized mAb targeting CD38, daratumumab, has certainly been the most exciting and successful treatment development in MM in recent years.

5.1. Daratumumab in Quadruplet VMP-Based Regimen

The anti-CD38 mAb has originally been approved in NTE NDMM in first line based on the results of the phase III ALCYONE trial [13]. The adjunction of daratumumab to VMP for 9 cycles followed by daratumumab alone until progression resulted in a significant improvement in outcome with an estimated 18-month PFS rate of 71.6% versus 50.2% in the VMP group ($p < 0.001$). The ≥ CR rate was greater in daratumumab-VMP, 42.6% versus 24.4% ($p < 0.001$). The safety of daratumumab appeared acceptable in the NTE population with most frequent ≥ grade 3 AEs being hematological and was comparable in both groups. The rate of treatment discontinuation was lower with daratumumab-VMP (4.9% versus 9% in the control group) even if the infection rate was higher (23.1% versus 4.7%) as well as infusion-related reactions (27.7% with 5% of grade ≥ 3 of grade 4). These infusion-related reactions are usually easily manageable with appropriate pre-medication with steroids, antipyretics, and leukotrien antagonists and tend to decrease after the first administrations, explaining the low rate (1.4%) of patients that stopped daratumumab because of this event.

Given the lack of improvement brought with the use of VMP regimen in NTE NDMM patients whose standard of care status was fading slowly over the years, the remarkable results of the quadruplet

Dara-VMP regimen clearly brings VMP back into the race. However, one would still hardly believe a quadruplet regimen could be administered to all NTE patients and particularly the frail ones.

5.2. Daratumumab-Lenalidomide-Dexamethasone (DRd)

The phase III open label MAIA study [37], compared **DRd** until progression in 28 days cycles to Rd. Daratumumab was administered at a dose of 16 mg/kg once weekly during cycles 1 and 2, then every 2 weeks during cycles 3 to 6, and every 4 weeks thereafter. The median age was 73 years old (range: 45–90) with 44% ≥75 years old. Another 15% had "high risk" cytogenetic (HRMM). After a median follow-up of 28 months, the estimated 30-months PFS rate was 70.6% versus 55.6% respectively, and median PFS was not reached for daratumumab, compared to 31.9 months for Rd. The risk of disease progression or death with daratumumab was reduced by 44% (HR 0.56; 95% CI 0.43–0.73). DRd deepened the depth of the response with three times more negative MRD at 10^{-5} (24.2% vs 7.3%, respectively). This PFS benefit was also observed for ≥75-year-old patients with a HR of 0.63 (CI 95% 0.44–0.92). In contrast, the PFS benefit was less present in HRMM (HR 0.83 compared to 0.49 in standard risk). The safety profile of DRd is similar to previous data from ALCYONE [13] with mainly neutropenia (50.0% and 35.3%, respectively) and respiratory infections (13.7% and 7.9%, respectively). The infusion related reactions occurred in 41% of patients with only 3% of grade ≥ 3. The DRd triplet Rd-based combination is about to become a new standard of care upfront in NTE NDMM patients, and for now shows the best data ever reported in this population, with the exception of the HRMM population.

On a side note, a subcutaneous daratumumab infusion version will soon be available, that will clearly improve the QoL of patients, based on the phase III COLUMBA study [38] (NCT03277105). This study showed in RRMM that SC daratumumab at a flat dose of 1800 mg was not inferior to IV with a comparable safety profile. Although this study was not specifically designed for NTE NDMM patients, SC infusion would surely provide these patients a major benefit, particularly concerning QoL.

5.3. Elotuzumab, anti SLAMF7 mAb

The ongoing ELOQUENT 1 (NCT01335399) study is evaluating the adjunction of elotuzumab to the Rd backbone in NTE NDMM but it is hardly expected that its results would match those of DRd.

6. Triplet-Based Regimens in RRMM

Although no phase III studies specifically designed to compare standards of care were run in RRMM NTE patients, NTE patients are often recruited into studies performed in the RRMM setting. We have therefore synthesized some of the main data provided recently on regimens that incorporated an immunotherapy into standards of care.

The choice of therapy at each relapse is guided by the response to prior lines of treatment and noticeably whether the patient is refractory to lenalidomide.

Then, if non refractory, lenalidomide-containing regimens can be proposed at relapse. Randomized trials have already demonstrated deeper responses and improved PFS with the addition of a PI to the lenalidomide and dexamethasone doublet (Rd) in RRMM such as carfilzomib + Rd (KRD) in ASPIRE phase III study [34] (median PFS of 26.3 versus 17.6 months; HR 0.66; 95% CI 0.55–0.78 and 32% of CR versus 9%) and ixazomib + Rd (IRD) until progression in TOURMALINE-MM1 trial [39] (median PFS of 20.6 vs. 14.7 months; HR 0.74, 95%; CI 0.59–0.94).

Next, antibody containing, lenalidomide-based triplets were tested. Daratumumab + Rd (DRD) has been first investigated in RRMM patients in the POLLUX trial [40]. It has shown an impressive MRD negativity rate at 10^{-4} and 10^{-5} of 22.4% and the median PFS was not reached with DRD versus 18.4 months with Rd alone, HR 0.37 (95% CI 0.27–0.52, $p < 0.01$).

Then, anti SLAMF7 mAb elotuzumab + Rd (EloRd) was also tested in the phase III ELOQUENT 2 trial [41] with notably 20% of ≥75-year-old patients included. Median PFS with EloRd was 19.4 months (HR 0.70, 95% CI 0.57–0.85) and the benefit was persistent for ≥65-year-old patients (HR 0.65, 95% CI

0.5–0.85). In addition, EloRd was well tolerated in a population with renal impairment [42], particularly useful in the comorbid elderly MM population.

Pomalidomide has shown to be a solid backbone for combinations at relapse for RRMM refractory to lenalidomide or if lenalidomide has been previously poorly tolerated.

Similarly to Rd, a randomized trial has already demonstrated deeper response and improved PFS with the addition of a PI to the pomalidomide and dexamethasone doublet (Pd) in RRMM. The bortezomib + Pd (VPD) triplet evaluated in phase III OPTIMISMM trial [43] has shown a median PFS of 11 versus 7 months (HR 0.61, 95% CI 0.49–0.77) and 12% of CR versus 3%. In addition, carfilzomib + Pd (KPD) was studied in a phase I dose escalation trial [44] and showed a median PFS of 7.2 months (95% CI 3–9) and 16% of VGPR with an acceptable tolerance profile.

Next, antibody containing pomalidomide-based triplets were tested with CD38 targeting. Therefore, daratumumab + Pd (DPd) has been evaluated in an open label non-randomized phase 1b EQUULEUS; MMY1001 study [45] and showed interesting MRD negativity rates of 29% at 10^{-5} and a PFS of 8.8 months (95% CI, 4.6–15.4).

Afterwards, the second generation anti CD38 mAb, isatuximab + Pd (Isa-Pom-Dex) was evaluated in the phase III open ICARIA-MM trial [46]. Median PFS with Isa-Pom-Dex was 11.53 months versus 6.47 months with Pd alone (HR 0.596, 95% CI 0.44–0.81, $p = 0.001$) and it is consistent in sub-groups of patients $\geq$ 75 years old or with renal impairment. MRD negativity at 10^{-5} is reached in 5.2% with isatuximab.

Finally, elotuzumab + Pd (EloPd) was studied in the phase II ELOQUENT 3 study [47]. Noticeably, 63% of patients were ≥65 and even 22% ≥ 75 years old. Median PFS with EloRd was 10.3 months versus 4.7 with Pd alone (HR 0.54, 95% CI 0.34–0.86; $p = 0.008$). The tolerability of elotuzumab in association with Pd was excellent as serious adverse events (SAEs) were similar in both groups (53% with EloPd versus 55% with Pd alone).

In the RRMM setting, it is also possible to omit IMID drugs and so the challenge is to improve a PI backbone whether being bortezomib-based (Vd) or carfilzomib-based (Kd). Accordingly, the adjunction of a monoclonal antibody to the PI-dexamethasone doublet has been widely studied. The phase III CASTOR trial [48] evaluating daratumumab + Vd (DVd) has shown an improved survival with a median PFS of 16.7 versus 7.1 months (HR 0.31, 95% CI 0.25–0.40) and deeper response with 29% of CR versus 10%. However, if patients were already refractory to lenalidomide, the results are slightly disappointing with a median PFS under 12 months. On the contrary, the adjunction of elotuzumab to the Vd backbone (EloVd) failed to reach statistical significance in the improvement of PFS (HR 0.72, 95% CI 0.49–1.06) in a phase II study [49].

The daratumumab + Kd (DKD) triplet in the CANDOR study [50] has shown an improved survival rate with a median PFS at 17 months which is not reached in the DKD group versus 15.8 months with Kd alone (HR 0.63, 95% CI 0.46–0.85). However, it enrolled younger and fitter patients with a median age of 64 years old. DKD has also been evaluated in the phase 1b EQUULEUS (MMY1001) trial [51] with a notable weekly 20/70 mg/m^2 schedule for carfilzomib. PFS was also not reached with DKD and seemed well tolerated, allowing further weekly schedule of carfilzomib with anti CD38 mAb.

Isatuximab + Kd (IsaKd) triplet evaluated in the phase III IKEMA study [52] showed, at a median follow-up of 20.7 months, a median PFS that was not reached with IsaKd versus 19.2 months with Kd (HR 0.531, 99% CI 0.318–0.889, $p = 0.0007$) and MRD negativity at 10^{-5} is reached in 29.6% with IsaKd.

7. Continuous Treatment Until Progression

One important growing concept in the field of myeloma care has been the increasing use of continuous treatment until disease progression with fixed duration regimen. The objective is to prolong the response or to improve its depth in order to delay the relapse and eventually lengthen the PFS and OS. This also focuses on the need to tailor medication management to improve the tolerability of treatment and avoid the negative impact of the dose intensity over time. To determine and to tailor the optimal duration of therapy has become another crucial point in the care of NTE MM patients more likely to suffer from the continuous triplet-based regimen approach. The demonstration of the role of continuous treatment until progression was first supported by the results of the FIRST study [25]. The PFS benefit of continuous over fixed duration of Rd for 18 cycles was demonstrated with a gain of almost 5 months. However, it failed to show any advantage on OS and could be related to the long use of corticosteroids and related adverse events such as infections and metabolic complications. However, maintenance with lenalidomide alone as in the UK Myeloma XI phase III study [53] also failed to show a benefit in OS over observation in the NTE NDMM arm with 3 years OS of 66.8% versus 69.8% (HR 1.02, 95% CI 0.80–1.29, $p = 0.88$). On the other hand, continuous triplet therapy in the NTE population could appear perilous with some drugs.

Various approaches have been studied to look into this 'how to manage continuous treatment in NTE' question. The first option would be to propose single agent maintenance to patients following triplet therapy, and several attempts were run in NTE patients. For instance, Kumar et al. have also evaluated the efficacy and the feasibility to continue ixazomib as a single agent maintenance after 12 cycles of IRd as a first line induction therapy for NTE NDMM [31]. They demonstrated that one third (32%) deepened their response with maintenance and the rate ≥ CR rate increased from 28% at the start of maintenance to 44% as best response on maintenance. This improvement in depth of response during maintenance was translated into prolonged outcome. Indeed, the median PFS was 37.2 months in NTE patients receiving maintenance versus 29.4 months in NTE patients not receiving maintenance. These results were persistent in the ≥65-year-old population with a gain in PFS even greater with 37 versus 21.5 months, respectively. The long-term tolerability of ixazomib is excellent with no treatment discontinuation due to AEs during maintenance and only 12% dose reductions. So continuous ixazomib compared favorably on toxicity profile to continuous Rd (in the FIRST trial) with a longer median duration of therapy with ixazomib. This highlights once more the limitations with steroids tolerance in elderly patients overall and the adverse impact on survival. This data was validated in the double-blind phase III TOURMALINE-MM4 trial (NCT02312258) of randomized single agent ixazomib maintenance versus placebo after 6 to 12 months of mainly PI-based induction in 706 NTE NDMM. Median age was 73 with 38% ≥ 75 years old [54]. Ixazomib maintenance has shown a 34% reduction in risk of progression or death and so, a PFS gain of 8 months with a median PFS of 17.4 months with ixazomib versus 9.4 months with placebo (HR 0.66, CI 95% 0.54–0.80, $p < 0.001$) at a median follow-up of 21.1 months. AEs during maintenance were mainly grade 1 or 2 and similar to previous studies, confirming a rather well tolerated safety profile. Ixazomib appears an interesting oral PI maintenance for NTE NDMM following cycles of triplet-based induction regimens.

The benefit of immunotherapy (IT) as monotherapy in maintenance has also been described in NTE NDMM in the ALCYONE trial [13]. It showed that the daratumumab maintenance increased the benefits of PFS following the quadruplet MPV + daratumumab regimen as induction. Indeed, the estimated PFS at 12 months (at the end of VMP induction) was 87% with Dara-VMP versus 76% with VMP alone and 72% versus 50% at 18 months, respectively.

So, maintenance therapy with PI or IT alone, namely oral ixazomib and daratumumab respectively, following triplet and even quadritherapy induction regimen in NTE NDMM patients has shown benefits in response rate and translated into prolonged outcomes with a suitable tolerability. However, relapse while on these continuous therapies, e.g., refractory disease to the given therapy, indicates the impossibility of reuse of these drugs at relapse.

The second option would be to favor the continuous triplet-based regimen, but this option cannot be offered to all regimens. The MAIA trial [40] has shown the possibility to continue triplet therapy until progressive disease (PD), independently of age and frailty condition, and in that regard is one of the unique regimens capable of managing triplet-based regimen until progression available to date. The development of IT-based triplet therapy manageable until progression could lead to further improvements of outcomes for NTE NDMM with a good tolerability and possibly have a lead across standards of care for NTE NDMM including for frail patients.

8. Future Perspectives for NTE NDMM

8.1. Triplet Combinations are Already Challenged by Quadritherapies with the Adjunction of Immunotherapy (IT) to a Triplet Regimen

With the previously discussed daratumumab + VMP (in the ALCYONE trial [13]) or in ongoing phase III studies evaluating daratumumab + VRd (CEPHEUS trial, NCT03652064) or isatuximab + VRD (IMROZ trial, NCT03319667). Daratumumab + ixazomib Rd is also investigated in a phase II (NCT04009109). Finally, elotuzumab + KRD (NCT02969837) is evaluated for NDMM in both transplant and non-transplant eligible patients.

These quadruplets carry the hope to improve the outcomes of HR NTE NDMM. However, there are several limitations already identified. First, VMP and VRd do not seem as appealing compared to DRd as a control arm. Secondly, quadruplets might be dedicated to non-frail NTE NDMM only due to the increased risk of toxicity. Thirdly, quadruplets will hardly be given for a very prolonged time. Other approaches will have to be anticipated.

8.2. Improving Safety of Frail NTE NDMM

The current trend of continuous therapy with Rd is also challenged due to the well-known toxicity related to the long-term use of dexamethasone in NTE MM [55]. A growing concept in the care of NTE MM is the early discontinuation of dexamethasone to favor compliance with other drugs, but the Rd regimen then becomes R monotherapy. Therefore, the search for a new continuous association with lenalidomide has led to the evaluation of an anti-CD38 mAb to lenalidomide association in the continuous setting; phase III IFM-2017-03 (NCT03993912) is evaluating SC daratumumab + lenalidomide (DR) versus Rd for NTE NDMM frail patients.

It is appealing to imagine an association of an anti-CD38 mAb and lenalidomide as a new maintenance standard after an induction therapy of a triple or quadruple association with PI, IMID, and IT in the care of fit NTE NDMM patients in order to spare the use of corticosteroids while lengthening the response or even improving its depth.

8.3. The Field of Immunotherapy is Expending in RRMM

With chimeric antigen receptor T cell (CAR-T), bispecific T-cell engagers (BiTEs), and antibody-drug conjugate (ADC) with belantamab mafodotin [56]. Concerning trending CAR-Ts, data on efficacity and safety in the older population are sparse. However, in a phase I study using bb2121 [57], an anti-BCMA CAR-T cell, inclusion criteria went up to 75 years old. So at least non-frail NTE NDMM patients should benefit from it. These new treatment options aim to obtain the quickest deepest response achievable, hopefully including HR.

8.4. Treatment Adaptation Depending on the MRD Status is Currently under Evaluation

The underlying hope is, in case of MRD negativity, the possibility of treatment discontinuation to avoid long term toxicity. Deepening the response could put an end to prolonged therapy which has real negative impact on QoL of patients.

9. Conclusions

NTE MM, historically called elderly MM, is the most represented, and highly heterogeneous population in MM. Therefore, it deserves specific standards of care, adapted to the frailty or fitness profile of each individual, with an aim to maintain the balance between safety and disease control.

In this population, patients' characteristics, e.g., frailty evaluation and MM characteristics with biological prognosis at diagnosis (ISS and R ISS scores, high risk cytogenetic features) are equally important. In recent years there have been several publications to draw attention to the management of frail NTE and their greater risk of drug related toxicity due to their comorbidities and therefore the need for more personalized therapy [58] and prolonged EFS, a more optimal survival indicator over PFS.

With the potential for increasing disease-free life expectancy, the aim of deepening the response to treatments and therefore prolonging outcomes should be the goal in the care of non-frail/fit NTE NDMM, similarly to younger patients [58]. The emergence of new drug families, particularly immunotherapy, with front runners such as the anti-CD38 mAbs, and soon to come the CAR T cells, TCE/BITEs, etc., the objective of MM being a chronic disease and for some patients with "cure" is close.

The high-risk MM will remain the greater challenge to face despite all this progress, and the treatment paradigm shift to see a significant improvement to the outcome of these patients has yet to be discovered.

Although NTE NDMM including frail patients is the group of patients with the worse outcomes and with least progress, knowing the improvements in treatment exposed above, their outcomes might soon significantly improve and even become as good as for younger patients.

Author Contributions: H.G. and X.L. wrote the manuscript. H.G., A.B., C.G., F.S., A.L., L.N., L.C., C.T., J.T., N.M., C.H., X.L. and S.G. critically reviewed the manuscript. All authors have read and agreed to the published version of the manuscript.

References

1. Palumbo, A.; Bringhen, S.; Ludwig, H.; Dimopoulos, M.A.; Bladé, J.; Mateos, M.V.; Rosiñol, L.; Boccadoro, M.; Cavo, M.; Lokhorst, H.; et al. Personalized therapy in multiple myeloma according to patient age and vulnerability: A report of the European Myeloma Network (EMN). *Blood* **2011**, *118*, 4519–4529. [CrossRef]
2. Brenner, H.; Gondos, A.; Pulte, D. Recent major improvement in long-term survival of younger patients with multiple myeloma. *Blood* **2008**, *111*, 2521–2526. [CrossRef]
3. Zweegman, S.; Engelhardt, M.; LaRocca, A. Elderly patients with multiple myeloma. *Curr. Opin. Oncol.* **2017**, *29*, 315–321. [CrossRef] [PubMed]
4. Avet-Loiseau, H.; Hulin, C.; Campion, L.; Rodon, P.; Marit, G.; Attal, M.; Royer, B.; Dib, M.; Voillat, L.; Bouscary, D.; et al. Chromosomal Abnormalities Are Major Prognostic Factors in Elderly Patients with Multiple Myeloma: The Intergroupe Francophone du Myélome Experience. *J. Clin. Oncol.* **2013**, *31*, 2806–2809. [CrossRef] [PubMed]
5. Bringhen, S.; Mateos, M.V.; Zweegman, S.; Larocca, A.; Falcone, A.P.; Oriol, A.; Rossi, D.; Cavalli, M.; Wijermans, P.; Ria, R.; et al. Age and organ damage correlate with poor survival in myeloma patients: Meta-analysis of 1435 individual patient data from 4 randomized trials. *Haematologica* **2013**, *98*, 980–987. [CrossRef] [PubMed]
6. Palumbo, A.; Bringhen, S.; Mateos, M.V.; Larocca, A.; Facon, T.; Kumar, S.K.; Offidani, M.; McCarthy, P.; Evangelista, A.; Lonial, S.; et al. Geriatric assessment predicts survival and toxicities in elderly myeloma patients: An International Myeloma Working Group report. *Blood* **2015**, *125*, 2068–2074. [CrossRef] [PubMed]
7. Engelhardt, M.; Domm, A.S.; Dold, S.M.; Ihorst, G.; Reinhardt, H.; Zober, A.; Hieke, S.; Baayen, C.; Müller, S.J.; Einsele, H.; et al. A concise revised Myeloma Comorbidity Index as a valid prognostic instrument in a large cohort of 801 multiple myeloma patients. *Haematologica* **2017**, *102*, 910–921. [CrossRef] [PubMed]
8. Facon, T.; Dimopoulos, M.A.; Meuleman, N.; Belch, A.; Mohty, M.; Chen, W.M.; Kim, K.; Zamagni, E.; Rodriguez-Otero, P.; Renwick, W.; et al. A simplified frailty scale predicts outcomes in transplant-ineligible patients with newly diagnosed multiple myeloma treated in the FIRST (MM-020) trial. *Leukemia* **2020**, *34*, 224–233. [CrossRef] [PubMed]
9. Cook, G.; Royle, K.L.; Pawlyn, C.; Hockaday, A.; Shah, V.; Kaiser, M.F.; Brown, S.R.; Gregory, W.M.; Child, J.A.; E Davies, F.; et al. A clinical prediction model for outcome and therapy delivery in transplant-ineligible patients with myeloma (UK Myeloma Research Alliance Risk Profile): A development and validation study. *Lancet Haematol.* **2019**, *6*, e154–e166. [CrossRef]
10. Hinton, R.; Levy, S.; Szydlo, R.; Deplano, S. A novel Haemato-oncology Frailty (HOF) score tool predicts survival in over 80s with Multiple Myeloma. *Br. J. Haematol.* **2019**, *187*, e72–e75. [CrossRef] [PubMed]

11. Palumbo, A.; Rajkumar, S.V.; Miguel, J.F.S.; LaRocca, A.; Niesvizky, R.; Morgan, G.; Landgren, O.; Hajek, R.; Einsele, H.; Anderson, K.C.; et al. International Myeloma Working Group Consensus Statement for the Management, Treatment, and Supportive Care of Patients With Myeloma Not Eligible for Standard Autologous Stem-Cell Transplantation. *J. Clin. Oncol.* **2014**, *32*, 587–600. [CrossRef]
12. Gay, F.; LaRocca, A.; Wijermans, P.; Cavallo, F.; Rossi, D.; Schaafsma, R.; Genuardi, M.; Romano, A.; Liberati, A.M.; Siniscalchi, A.; et al. Complete response correlates with long-term progression-free and overall survival in elderly myeloma treated with novel agents: Analysis of 1175 patients. *Blood* **2011**, *117*, 3025–3031. [CrossRef]
13. Mateos, M.V.; Dimopoulos, M.A.; Cavo, M.; Suzuki, K.; Jakubowiak, A.; Knop, S.; Doyen, C.; Lúcio, P.; Nagy, Z.; Kaplan, P.; et al. Daratumumab plus Bortezomib, Melphalan, and Prednisone for Untreated Myeloma. *N. Engl. J. Med.* **2018**, *378*, 518–528. [CrossRef]
14. Muchtar, E.; Dingli, D.; Kumar, S.; Buadi, F.K.; Dispenzieri, A.; Hayman, S.R.; Wolf, R.C.; A Gastineau, D.; Chakraborty, R.; Hogan, W.J.; et al. Autologous stem cell transplant for multiple myeloma patients 70 years or older. *Bone Marrow Transplant.* **2016**, *51*, 1449–1455. [CrossRef] [PubMed]
15. Badros, A.; Barlogie, B.; Siegel, E.; Morris, C.; Desikan, R.; Zangari, M.; Fassas, A.; Anaissie, E.; Munshi, N.; Tricot, G. Autologous stem cell transplantation in elderly multiple myeloma patients over the age of 70 years. *Br. J. Haematol.* **2001**, *114*, 600–607. [CrossRef]
16. Marini, C.; Maia, T.; Bergantim, R.; Pires, J.; Aguiar, E.; Guimarães, J.E.; Trigo, F. Real-life data on safety and efficacy of autologous stem cell transplantation in elderly patients with multiple myeloma. *Ann. Hematol.* **2018**, *98*, 369–379. [CrossRef]
17. Sharma, M.; Zhang, M.J.; Zhong, X.; Abidi, M.H.; Akpek, G.; Bacher, U.; Callander, N.S.; Dispenzieri, A.; Freytes, C.O.; Fung, H.C.; et al. Older Patients with Myeloma Derive Similar Benefit from Autologous Transplantation. *Biol. Blood Marrow Transplant.* **2014**, *20*, 1796–1803. [CrossRef] [PubMed]
18. Auner, H.W.; Szydlo, R.; Hoek, J.; Goldschmidt, H.; Stoppa, A.M.; Morgan, G.J.; Moreau, P.; Attal, M.; Marit, G.; Russell, N.; et al. Trends in autologous hematopoietic cell transplantation for multiple myeloma in Europe: Increased use and improved outcomes in elderly patients in recent years. *Bone Marrow Transplant.* **2015**, *50*, 209–215. [CrossRef]
19. Facon, T.; Mary, J.Y.; Hulin, C.; Benboubker, L.; Attal, M.; Pegourie, B.; Renaud, M.; Harousseau, J.L.; Guillerm, G.; Chaleteix, C.; et al. Melphalan and prednisone plus thalidomide versus melphalan and prednisone alone or reduced-intensity autologous stem cell transplantation in elderly patients with multiple myeloma (IFM 99–06): A randomised trial. *Lancet* **2007**, *370*, 1209–1218. [CrossRef]
20. Miguel, J.F.; Schlag, R.; Khuageva, N.K.; Dimopoulos, M.A.; Shpilberg, O.; Kropff, M.; Spicka, I.; Petrucci, M.T.; Palumbo, A.; Samoilova, O.S.; et al. Continued Overall Survival Benefit After 5 Years' Follow-up with Bortezomib-Melphalan-Prednisone (VMP) Versus Melphalan-Prednisone (MP) in Patients with Previously Untreated Multiple Myeloma, and No Increased Risk of Second Primary Malignancies: Final Results of the Phase 3 VISTA Trial. *Blood* **2011**, *118*, 476.
21. Facon, T.; Lee, J.H.; Moreau, P.; Niesvizky, R.; Dimopoulos, M.; Hajek, R.; Pour, L.; Jurczyszyn, A.; Qiu, L.; Klippel, Z.; et al. Carfilzomib or bortezomib with melphalan-prednisone for transplant-ineligible patients with newly diagnosed multiple myeloma. *Blood* **2019**, *133*, 1953–1963. [CrossRef]
22. Richez, V.; Gruchet, C.; Guidez, S.; Fouquet, G.; Azais, I.; Durand, G.; Javaugue, V.; Brigaud, A.; Plasse, F.; Diolez, J.; et al. Carfilzomib weekly 20/56 mg/m2, lenalidomide and dexamethasone for early relapsed refractory multiple myeloma. *Am. J. Hematol.* **2019**, *94*, E17–E20. [CrossRef]
23. Moreau, P.; Kolb, B.; Attal, M.; Caillot, D.; Benboubker, L.; Tiab, M.; Touzeau, C.; Leleu, X.; Roussel, M.; Chaleteix, C.; et al. Phase 1/2 study of carfilzomib plus melphalan and prednisone in patients aged over 65 years with newly diagnosed multiple myeloma. *Blood* **2015**, *125*, 3100–3104. [CrossRef] [PubMed]
24. Leleu, X.; Fouquet, G.; Richez, V.; Guidez, S.; Duhamel, A.; Machuron, F.; Karlin, L.; Kolb, B.; Tiab, M.; Araujo, C.; et al. Carfilzomib Weekly plus Melphalan and Prednisone in Newly Diagnosed Transplant-Ineligible Multiple Myeloma (IFM 2012-03): A Phase I Trial. *Clin. Cancer Res.* **2019**, *25*, 4224–4230. [CrossRef] [PubMed]
25. Facon, T.; Dimopoulos, M.A.; Dispenzieri, A.; Catalano, J.V.; Belch, A.; Cavo, M.; Pinto, A.; Weisel, K.; Ludwig, H.; Bahlis, N.J.; et al. Final analysis of survival outcomes in the phase 3 FIRST trial of up-front treatment for multiple myeloma. *Blood* **2018**, *131*, 301–310. [CrossRef]

26. Weisel, K.; Doyen, C.; Dimopoulos, M.; Yee, A.; Lahuerta, J.J.; Martin, A.; Travers, K.; Druyts, E.; Toor, K.; Abildgaard, N.; et al. A systematic literature review and network meta-analysis of treatments for patients with untreated multiple myeloma not eligible for stem cell transplantation. *Leuk. Lymphoma* **2016**, *58*, 153–161. [CrossRef] [PubMed]
27. LaRocca, A.; Mina, R.; Offidani, M.; Liberati, A.M.; Ledda, A.; Patriarca, F.; Evangelista, A.; Spada, S.; Benevolo, G.; Oddolo, D.; et al. First-line therapy with either bortezomib-melphalan-prednisone or lenalidomide-dexamethasone followed by lenalidomide for transplant-ineligible multiple myeloma patients: A pooled analysis of two randomized trials. *Haematologica* **2019**, *105*, 1074–1080. [CrossRef]
28. Durie, B.G.M.; Hoering, A.; Abidi, M.H.; Rajkumar, S.V.; Epstein, J.; Kahanic, S.P.; Thakuri, M.; Reu, F.; Reynolds, C.M.; Sexton, R.; et al. Bortezomib with lenalidomide and dexamethasone versus lenalidomide and dexamethasone alone in patients with newly diagnosed myeloma without intent for immediate autologous stem-cell transplant (SWOG S0777): A randomised, open-label, phase 3 trial. *Lancet* **2017**, *389*, 519–527. [CrossRef]
29. O'Donnell, E.K.; Laubach, J.P.; Yee, A.J.; Chen, T.; Huff, C.A.; Basile, F.G.; Wade, P.M.; Paba-Prada, C.E.; Ghobrial, I.M.; Schlossman, R.L.; et al. A phase 2 study of modified lenalidomide, bortezomib and dexamethasone in transplant-ineligible multiple myeloma. *Br. J. Haematol.* **2018**, *182*, 222–230. [CrossRef]
30. Dempsey, J.L.; Johns, A.; Rosko, A.E.; Lazarus, H.M. The pharmacologic management of multiple myeloma in older adults. *Expert Opin. Pharmacother.* **2019**, *20*, 887–902. [CrossRef]
31. Kumar, S.K.; Berdeja, J.G.; Niesvizky, R.; Lonial, S.; Laubach, J.P.; Hamadani, M.; Stewart, A.K.; Hari, P.; Roy, V.; Vescio, R.; et al. Ixazomib, lenalidomide, and dexamethasone in patients with newly diagnosed multiple myeloma: Long-term follow-up including ixazomib maintenance. *Leukemia* **2019**, *33*, 1736–1746. [CrossRef] [PubMed]
32. Richardson, P.G.; Hofmeister, C.C.; Rosenbaum, C.A.; Htut, M.; Vesole, D.H.; Berdeja, J.G.; Liedtke, M.; Chari, A.; Smith, S.D.; Lebovic, D.; et al. Twice-weekly ixazomib in combination with lenalidomide-dexamethasone in patients with newly diagnosed multiple myeloma. *Br. J. Haematol.* **2018**, *182*, 231–244. [CrossRef]
33. Takeda Provides Update on TOURMALINE-MM2 Phase 3 Trial. Available online: https://www.takeda.com/newsroom/newsreleases/2020/takeda-provides-update-on-tourmaline-mm2-phase-3-trial/ (accessed on 28 April 2020).
34. Dimopoulos, M.; Wang, M.; Maisnar, V.; Minarik, J.; Bensinger, W.; Mateos, M.V.; Obreja, M.; Blaedel, J.; Moreau, P. Response and progression-free survival according to planned treatment duration in patients with relapsed multiple myeloma treated with carfilzomib, lenalidomide, and dexamethasone (KRd) versus lenalidomide and dexamethasone (Rd) in the phase III ASPIRE study. *J. Hematol. Oncol.* **2018**, *11*, 49. [CrossRef] [PubMed]
35. Gay, F.; Cerrato, C.; Scalabrini, D.R.; Galli, M.; Belotti, A.; Zamagni, E.; Ledda, A.; Grasso, M.; Angelucci, E.; Liberati, A.M.; et al. Carfilzomib-Lenalidomide-Dexamethasone (KRd) Induction-Autologous Transplant (ASCT)-Krd Consolidation vs. KRd 12 Cycles vs. Carfilzomib-Cyclophosphamide-Dexamethasone (KCd) Induction-ASCT-KCd Consolidation: Analysis of the Randomized Forte Trial in Newly Diagnosed Multiple Myeloma (NDMM). *Blood* **2018**, *132*, 121. [CrossRef]
36. Kumar, S.; Jacobus, S.J.; Cohen, A.D.; Weiss, M.; Callander, N.S.; Singh, A.A.; Parker, T.L.; Menter, A.R.; Yang, X.; Parsons, B.M.; et al. Carfilzomib, lenalidomide, and dexamethasone (KRd) versus bortezomib, lenalidomide, and dexamethasone (VRd) for initial therapy of newly diagnosed multiple myeloma (NDMM): Results of ENDURANCE (E1A11) phase III trial. *J. Clin. Oncol.* **2020**, *38*, LBA3. [CrossRef]
37. Dimopoulos, M.A.; Oriol, A.; Nahi, H.; San-Miguel, J.; Bahlis, N.J.; Usmani, S.Z.; Rabin, N.; Orlowski, R.Z.; Komarnicki, M.; Suzuki, K.; et al. Daratumumab, Lenalidomide, and Dexamethasone for Multiple Myeloma. *N. Engl. J. Med.* **2016**, *375*, 1319–1331. [CrossRef]
38. Mateos, M.V.; Nahi, H.; Legiec, W.; Grosicki, S.; Vorobyev, V.; Spicka, I.; Hungria, V.T.; Korenkova, S.; Bahlis, N.J.; Flogegard, M.; et al. Efficacy and safety of the randomized, open-label, non-inferiority, phase 3 study of subcutaneous (SC) versus intravenous (IV) daratumumab (DARA) administration in patients (pts) with relapsed or refractory multiple myeloma (RRMM): COLUMBA. *J. Clin. Oncol.* **2019**, *37*, 8005. [CrossRef]
39. Moreau, P.; Masszi, T.; Grzasko, N.; Bahlis, N.J.; Hansson, M.; Pour, L.; Sandhu, I.; Ganly, P.S.; Baker, B.W.; Jackson, S.R.; et al. Oral Ixazomib, Lenalidomide, and Dexamethasone for Multiple Myeloma. *N. Engl. J. Med.* **2016**, *374*, 1621–1634. [CrossRef] [PubMed]

40. Facon, T.; Kumar, S.; Plesner, T.; Orlowski, R.Z.; Moreau, P.; Bahlis, N.; Basu, S.; Nahi, H.; Hulin, C.; Quach, H.; et al. Daratumumab plus Lenalidomide and Dexamethasone for Untreated Myeloma. *N. Engl. J. Med.* **2019**, *380*, 2104–2115. [CrossRef]
41. Lonial, S.; A Dimopoulos, M.; Palumbo, A.; White, D.; Grosicki, S.; Spicka, I.; Walter-Croneck, A.; Moreau, P.; Mateos, M.V.; Magen, H.; et al. Elotuzumab Therapy for Relapsed or Refractory Multiple Myeloma. *N. Engl. J. Med.* **2015**, *373*, 621–631. [CrossRef]
42. Berdeja, J.; Jagannath, S.; Zonder, J.; Badros, A.; Kaufman, J.L.; Manges, R.; Gupta, M.; Tendolkar, A.; Lynch, M.; Bleickardt, E.; et al. Pharmacokinetics and Safety of Elotuzumab Combined With Lenalidomide and Dexamethasone in Patients With Multiple Myeloma and Various Levels of Renal Impairment: Results of a Phase Ib Study. *Clin. Lymphoma Myeloma Leuk.* **2016**, *16*, 129–138. [CrossRef]
43. Richardson, P.G.; Oriol, A.; Beksac, M.; Liberati, A.M.; Galli, M.; Schjesvold, F.; Lindsay, J.; Weisel, K.; White, D.; Facon, T.; et al. Pomalidomide, bortezomib, and dexamethasone for patients with relapsed or refractory multiple myeloma previously treated with lenalidomide (OPTIMISMM): A randomised, open-label, phase 3 trial. *Lancet Oncol.* **2019**, *20*, 781–794. [CrossRef]
44. Sonneveld, P.; Zweegman, S.; Cavo, M.; Nasserinejad, K.; Troia, R.; Pour, L.; Croockewit, S.; Corradini, P.; Patriarca, F.; Wu, K.; et al. Carfilzomib, Pomalidomide and Dexamethasone (KPd) in Patients with Multiple Myeloma Refractory to Bortezomib and Lenalidomide. the EMN011 Trial. *Blood* **2018**, *132*, 801. [CrossRef]
45. Chari, A.; Suvannasankha, A.; Fay, J.W.; Arnulf, B.; Kaufman, J.L.; Ifthikharuddin, J.J.; Weiss, B.M.; Krishnan, A.; Lentzsch, S.; Comenzo, R.; et al. Daratumumab plus pomalidomide and dexamethasone in relapsed and/or refractory multiple myeloma. *Blood* **2017**, *130*, 974–981. [CrossRef]
46. Attal, M.; Richardson, P.G.; Rajkumar, S.V.; San-Miguel, J.; Beksac, M.; Spicka, I.; Leleu, X.; Schjesvold, F.; Moreau, P.; A Dimopoulos, M.; et al. Isatuximab plus pomalidomide and low-dose dexamethasone versus pomalidomide and low-dose dexamethasone in patients with relapsed and refractory multiple myeloma (ICARIA-MM): A randomised, multicentre, open-label, phase 3 study. *Lancet* **2019**, *394*, 2096–2107. [CrossRef]
47. Dimopoulos, M.A.; Dytfeld, D.; Grosicki, S.; Moreau, P.; Takezako, N.; Hori, M.; Leleu, X.; Leblanc, R.; Suzuki, K.; Raab, M.S.; et al. Elotuzumab plus Pomalidomide and Dexamethasone for Multiple Myeloma. *N. Engl. J. Med.* **2018**, *379*, 1811–1822. [CrossRef]
48. Palumbo, A.; Chanan-Khan, A.; Weisel, K.; Nooka, A.K.; Masszi, T.; Beksac, M.; Spicka, I.; Hungria, V.; Munder, M.; Mateos, M.V.; et al. Daratumumab, Bortezomib, and Dexamethasone for Multiple Myeloma. *N. Engl. J. Med.* **2016**, *375*, 754–766. [CrossRef]
49. Jakubowiak, A.; Offidani, M.; Pégourie, B.; de la Rubia, J.; Garderet, L.; Laribi, K.; Bosi, A.; Marasca, R.; Laubach, J.; Mohrbacher, A.; et al. Randomized phase 2 study: Elotuzumab plus bortezomib/dexamethasone vs. bortezomib/dexamethasone for relapsed/refractory MM. *Blood* **2016**, *127*, 2833–2840. [CrossRef]
50. Dimopoulos, M.; Quach, H.; Mateos, M.V.; Landgren, O.; Leleu, X.; Siegel, D.; Weisel, K.; Yang, H.; Klippel, Z.; Zahlten-Kumeli, A.; et al. Carfilzomib, dexamethasone, and daratumumab versus carfilzomib and dexamethasone for patients with relapsed or refractory multiple myeloma (CANDOR): Results from a randomised, multicentre, open-label, phase 3 study. *Lancet* **2020**, *396*, 186–197. [CrossRef]
51. Chari, A.; Martinez-Lopez, J.; Mateos, M.V.; Bladé, J.; Benboubker, L.; Oriol, A.; Arnulf, B.; Rodriguez-Otero, P.; Pineiro, L.; Jakubowiak, A.; et al. Daratumumab plus carfilzomib and dexamethasone in patients with relapsed or refractory multiple myeloma. *Blood* **2019**, *134*, 421–431. [CrossRef] [PubMed]
52. Moreau, P. Inc MG. Isatuximab Plus Carfilzomib and Dexamethasone vs. Carfilzomib and Dexamethasone in Relapsed/Refractory Multiple Myeloma (IKEMA): Interim Analysis of a Phase 3, Randomized, Open-Label Study. EHA25 Virtual Congress. Abstract LB2603.
53. Jackson, G.H.; E Davies, F.; Pawlyn, C.; A Cairns, D.; Striha, A.; Collett, C.; Hockaday, A.; Jones, J.R.; Kishore, B.; Garg, M.; et al. Lenalidomide maintenance versus observation for patients with newly diagnosed multiple myeloma (Myeloma XI): A multicentre, open-label, randomised, phase 3 trial. *Lancet Oncol.* **2019**, *20*, 57–73. [CrossRef]
54. Dimopoulos, M.A.; Spicka, I.; Quach, H.; Oriol, A.; Hajek, R.; Garg, M.; Beksac, M.; Bringhen, S.; Katodritou, E.; Chng, W.J.; et al. Ixazomib vs. placebo maintenance for newly diagnosed multiple myeloma (NDMM) patients not undergoing autologous stem cell transplant (ASCT): The phase III TOURMALINE-MM4 trial. *J. Clin. Oncol.* **2020**, *38*, 8527. [CrossRef]

55. Biran, N.; Jacobus, S.; Vesole, D.H.; Callander, N.S.; Fonseca, R.; Williams, M.E.; Abonour, R.; Katz, M.S.; Rajkumar, S.V.; Greipp, P.R.; et al. Outcome with lenalidomide plus dexamethasone followed by early autologous stem cell transplantation in patients with newly diagnosed multiple myeloma on the ECOG-ACRIN E4A03 randomized clinical trial: Long-term follow-up. *Blood Cancer J.* **2016**, *6*, e466. [CrossRef]
56. Lonial, S.; Lee, H.C.; Badros, A.; Trudel, S.; Nooka, A.K.; Chari, A.; Abdallah, A.O.; Callander, N.; Lendvai, N.; Sborov, D.; et al. Belantamab Mafodotin for Relapsed or Refractory Multiple Myeloma (DREAMM-2): A Two-Arm, Randomised, Open-Label, Phase 2 Study. *Lancet Oncol.* **2020**, *21*, 207–221. Available online: https://pubmed.ncbi.nlm.nih.gov/31859245/ (accessed on 28 May 2020). [CrossRef]
57. Raje, N.; Berdeja, J.; Lin, Y.; Siegel, D.; Jagannath, S.; Madduri, D.; Liedtke, M.; Rosenblatt, J.; Maus, M.V.; Turka, A.; et al. Anti-BCMA CAR T-Cell Therapy bb2121 in Relapsed or Refractory Multiple Myeloma. *N. Engl. J. Med.* **2019**, *380*, 1726–1737. [CrossRef]
58. LaRocca, A.; Dold, S.M.; Zweegman, S.; Terpos, E.; Wäsch, R.; D'Agostino, M.; Scheubeck, S.; Goldschmidt, H.; Gay, F.; Cavo, M.; et al. Patient-centered practice in elderly myeloma patients: An overview and consensus from the European Myeloma Network (EMN). *Leukemia* **2018**, *32*, 1697–1712. [CrossRef]

2

Managing Bladder Cancer Care during the COVID-19 Pandemic Using a Team-Based Approach

Tina Wang, Sariah Liu, Thomas Joseph and Yung Lyou *

Department of Medical Oncology & Experimental Therapeutics, City of Hope Comprehensive Cancer Center, Duarte, CA 91010, USA; tinawang@coh.org (T.W.); sarliu@coh.org (S.L.); thojoseph@coh.org (T.J.)
* Correspondence: ylyou@coh.org

Abstract: The recent novel coronavirus, named coronavirus disease 2019 (COVID-19), has developed into an international pandemic affecting millions of individuals with hundreds of thousands of deaths worldwide. The highly infectious nature and widespread prevalence of this disease create a new set of obstacles for the bladder cancer community in both delivering and receiving care. In this manuscript, we address the unique issues regarding treatment prioritization for the patient with bladder cancer and how we at City of Hope have adjusted our clinical practices using a team-based approach that utilizes shared decision making with all stakeholders (physicians, patients, caregivers) to optimize outcomes during this difficult time. In addition to taking standard precautions for minimizing COVID-19 risk of exposure for those entering a healthcare facility (screening all personnel upon entry and donning facemasks at all times), we suggest the following three measures: (1) delay post-treatment surveillance visits until there is a decrease in local COVID-19 cases, (2) continue curative intent treatments for localized bladder cancer with COVID-19 precautions (i.e., choosing gemcitabine/cisplatin (GC) over dose-dense methotrexate, vinblastine, doxorubicin, cisplatin (ddMVAC) neoadjuvant chemotherapy), and (3) increase the off-treatment period between cycles of palliative systemic therapy in metastatic urothelial carcinoma patients.

Keywords: bladder cancer; urothelial carcinoma; COVID-19; team-based medicine

---

1. Introduction

Recently, a novel coronavirus, named severe acute respiratory syndrome coronavirus 2 (SARS-CoV-2), has developed into an international pandemic affecting millions of individuals in more than 150 countries with hundreds of thousands of deaths worldwide [1,2]. This disease has been named coronavirus disease 2019 (COVID-19) by the World Health Organization (WHO) [1]. Patients with this disease are at high risk for developing septic shock and hypoxemia, which can frequently progress to acute respiratory distress syndrome (ARDS) and death [3]. This disease creates a new set of obstacles for the bladder cancer community in both delivering and receiving care. In this manuscript, we address the unique issues regarding treatment prioritization for the patient with bladder cancer and how we at City of Hope have adjusted our clinical practices using a team-based, shared decision approach with all stakeholders (patients, caregivers, and physicians) to optimize outcomes during this difficult time.

2. Balancing the Need for Bladder Cancer Treatments and Risk of Exposure to COVID-19

2.1. Patients with Bladder Cancer Undergoing Treatments Are at a Higher Risk for COVID-19 Infections and Worse Outcomes Compared to the General Population without Cancer

For the patient with bladder cancer undergoing treatment, there are several safety issues that place them at higher risk of infection for COVID-19 compared to the general population without cancer.

First, patients must physically leave the safety of their residences to go to the clinic, infusion center, or imaging facility where they could potentially be exposed to COVID-19. Second, the platinum-based chemotherapy regimens commonly used in bladder cancer treatments are immunosuppressive and place them at a higher risk for infection. Third, many bladder cancer patients tend to be of older age and also have multiple medical comorbidities, which has been shown to place them in a group with worse outcomes for COVID-19 [2,4]. A retrospective study that examined the outcomes of approximately 72,000 patients with COVID-19 found that those with older age and presence of medical comorbidities were associated with adverse outcomes [2,4]. In another retrospective study by Liang and colleagues, it was suggested that patients with a history of cancer itself may be associated with worse outcomes from COVID-19 [5,6]. However, it should be noted that this particular retrospective study was limited in that only 18 of the 1590 patients who were studied had a history of cancer, making it difficult to form a general conclusion from such a small sample size [5,6]. Regardless, based on the other reasons discussed above, it is clear that patients with bladder cancer undergoing active therapy or post-treatment surveillance are at a higher risk for COVID-19 exposure and could potentially suffer worse outcomes compared to the general population.

2.2. Prioritizing Treatments Appropriately and Applying Social Distancing

Ensuring patient safety is the key principle when it comes to delivering medical care among all healthcare professions. In the setting of the COVID-19 pandemic, the central question we have asked ourselves as providers while managing each patient's care has been: Will delaying the patient's bladder cancer treatment in accordance with current COVID-19 social distancing measures lead to a worse long-term outcome? Current models suggest that this pandemic may proceed until herd immunity or a vaccine is developed, with repeated waves of infections, which some experts estimate could continue for another 18 months. Since it is not feasible to delay bladder cancer treatments for another 18 months, we at City of Hope have developed a consensus framework to help balance these competing risks (Figure 1). By utilizing this framework, we have been able to guide our clinicians within the network on how to make a shared decision with the patient that can prioritize bladder cancer treatments appropriately while minimizing the risk for COVID-19 exposure (Figure 1).

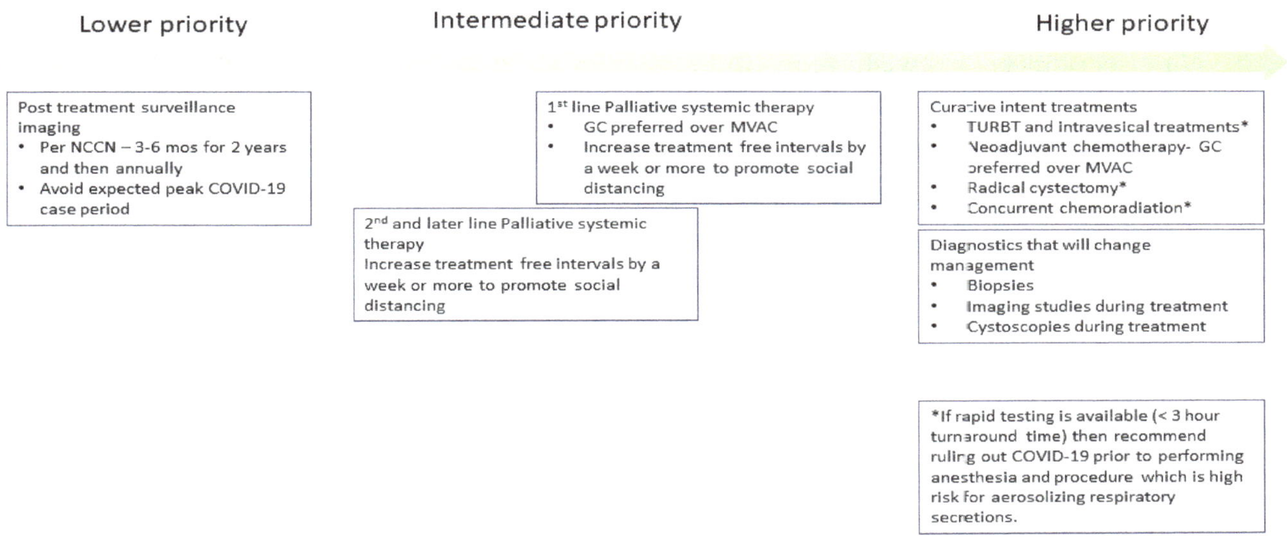

Figure 1. Conceptual framework for prioritizing bladder cancer treatments during the COVID-19 pandemic. This framework provides guidance on key treatments that should still be offered in order to ensure optimal bladder cancer outcomes if possible. We recommend that these listed priorities can be modified based on available local resources and the patient's overall medical status.

2.3. *Applying COVID-19 Risk Mitigation Measures for Bladder Cancer Treatment*

In the state of California, there is a "shelter in place" order that was initiated on 19 March 2020 along with other social distancing measures due to the concern that individuals may be at high risk of becoming infected and could also infect others, further propagating this pandemic. Current epidemiology modeling suggests that the peak incidence of COVID-19 will have occurred sometime in mid-to-late April in the state of California. This framework assumes that the number of new cases will start to decrease in the months of May and June 2020. In the case that there is indeed a second wave of infections later during the fall and winter months of 2020, one could reapply this framework based on the expected peaks. As a result, we suggest the following framework to assist the practicing oncologist in determining optimal treatment strategies for the patient with bladder cancer.

2.3.1. Delay Post-Treatment Surveillance Visits until There Is a Decrease in COVID-19 Cases

For patients undergoing surveillance imaging after completion of cystectomy or other definitive therapies, the National Comprehensive Cancer Network (NCCN) guidelines currently recommend imaging every 6–12 months [7]. Keeping these guidelines in mind, we have rescheduled the patient's clinic and imaging visit to avoid the expected COVID-19 peak period (April–May) so that it will take place during the next 2–3 months in June or July as a way to minimize risk of exposure.

2.3.2. Continue Curative Intent Treatments for Localized Bladder Cancer with COVID-19 Precautions

Even in these difficult times, urothelial bladder cancer is an aggressive disease with poor prognosis when it progresses to metastatic disease. Therefore, we have been vigilant in continuing to deliver curative intent treatments when patients have localized urothelial carcinoma, if possible in a timely manner. A meta-analysis of 13 studies suggested that a delay of more than 12 weeks from time of diagnosis to execution of radical cystectomy, only in muscle invasive urothelial cancer, was associated with worse outcomes [8]. Another study showed that initiating neoadjuvant chemotherapy (NAC) with a delay of more than 8 weeks from time of diagnosis led to worse outcomes [9]. Therefore, we have continued to offer cisplatin-eligible patients NAC within 8 weeks and cisplatin-ineligible patients radical cystectomy within 12 weeks from time of diagnosis, while the infusion center and operating room resources are available for those patients with localized disease since there is a limited window of curative treatment opportunity.

The first set of measures we have instituted to minimize potential risk for COVID-19 exposure for all on-site people (visitors and healthcare workers) is to create a single, separate point of entry to the active clinical areas and institute a strict policy limiting visitors to patients only. Prior to entering the clinical area, all personnel (including patients and healthcare workers) are screened for COVID-19 symptoms (i.e., cough, dyspnea, and fever) and have their temperatures measured. People determined to be asymptomatic and afebrile are then required to don a face mask and are issued an entrance band indicating they have passed screening measures for that day. If someone is found to be symptomatic, we then refer this individual to an on-site "fever clinic" staffed by designated clinical personnel who have been trained and equipped with the appropriate personal protective equipment (PPE) to perform a nasopharyngeal swab for in-house COVID-19 testing. We have also repurposed one of our hospital wards with negative pressure rooms to serve as the COVID-19 unit with its own set of designated staff to decrease exposure within the facility. In both the inpatient and outpatient areas, all people (patients and healthcare workers) are required to don a face mask at all times, which has been suggested as a way to prevent sustained exposure to COVID-19 and reduce risk for infection [10].

The second set of COVID-19 risk mitigation measures specifically pertain to treatments used for urothelial bladder cancer. Current NCCN guidelines recommend neoadjuvant chemotherapy in muscle invasive bladder cancer [7]. In the choice of regimen, the two most commonly used regimens are dose-dense methotrexate, vinblastine, doxorubicin, cisplatin (ddMVAC) and gemcitabine/cisplatin (GC) [7,11,12]. During this time, we have advocated for using gemcitabine/cisplatin over ddMVAC for the following reasons. Although there is some discussion suggesting that ddMVAC may have a trend towards higher efficacy, it has yet to be definitively supported in a head-to-head prospective trial and retrospective studies have shown similar amounts of efficacy between these two regimens [11,12]. In addition, ddMVAC tends to be more myelosuppressive than GC, placing patients at higher risk for infections due to the neutropenia and symptomatic anemia requiring blood transfusions, which during this time have been especially challenging due to a steep drop in blood donations [11,12]. Finally, ddMVAC is given as a 14-day cycle whereas GC is given as a 21-day cycle. The 14-day cycle of ddMVAC allows a patient to proceed sooner to radical cystectomy compared to GC, but during this time we would recommend GC because it allows the oncologist to space out the patient visits and can help adhere better to the principle of social distancing [11,12]. Another measure we have taken is to implement weekly telephone checks with patients undergoing active systemic therapy. This allows us to determine if a patient is having any significant chemotherapy-related adverse effects or other acute medical issues, for which they could potentially be treated as an outpatient before they progress to needing emergency room or acute inpatient care. For example, if a patient is experiencing significant dysuria due to a potential urinary tract infection, one can prescribe antibiotics empirically at their local pharmacy and help them avoid the need to seek emergency room care, which is most likely to be overcrowded during this pandemic. For those patients that are undergoing concurrent radiation and chemotherapy with curative intent, we have continued their treatments while taking the abovementioned general COVID-19 precautions (i.e., screening at entry, donning facemasks, and weekly telephone checks).

2.3.3. Increasing Off-Treatment Period between Cycles for Palliative Systemic Therapy in Metastatic Urothelial Carcinoma Patients

For those patients already undergoing palliative first-line systemic therapy, we have continued their treatments as those regimens provide overall survival benefit. In this situation, if chemotherapy needs to be started we would recommend, as discussed above, to prescribe anti-emetics and pain medications for the patient to have immediately available at home as an outpatient. Additionally, weekly telephone checks would be conducted to prevent any chemotherapy-related complications early. Another important factor to consider, as discussed above, is lengthening the period of time between treatments. Normally, gemcitabine/cisplatin or gemcitabine/carboplatin is administered as a two weeks on, 1 week off schedule. In this case, it is reasonable to do 2 weeks on, 2 weeks off to help spread out the treatment duration as much as possible to maximize social distancing. Second-line treatment usually involves the use of immune checkpoint inhibitors such as pembrolizumab or atezolizumab. Pembrolizumab is dosed every 3 weeks, but in order to maximize social distancing for the patient, it is reasonable to stretch it to every 4 weeks during this period since it is unlikely the cancer will grow significantly during the extra week off. In this setting, atezolizumab and nivolumab already has an Federal Drug Administration (FDA)-approved every-4-week dosing, which would also make it a viable alternative. The use of third-line treatment with enfortumab vedotin requires administration once every week for 3 weeks straight and then taking the fourth week off. Again, to provide more space between visits, it would be reasonable to increase the off-treatment period from 1 week to 2 weeks to provide the patient more social distancing.

Even during these difficult times, it is crucial to continue clinical trials to the best of our ability and help advance the field of oncology. In order to preserve needed resources for COVID-19 prevention and treatment within our institution, we have focused our efforts on continuing current open clinical trials and slowing down the pace of opening new trials.

3. Conclusions

COVID-19 has developed into an international pandemic affecting millions of individuals and has created a new set of obstacles for the bladder cancer community in both delivering and receiving care. Because patients with bladder cancer require treatment even in these difficult times, we have developed a framework that utilizes a team-based approach with shared decision making among all stakeholders involved (physicians, patients, caregivers) to optimize outcomes during this difficult time. It is our hope that the conceptual framework presented above and institutional experience can be adjusted to fit the available local resources for others that are looking to balance these two competing needs when treating patients with bladder cancer during the COVID-19 pandemic.

Author Contributions: Y.L. conceived the article; T.W., S.L., and T.J. wrote the manuscript with input from Y.L. All authors have read and agreed to the published version of the manuscript.

Abbreviations

COVID-19	coronavirus disease 2019
FDA	Federal Drug administration
GC	gemcitabine/cisplatin
ddMVAC	dose-dense methotrexate, vinblastine, doxorubicin, cisplatin
NCCN	National Comprehensive Cancer Network

References

1. Novel Coronavirus (2019-nCoV) Situation Reports. Available online: https://www.who.int/emergencies/diseases/novel-coronavirus-2019/situation-reports (accessed on 4 April 2020).
2. Wu, Z.; McGoogan, J.M. Characteristics of and Important Lessons from the Coronavirus Disease 2019 (COVID-19) Outbreak in China: Summary of a Report of 72 314 Cases from the Chinese Center for Disease Control and Prevention. *JAMA* **2020**, *323*, 1239–1242. [CrossRef] [PubMed]
3. Alhazzani, W.; Møller, M.H.; Arabi, Y.M.; Loeb, M.; Gong, M.N.; Fan, E.; Oczkowski, S.; Levy, M.M.; Derde, L.; Dzierba, A.; et al. Surviving Sepsis Campaign: Guidelines on the management of critically ill adults with Coronavirus Disease 2019 (COVID-19). *Intensive Care Med.* **2020**, *46*, 854–887. [CrossRef] [PubMed]
4. Zhou, F.; Yu, T.; Du, R.; Fan, G.; Liu, Y.; Liu, Z.; Xiang, J.; Wang, Y.; Song, B.; Gu, X.; et al. Clinical course and risk factors for mortality of adult inpatients with COVID-19 in Wuhan, China: A retrospective cohort study. *Lancet* **2020**, *395*, 1054–1062. [CrossRef]
5. Wang, H.; Zhang, L. Risk of COVID-19 for patients with cancer. *Lancet Oncol.* **2020**, *21*, e181. [CrossRef]
6. Xia, Y.; Jin, R.; Zhao, J.; Li, W.; Shen, H. Risk of COVID-19 for patients with cancer. *Lancet Oncol.* **2020**, *21*, e180. [CrossRef]
7. Flaig, T.W.; Spiess, P.E.; Agarwal, N.; Bangs, R.; Boorjian, S.A.; Buyyounouski, M.K.; Chang, S.; Downs, T.M.; Efstathiou, J.A.; Friedlander, T.; et al. Bladder Cancer, Version 3.2020, NCCN Clinical Practice Guidelines in Oncology. *J. Natl. Compr. Cancer Netw.* **2020**, *18*, 329–354. [CrossRef] [PubMed]
8. Fahmy, N.M.; Mahmud, S.; Aprikian, A.G. Delay in the surgical treatment of bladder cancer and survival: Systematic review of the literature. *Eur. Urol.* **2006**, *50*, 1176–1182. [CrossRef] [PubMed]
9. Audenet, F.; Sfakianos, J.P.; Waingankar, N.; Ruel, N.H.; Galsky, M.D.; Yuh, B.E.; Gin, G.E. A delay ≥8 weeks to neoadjuvant chemotherapy before radical cystectomy increases the risk of upstaging. *Urol. Oncol.* **2019**, *37*, 116–122. [CrossRef] [PubMed]
10. Gawande, A. Keeping the Coronavirus from Infecting Health-Care Workers. Available online: https://www.newyorker.com/news/news-desk/keeping-the-coronavirus-from-infecting-health-care-workers (accessed on 12 April 2020).

11. Dash, A.; Pettus, J.A.; Herr, H.W.; Bochner, B.H.; Dalbagni, G.; Donat, S.M.; Russo, P.; Boyle, M.G.; Milowsky, M.I.; Bajorin, D.F. A Role for Neoadjuvant Gemcitabine Plus Cisplatin in Muscle-Invasive Urothelial Carcinoma of the Bladder: A Retrospective Experience. *Cancer* **2008**, *113*, 2471–2477. [CrossRef] [PubMed]

12. Choueiri, T.K.; Jacobus, S.; Bellmunt, J.; Qu, A.; Appleman, L.J.; Tretter, C.; Bubley, G.J.; Stack, E.C.; Signoretti, S.; Walsh, M.; et al. Neoadjuvant dose-dense methotrexate, vinblastine, doxorubicin, and cisplatin with pegfilgrastim support in muscle-invasive urothelial cancer: Pathologic, radiologic, and biomarker correlates. *J. Clin. Oncol.* **2014**, *32*, 1889–1894. [CrossRef] [PubMed]

3

Careful Breakthrough Cancer Pain Treatment through Rapid-Onset Transmucosal Fentanyl Improves the Quality of Life in Cancer Patients: Results from the BEST Multicenter Study

Arturo Cuomo [1,†], Marco Cascella [1,*,†], Cira Antonietta Forte [1,†], Sabrina Bimonte [1], Gennaro Esposito [1], Stefano De Santis [2], Luigi Cavanna [3], Flavio Fusco [4], Mario Dauri [5], Silvia Natoli [5], Marco Maltoni [6], Alessandro Morabito [7], Rocco Domenico Mediati [8], Vito Lorusso [9], Sandro Barni [10], Giampiero Porzio [11], Sebastiano Mercadante [12] and Anna Crispo [13]

1 Division of Anesthesia and Pain Medicine, Istituto Nazionale Tumori, IRCCS. Fondazione G. Pascale, 80131 Napoli, Italy; a.cuomo@istitutotumori.na.it (A.C.); c.forte@istitutotumori.na.it (C.A.F.); s.bimonte@istitutotumori.na.it (S.B.); gennaro.esposito@istitutotumori.na.it (G.E.)

2 Palliative Care and Oncologic Pain Service, S. Camillo-Forlanini Hospital, 00149 Rome, Italy; sdesantis@scamilloforlanini.rm.it

3 Department of Oncology-Hematology, G. da Saliceto Hospital, 29121 Piacenza, Italy; l.cavanna@ausl.pc.it

4 Palliative Home Care Unit, ASL 3, 16153 Genova, Italy; flavio.fusco@asl3.liguria.it

5 Department of Anesthesiology and Resuscitation, II University of Rome, Tor Vergata, 00133 Roma, Italy; mario.dauri@uniroma2.it (M.D.); silvia.natoli@uniroma2.it (S.N.)

6 Palliative Care Unit, Istituto Scientifico Romagnolo per lo Studio e la Cura dei Tumori (IRST) IRCCS, 47014 Meldola, Italy; ma.maltoni@ausl.fo.it

7 Medical Oncology Unit, Istituto Nazionale Tumori, IRCCS. Fondazione G. Pascale, 80131 Napoli, Italy; a.morabito@istitutotumori.na.it

8 Palliative Care and Pain Therapy Unit, University Hospital Careggi, 50134 Firenze, Italy; mediatir@aou-careggi.toscana.it

9 UO Oncologia Medica, Istituto Tumori "G Paolo II", 70124 Bari, Italy; vitolorusso@me.com

10 Oncology Unit, ASST Bergamo Ovest, 24047 Treviglio, Italy; sandro_barni@asst-bgovest.it

11 Medical Oncology Unit, San Salvatore Hospital, University of L'Aquila, 67100 L'Aquila, Italy; terapiesupportoaq@interfree.it

12 Main regional center for Pain Relief & Supportive Care, La Maddalena Cancer Center, 90146 Palermo, Italy; terapiadeldolore@lamaddalenanet.it

13 Epidemiology and Biostatistics Unit, Istituto Nazionale Tumori, IRCCS. Fondazione G. Pascale, 80131 Napoli, Italy; a.crispo@istitutotumori.na.it

* Correspondence: m.cascella@istitutotumori.na.it

† These authors contributed equally to this work.

Abstract: Objectives: To explore the effect of breakthrough cancer pain (BTcP) treatment on quality of sleep and other aspects of the health-related quality of life (HRQoL) in patients with cancer pain. Methods: In an observational, multicenter, cohort study, cancer patients from palliative care units, oncology departments, and pain clinics and affected by BTcP were included. Enrolled patients were assessed at the four visits: T0 (baseline), T7, T14, and T28. Stable chronic background pain (numeric rating scale, NRS ≤ 4) during the whole study period was mandatory. BTcP was treated through transmucosal fentanyl. Three questionnaires were used to measure the HRQoL: EORTC QLQ-C15-PAL, Pittsburgh Sleep Quality Index (PSQI), and the Edmonton Symptom Assessment System (ESAS). RESULTS: In 154 patients, the HRQoL showed a significant improvement for all physical and emotional characteristics in the EORTC QLQ-C15-PAL, except for nausea and vomiting (linear p-value = 0.1) and dyspnea (Linear p-value = 0.05). The ESAS and PSQI questionnaires confirmed these positive results ($p < 0.0001$ and $p = 0.002$, respectively). Conclusions: This prospective investigation by an Italian expert group, has confirmed that careful management of BTcP induces a paramount improvement on the HRQoL. Because in cancer patients there is a high prevalence of BTcP and this severe acute pain has deleterious consequences, this information can have an important clinical significance.

Keywords: breakthrough cancer pain; cancer-associated pain; cancer; health-related quality of life; sleep disorders; transmucosal fentanyl

---

1. Introduction

Pain is one of the most frequent symptoms in cancer patients as it occurs in 20–30% of cases during the initial stages and in up to 75% of patients in advanced disease. The prevalence of cancer pain at any stage of the disease is over 50%. Concerning pain intensity, moderate to severe pain can affect up to 40% of all patients. Furthermore, this symptom strongly affects the patient's health-related quality of life (HRQoL) and daily activities throughout the cancer disease [1]. As a consequence, in this clinical setting, it is mandatory to relieve pain and other symptoms and to improve the HRQoL at any stage of the disease [2]. Despite the clear validity of this statement, the availability of several guidelines on the topic [3], and evidence that effective pain-relieving strategies can improve HRQoL and adherence to anticancer treatment [4], cancer-pain management remains an impressive challenge in medicine.

Assessment and management of cancer pain become particularly critical when the patient faces temporary exacerbations of pain despite adequate control with opioids. This phenomenon, termed as breakthrough cancer pain (BTcP), is a very frequent condition as approximately 70% of patients suffering from chronic pain of oncological nature report episodes of BTcP [5]. Typical BTcP episodes are of short duration (15–30 min/episode), moderate to severe intensity and with rapid onset (maximum peak between 3–15 min). Our recent investigations conducted on a large sample of patients ($n = 4016$), dissected the features of this painful phenomenon and demonstrated that in 86% of patients the occurrence of BTcP induced a marked interference with their daily activities [6]. Moreover, several pieces of evidence demonstrated that BTcP is associated with negative outcomes for both patients and healthcare providers [7]. Thus, during the IOPS study, we realized that the impact of pain therapy on some aspects of the HRQoL required further investigation. Because previous studies showed that cancer-related poor sleep quality can lead to a worsening in psychological, and physical functions [8], the next step was to evaluate whether an effective background analgesia control combined with proper management of the BTcP could lead to an improvement of the sleep quality and the overall HRQoL.

The present observational study—indicated as breakthrough cancer pain evaluation study (BEST-Study)—aimed at assessing the impact of BTcP management on HRQoL, sleep and daily activities in patients from different clinical settings and with adequately controlled background pain through strong opioids.

2. Materials and Methods

2.1. Study Population and Design

This clinical study was conducting by following the Declaration of Helsinki's ethical principles. Individuals with a diagnosis of any type of solid cancer and affected by chronic pain effectively controlled—numeric rating scale (NRS) ≤4—by around-the-clock (ATC) opioid maintenance therapy through ≥ 60 mg of oral morphine equivalent daily doses (OMEDD) on the day of enrollment, were included in this national multicenter prospective cohort study, from March 2015 to August 2017. Approval from the Institutional Medical Ethical Committee (protocol 32/14 OSS) of the Istituto Nazionale Tumori-Fondazione Pascale, Naples was obtained, and patients signed informed consent before enrolling in the study. The Strengthening Reporting of Observational Studies in Epidemiology (STROBE) guidelines were followed [9].

Patients' eligibilities were evaluated by an oncologist or pain specialist or palliative care specialist and in-hospital patients, outpatients, and those in home-care settings, were included. Each participating patient was observed for a maximum of 28 days. During the study, patients underwent to four consultations starting from baseline examination (T0) for enrolment and data collection. In particular, in this initial step demographic characteristics, settings, tumor type, background pain characterization (the type of pain and pain intensity), and performance status through the Eastern Cooperative Oncology Group (ECOG) 0–5 scale, were collected. Each participating patient was then evaluated after 7 days (T7), 14 days (T14), and 28 days from baseline (T28), (Figure 1).

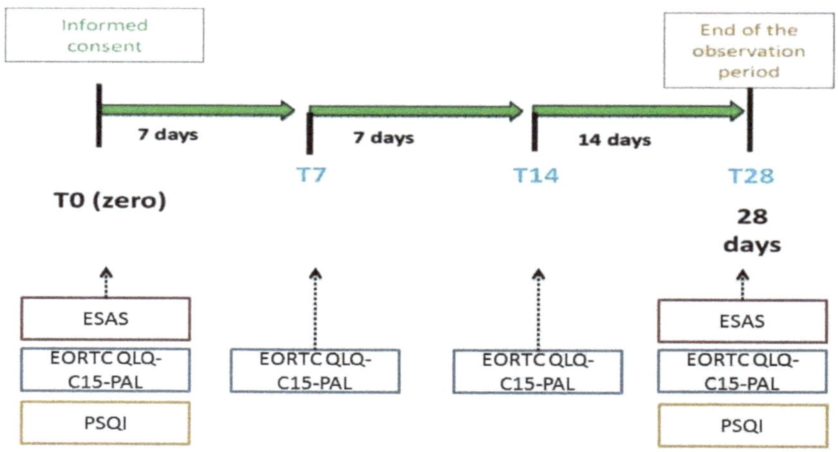

Figure 1. Study design. Legend: EORTC QLQ-C15-PAL, European Organization of Research and Treatment Quality of Life Questionnaire-Cancer 15; PSQI, Pittsburgh Sleep Quality Index; ESAS, Edmonton Symptom Assessment System.

Data were collected from the patient's medical records and summarized in e-CRF (electronic Case Report Form). The definition of BTcP was: a transitory pain exacerbation of moderate to severe intensity that occurs spontaneously or predictably [10], well distinguished from a stable background pain (NRS ≤ 4) [11]. BTcP treatment was carried out through one of the available rapid-onset transmucosal formulations. Inclusion and exclusion criteria are summarized in Table 1.

Table 1. Inclusion and exclusion criteria.

Inclusion Criteria	Exclusion Criteria
• Adult male and female patients (≥18 years) of any ethnic origin with solid malignancy (any stage) • Stable chronic background pain: baseline NRS ≤4 for more than 12 h a day in the previous week through ATC opioid therapy • Patients who report suffering from BTcP crisis: 1 to 4 times a day in at least 1 of the 3 days before the start of the study • Prescription of transmucosal fentanyl (any formulation) for the treatment of BTcP in doses effective according to the best supportive therapy and in accordance with the provisions of the relative SmPC, in absence of specific contraindications • Basic therapy of chronic background pain through OMEDD of ≥60 mg • Patient's ability to understand and sign the informed consent • Life expectancy of at least 30 days • ECOG Performance Status 0 to 3	• Intense episodic pain of a non-oncological nature • Intense no-BTcP * • ECOG Performance Status 4 • Altered patient's state of consciousness and/or inability to fill in the evaluation questionnaires • Participation in an intervention clinical study • Pregnancy or breastfeeding • Contraindications to the use of opioids • BTcP treatment already in place • Patients with previous or current history of neurological/psychiatric disorder and/or any substance abuse (or dependence) ^ • Any medical condition or situation complicating the collection of study data, as determined by the Investigator

Notes: * End-dose pain or pain during titration of the opioid dose; ^ patients treated with antidepressants have been not excluded. Abbreviations: NRS, Numeric Rating Scale; ATC, around-the-clock; OMEDD, oral morphine equivalent daily doses; BTcP, breakthrough cancer pain; SmPC, summary of product characteristics; ECOG, Eastern Cooperative Oncology Group.

2.2. *Study Endpoints and HRQoL Assessments*

The primary objective of the study was to define:

- The impact on BTcP treatment through transmucosal fentanyl on HRQoL, sleep quality and daily activities in patients with background pain adequately controlled by ATC opioids as maintenance therapy.

The HR quality of life (QoL) was measured by the European Organization of Research and Treatment Quality of Life Questionnaire-Cancer 15 (EORTC QLQ-C15-PAL) [12] and the Edmonton Symptom Assessment System (ESAS) [13] whereas sleep quality was assessed by the Pittsburgh Sleep Quality Index (PSQI) [14]. EORTC QLQ-C15-PAL was administered at the four visits: T0 (baseline), T7, T14, and T28, whereas ESAS and PSQI were adopted at the baseline (T0) and the end of the observation period (T28).

The secondary objective was to evaluate the:

- Baseline background pain characteristics;
- BTcP features including type (spontaneous, incident), and the number of episodes. Differences according to visits (T0, T7, T14, T28) on number of BTcP episodes were evaluated;
- BTcP management in terms of median time to pain relief.

Any serious adverse event related to background pain therapy and for BTcP management was reported.

2.3. *Statistical Analyses*

2.3.1. General Linear Model

Categorical variables were presented by frequencies and percentages. The general linear model (GLM) for repeated measures analysis was used. This statistical approach is mathematically identical to multiple regression analysis and it is particularly useful for the correlation of multiple qualitative and quantitative variables. According to this strategy, the mean-scores for HRQoL parameters in T0, T7, T14, and T28 were evaluated: the linear *p*-value indicates the statistical trend for the four measures, while the square *p*-value shows the statistical change from the last visit to the baseline (T28 vs. T0).

Results were only based on non-missing data (i.e., no replacement of missing observations was applied), unless specified otherwise; in particular, the number of patients that completed each visit was taken into account: T0 = 154 pts; T7 = 136 pts; T14 = 124 pts and T28 = 100 pts.

The Bonferroni's method can be used to compare different groups at the baseline. It provides a pairwise comparison of the means, investigates on the relationship between variables, or examines one or more endpoints in clinical trials. To obtain effect size, partial eta-squared ($\eta 2p$) was calculated. Estimates of effect size give a partial eta squared ($\eta 2p$) value for each effect and each parameter considered. The partial eta-squared statistic describes the proportion of the total variability attributable to a factor (small = 0.01, medium = 0.06, and large = 0.14).

Statistical analyses were performed using IBM® SPSS® Statistics, version 25 (IBM Corp., Armonk, NY, USA). All statistical tests were two-sided, and *p* values of less than 0.05 were considered significant.

2.3.2. Quality of Life Analysis

We used a mathematical approach that could allow us to obtain the greatest amount of information despite the reduced sample size. In particular, since each score represented a continuous quantity, to make the variable discrete, we applied a statistical approach proposed by Osaba et al. [15] which allows establishing the improvement or the worsening, setting in advance what the variation of the score must be (e.g., of 10 points). In short, each patient represents his control. According to this method, the best HRQoL response from baseline for each domain or symptom was estimated as a change of the score of at least 10 points from baseline to be clinically relevant. Subjects were intended as improved if they achieved a score ≥10 points than baseline anytime, and were judged worsened with a score ≥10 points lower than baseline without having improved at any time; those with scores fluctuating less than 10 points from baseline were intended stable. A Chi-square test was used to test statistical significance.

An adjusted logistic regression analysis was performed to assess the association between the best response of HRQoL questionnaires (EORTC; PSQI and ESAS) and some covariates. Odds ratios (ORs) and 95% confidence intervals (95% CI) were estimated.

3. Results

Table 2 summarizes demographic and clinical data for the population under study. Among the eligible patients, 154 who referred to control cancer pain by ATC opioid therapy maintenance and suffering from BTcP were included in the analysis. The mean age was 63 ± 11 years, 56% were men and 44% women. A total of 92 patients were treated in an oncological department, 36 by pain therapists, and 26 in a palliative care setting. Background pain was nociceptive in 37% of patients and mixed (nociceptive plus neuropathic) in the remaining 63%.

Table 2. Baseline demographic and clinical data (n = 154).

Sex	*N* (%)
Male	86 (55.8)
Female	68 (44.2)
Age (mean ± SD)	63.5 ± 11.2
Tumor type, *n* (%)	
Lung	51 (33.1)
Breast/Gynecological	12 (7.8)
Gastrointestinal	20 (13.0)
Others #	71 (46.1)
Pain management	
Oncology	92 (59.7)
Pain therapy	36 (23.4)
Palliative care	26 (16.9)
Settings	
Hospital patients	88 (57.1)
Outpatients	61 (39.6)
Home-care settings	5 (3.2)
Background pain	
Nociceptive	62 (37.1)
Mixed pain	105 (62.9)

Legend: # sarcomas, melanomas and other skin cancers, bone tumors, urological tumors.

3.1. *Quality of Life*

The HRQoL analysis through GLM showed a significant improvement for all physical and emotional characteristics in the EORTC QLQ-C15-PAL, except for nausea and vomiting (linear p-value = 0.1), and dyspnea (linear p-value = 0.05). Moreover, there was a significant improvement in the global health status at the end of the study (p = 0.002) (Figure 2).

PSQI and ESAS questionnaires confirmed a significant improvement in the quality of sleep (PSQI), and in all domains of the HRQoL including psychological outcomes (ESAS), after 28 days of observation (p = 0.002, and $p < 0.0001$ respectively) (Table 3). Concerning effect size of GLM analysis, Table 3 compares each follow-up (T7, T14, T28) at baseline for each tool administered. Significant results with largest effect size were observed for Global health status/QoL, pain and ESAS ($\eta 2p$ = 0.14; 0.26 and 0.14, respectively).

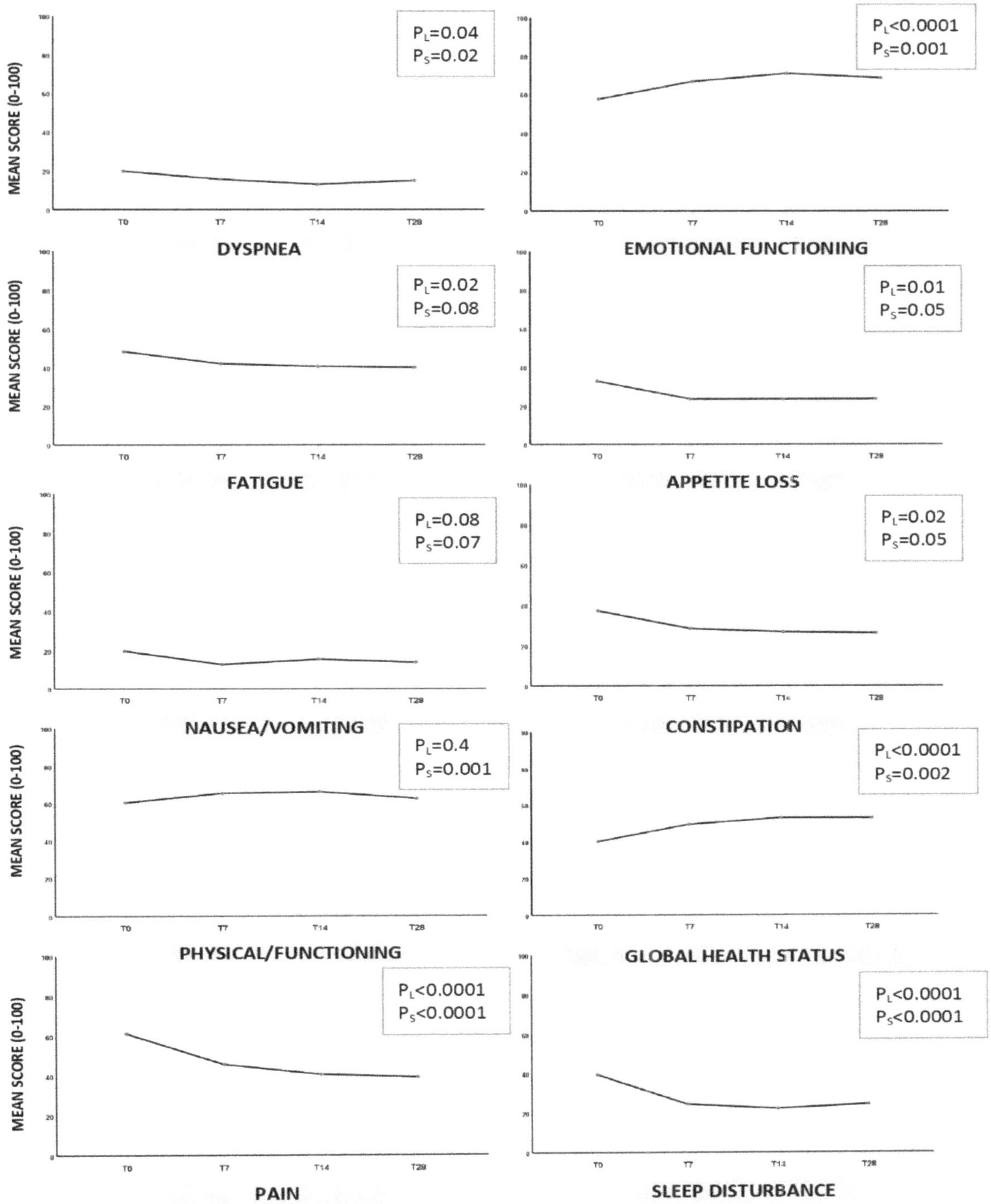

Figure 2. EORTC QLQ-C15-PAL results. Legend: P_L = Linear p-value indicates the statistical trend for the 4 visits; P_S = square p-value indicates the statistical change from T28 to T0. $p < 0.05$ was considered statistically significant for both.

Consistent results were found when QoL best response was calculated (Table 4A). The improved were 55% for the Global health status of the EORTC tool; about 40% for PSQI, and 62% for ESAS. Interestingly, the female gender was associated with an improvement in global health status (68%) (Table 4B). On the other hand, the lowest number of improved were observed for nausea/vomiting, and dyspnea (27% and 29%, respectively), confirming the significant results from GLM analysis (Figure 2 and Table 3).

Table 3. General linear model analyses: mean score of quality of life at baseline until last follow-up.

	Baseline Mean (I) ± SD	Follow-Up T7 Mean (J) ± SD	Follow-Up T14 Mean (J) ± SD	Follow-Up T28 Mean (J) ± SD	Partial Square Eta (η^2_p) **
EORTC Global health status/QoL	40.06 ± 20.4	49.36 ± 18.7	52.88 ± 22.2	52.72 ± 23.7	
Mean differences (I-J) (*p*-value) *		−9.30 (<0.0001)	−12.82 (<0.0001)	−12.66 (<0.0001)	0.14
Physical functioning	60.25 ± 28.3	65.27 ± 24.6	66.03 ± 26.9	62.4 ± 30.1	
Mean differences (I-J) (*p*-value) *		−5.02 (0.06)	−5.76 (0.05)	−2.14 (0.9)	0.03
Emotional functioning	57.53 ± 25.2	66.66 ± 24.1	70.83 ± 25.1	68.58 ± 26.4	
Mean differences (I-J) (*p*-value) *		−9.13 (0.001)	−13.3 (<0.0001)	−11.06 (0.001)	0.10
Fatigue	48.39 ± 28.3	42.15 ± 25.7	40.7 ± 26.7	40.22 ± 28.3	
Mean differences (I-J) (*p*-value) *		6.25 (0.1)	7.69 (0.02)	8.17 (0.08)	0.04
Nausea/vomiting	19.74 ± 25.3	12.94 ± 19.9	15.53 ± 22.7	13.91 ± 22.1	
Mean differences (I-J) (*p*-value) *		6.79 (0.01)	4.20 (0.4)	5.82 (0.2)	0.03
Pain	61.21 ± 22.8	45.67 ± 22.5	40.54 ± 25.4	39.10 ± 22.5	
Mean differences (I-J) (*p*-value) *		15.54 (<0.0001)	20.67 (<0.0001)	22.11 (<0.0001)	0.26
Dyspnea	19.87 ± 25.2	15.7 ± 21.3	13.14 ± 22.5	15.1 ± 23.6	
Mean differences (I-J) (*p*-value) *		4.17 (0.1)	6.73 (0.01)	4.80 (0.4)	0.03
Sleeping disturbance	39.4 ± 35.9	24.35 ± 27.2	22.11 ± 27.3	24.35 ± 28.3	
Mean differences (I-J) (*p*-value) *		15.06 (<0.0001)	17.3 (<0.0001)	15.06 (<0.0001)	0.13
Appetite loss	33.01 ± 31.6	23.71 ± 28.1	23.71 ± 30.3	23.71 ± 29.9	
Mean differences (I-J) (*p*-value) *		9.29 (0.008)	9.29 (0.03)	9.29 (0.04)	0.05
Constipation	37.22 ± 32.7	28.48 ± 27.7	26.89 ± 27.2	26.21 ± 29.01	
Mean differences (I-J) (*p*-value) *		8.74 (0.002)	2.9 (0.003)	11.0 (0.008)	
PSQI Sleep disorders	9.54 ± 4.3	-	-	8.29 ± 4.6	
Mean differences (I-J) (*p*-value) *				1.25 (0.001)	0.10
ESAS	29.95 ± 16.1	-	-	23.1 ± 16.9	
Mean differences (I-J) (*p*-value) *				6.86 (<0.0001)	0.14

Notes: * Bonferroni's method (*p*-value); ** Partial eta-squared (η^2_p) small = 0.01, medium = 0.06, and large = 0.14. Abbreviations: EORTC QLQ-C15-PAL, European Organization of Research and Treatment Quality of Life Questionnaire-Cancer 15; PSQI, Pittsburgh Sleep Quality Index; ESAS, Edmonton Symptom Assessment System.

Subsequently, the improved were compared with worse response to assess variables that contributed to explain this difference for the three questionnaires adopted (EORTC QLQ-C15-PAL, PSQI, and ESAS). Some covariates were also studied. Table 5 shows the results of the adjusted logistic regression analysis. A significant improvement for the global health status (EORTC) was found for female patients (OR = 0.17 95% CI 0.04–0.68), and the setting of patients treated by pain therapists compared with those managed by oncologists (OR = 0.11 95% CI 0.02–0.58). This latter significant result was confirmed either for the sleep quality (PSQI) or ESAS questionnaires (OR = 0.15 95% CI 0.03–0.77; OR = 0.27 95% CI 0.09–0.85, respectively). Furthermore, a significant association was found with the type of BTcP. In particular, the presence of mixed pain was associated with a better response in the global health status (OR = 0.17 95% CI 0.05–0.67) compared with the nociceptive pain alone

(p= 0.01). Finally, data from the PSQI questionnaire indicated that the older age (>70) is significantly associated with worse sleep quality (OR = 8.46 95% CI 2.46–29.11).

Table 4. Best quality of life response: overall data (**A**) and gender stratification (**B**).

	Overall Response						Gender Stratification					
	RESULT TREND ^											
SCALE/ITEM	Improved		Stable		Worsened		Improved		Stable		Worsened	
							M	F	M	F	M	F
	n	(%)	*n*	(%)	*n*	(%)	*n* (%)	*n* (%)	*n* (%)	*n* (%)	*n* (%)	*n* (%)
EORTC												
Global health status	55	(55)	27	(27)	18	(18)	28 (47)	27 (68)	17 (28)	10 (25)	15 (25)	3 (7)
Physical function.	39	(39)	26	(26)	35	(35)	22 (37)	17 (43)	16 (26)	10 (25)	22 (37)	13 (32)
Emotional function.	54	(54)	27	(27)	19	(19)	31 (52)	23 (58)	17 (28)	10 (25)	12 (20)	7 (17)
Fatigue	53	(53)	19	(19)	28	(28)	30 (50)	23 (58)	13 (22)	6 (15)	17 (28)	11 (27)
Nausea/vomiting	27	(27)	59	(59)	14	(14)	17 (28)	10 (25)	34 (57)	25 (63)	9 (15)	5 (12)
Pain	61	(61)	28	(28)	11	(11)	31 (52)	30 (75)	21 (35)	7 (18)	8 (13)	3 (7)
Dyspnea	29	(29)	60	(60)	11	(11)	23 (38)	6 (15)	32 (54)	28 (70)	5 (8)	6 (15)
Sleep disturbance	45	(45)	40	(40)	15	(15)	27 (45)	18 (45)	23 (38)	17 (43)	10 (17)	5 (12)
Appetite loss	38	(38)	42	(42)	20	(20)	20 (33)	18 (45)	26 (44)	16 (40)	14 (23)	6 (15)
Constipation	36	(36)	45	(45)	19	(19)	22 (37)	14 (35)	24 (40)	21 (53)	14 (23)	5 (12)
PSQI Sleep disorders	39	(40)	42	(43)	16	(17)	20 (34)	19 (50)	29 (49)	13 (34)	10 (17)	6 (16)
ESAS	62	(63)	6	(6)	31	(31)	37 (62)	25 (64)	4 (6)	2 (5)	19 (32)	12 (31)

Notes: ^ Improved=score ≥10 points were better than baseline anytime; worsened = sccre ≥10 points lower than baseline without having improved at any time; stable = score changes ≤ 10 points from baseline. Abbreviations: EORTC QLQ-C15-PAL, European Organization of Research and Treatment Quality of Life Questionnaire-Cancer 15; PSQI, Pittsburgh Sleep Quality Index; ESAS, Edmonton Symptom Assessment System.

Table 5. Adjusted logistic regression analysis on improved^ patients.

	Global health status *	PSQI	ESAS
	p-Value (OR 95% CI)	*p*-Value (OR 95% CI)	*p*-Value (OR 95% CI)
Sex	0.01	0.3	0.9
Male	1 †		
Female	0.17 (0.04–0.68)		
Age	0.7	0.002	0.4
<60		1 †	
61–70		1.68 (0.51–5.53)	
>70		8.46 (2.46–29.11)	
Department	0.03	0.07	0.02
Oncology	1 †	1 †	1 †
Pain therapy	0.11 (0.02–0.58)	0.15 (0.03–0.77)	0.27 (0.09–0.85)
Palliative care	0.53 (0.13–2.11)	0.81 (0.23–2.74)	0.46 (0.15–1.36)
Type of Pain	0.01	0.1	0.2
Nociceptive	1 †		
Neurop. /Nocic.	0.17 (0.05–0.67)		

Notes: ^ Score ≥ 10 points better than baseline anytime; * evaluated by the European Organization of Research and Treatment Quality of Life Questionnaire-Cancer 15 (EORTC QLQ-C15-PAL); † logistic regression adjusted for terms of sex, age. Abbreviations: PSQI, Pittsburgh Sleep Quality Index; ESAS, Edmonton Symptom Assessment System.

3.2. *Breakthrough Cancer Pain*

Figure 3 illustrates the features of BTcP in patients who completed the study (real percentage). At baseline, BTcP was mainly spontaneous/idiopathic (70% of all registered cases), the incident type (voluntary or non-voluntary) occurred in 21% of cases, while in the remaining 9% a procedural BTcP was found. In the course of the study, this distribution did not change (not significant, p = 0.2) (Figure 3A). At T0, the BTcP number of episodes (1 to 7; 8 to 14; 15 to 21; 22 to 28), showed that 1–7 BTcP episodes per week occurred in approximately 53% of all cases and a high number of events (22 to 28) were reported by 7.8% of patients. During the observation times, the number of patients with many episodes of BTcP (22 to 28) decreased (T7 4.4%; T14 2.4%) but returned to increase at the end of the study (7%). We also found that the amount of patients who were free from BTcP increased significantly during the study (from 0 to 13%) ($p < 0.001$). The reduction was also significant for the clusters 8-14 and 15-21 events. In particular, 15-21 episodes at baseline were reported for about 15% of patient to decrease to 7% at T28 ($p < 0.001$) (Figure 3B). Concerning the medium time to relief, while at T0 it was 30–60 minutes in about 20% of patients, at the end of the study the percentage of patients who responded in long times dropped to 7% ($p < 0.0001$). Furthermore, the number of patients who responded to treatment in 20–30 minutes also dropped significantly from about 29.2% to 15% ($p < 0.0001$). On the contrary, the response increased in ultra-short (<5 min) and short (5–10, 10–20) times. In addition, in these ranges, the variations were significant ($p < 0.0001$) (Figure 3C).

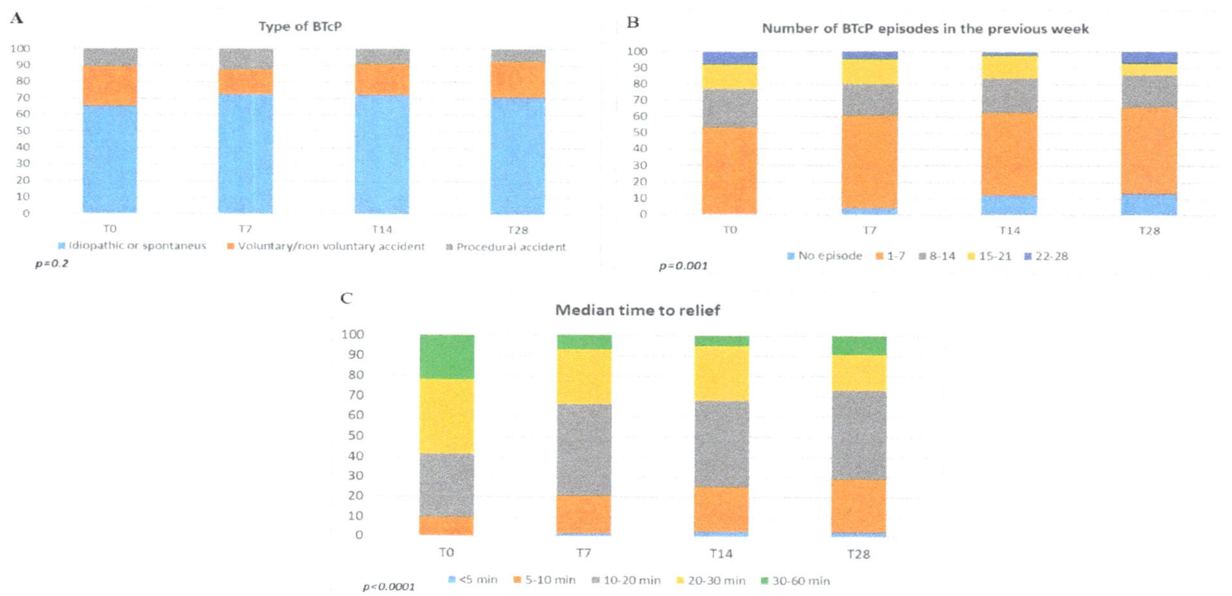

Figure 3. Breakthrough cancer pain (BTcP) results. (**A**) Features, (**B**) trend, and (**C**) response to therapy.

4. Study Limitations

The major limitation of the study seems to be the poor consistency of the sample size. For instance, the small size simple and the lack of a complete multivariate analysis, associated with the rapid-onset opioids (ROO) pharmacokinetics features (i.e., time limited activity) made it difficult to establish how the therapeutic variable was related—in a cause-effect relationship—with the type of response. However, thanks to the statistical approach adopted which combined the multivariate analysis with the careful interpretation of the changes in the HRQoL scores, we were able to measure the change in the four observation times for each patient enrolled, estimating, in turn, the trend. In other words, an 'outcome' variable was established making the analysis independent from the sample size. In addition, adjusted multivariate analysis was also applied to the three questionnaires.

Another limitation is the lack of data on the type of treatment of background pain (e.g., opioids and their doses, adjuvants, other pharmacological and non-pharmacological therapies). As a characterization of therapy was not the aim of the study, we considered all patients with OMEDD of ≥ 60 mg and well-controlled pain to be enrolled.

Finally, the lack of the control group due to the study design did not allow for a precise analysis of different dose response patterns. We hope that the data from this observational investigation can be used to design controlled studies.

5. Discussion

This study explored the effect of BTcP treatment on several aspects of the HRQoL in patients with cancer pain. The HRQoL was investigated through a battery of tools capable of evaluating the largest number of domains. General data were investigated by the EORTC QLQ-C15-PAL, the PSQI questionnaire served to evaluate sleep quality, and the ESAS one helped to explore general domains and psychological aspects of cancer pain including anxiety and depression.

In regards to BTcP management, we have chosen to treat BTcP through rapid-onset opioids (ROOs), drugs specifically indicated for this purpose. ROOs, indeed, have a pharmacodynamics that mirror the sudden start and brief duration of the pain event [3]. However, because the lack of comparative data, we have not indicated the type of formulation to be used. Furthermore, despite there is a debate on the starting dose of ROOs, i.e., if a titration dose is needed or these drugs must be administered in proportional to the regimen of opioid for background pain treatment [16], in this study we have adopted the ROOs administration strategy based on the following the provisions of the relative summary of product characteristics, and in absence of specific contraindications.

Although the HRQoL investigated through the EORTC QLQ-C15-PAL instrument showed a significant amelioration in the global health status at the end of the study and a significant improvement for all physical and emotional descriptors of the questionnaire, except for nausea and vomiting, and dyspnea. Concerning dyspnea, it is a symptom of advanced disease, whereas nausea and vomiting are mainly related to opioid therapy but can be also related to the cancer disease itself, and anticancer therapies. Having observed an improvement for constipation and not for nausea and vomiting, perhaps may indicate that during opioid therapy more attention is paid to constipation than to other adverse effects that only apparently have a lower impact on HRQoL.

Concerning quality of sleep, compared to the baseline we observed a significant improvement ($p < 0.0001$) at the end of the study. Nevertheless, the adjusted logistic regression analysis demonstrated that the elderly patients (>70 years) had a risk 8.5 fold higher than those observed in patients less than 60 years of age. These findings are not surprising as a recent cross-sectional multicenter study has highlighted that around 80% of cancer patients experienced poor sleep quality, and this issue mainly concerns older patients [17]. The clinical implication is that sleep quality must be better assessed and greater efforts must be made to ensure adequate treatment of sleep disturbances in these patients.

The ESAS questionnaire also showed a significant improvement between the end and the beginning of the study ($p < 0.0001$). However, the regression analysis failed to find a correlation between these positive results and age-related factors, gender, and type of underlying pain. Whatever the underlying correlation, we can assume that the treatment of cancer pain induces an important improvement of multiple patient's psychological aspects [18].

Further significant data came from the regression analysis. Female gender, for example, was associated with an improvement in global health status ($p < 0.01$). Several pieces of evidence suggested that different pain thresholds may exist between men and women. Physiologic factors such as ovarian hormone and increased serotonergic activity, and psychological dynamics (e.g., increased anxiety in women) have been called into question to explain this phenomenon which, in turn, must be better explained [19]. However, it seems to be difficult to explain a better therapeutic result in terms of pain relief in one sex compared to the other. Preclinical research in rodents showed different concentration of opioid receptors between male and female animals. Furthermore, morphine seems to induce more potent effects in female than in male [20]. Again, it was proved that female rats require almost twice as much morphine as males for obtaining comparable analgesic effects [21]. Probably, sex differences in opioids response must be better elucidated. Furthermore, the gender-related improvement concerned not only the symptom pain but involved other aspects of HRQoL, except for sleep (PSQI) and the domains of the ESAS tool.

Of note, the main finding that is found in all questionnaires is the paramount role of pain therapists as there was significant improvement in the setting of patients treated by these clinicians. Pain therapists are perhaps more likely to perform pain management through tailored therapies and by coordinating multidisciplinary strategies [22]. The improvement also affected patients treated in palliative care, although the result was not significant.

With regards to background pain, the best results have been achieved in patients with mixed pain, although only in the EORTC questionnaire. The data can be explained with probable greater attention towards forms of pain that represent a challenge for those who must treat chronic pain.

The analysis of BTcP and its trend during the investigation period showed interesting data. Our study suggested that adequate BTcP management can probably reverberate on the characteristics of BTcP by reducing the number of episodes. Of note, there was also an improved response to therapy. The phenomenon, however, requires further investigation as multiple factors such as type and course of cancer disease, clinical setting, and background pain therapy can influence the incidence and characteristics of BTcP. Furthermore, this unpredictable severe acute pain represents a heterogeneous condition and includes spontaneous forms and those induced by voluntary, or involuntary movements. Therefore, especially incident pain benefits from better therapy. In a longitudinal study, carried out on in-hospital patients, the incidence changed over time, falling from 87% to 32% after six months from the first detection. The greatest decrease in BTcP occurrence concerned the incident subtype [23]. Moreover, Mercadante et al. [24] found in home-care patients, that the prevalence of BTcP decreased after one month, possibly due to a progressive reduction in physical activity or as a consequence of a better background pain control. Thus, we have planned to carry out another multicenter research and a retrospective analysis on a large database, for evaluating potential associations between BTcP and several clinical variables.

6. Conclusions

BTcP treatment remains a great challenge in medicine. It requires, indeed, individualized treatment through the involvement of a multidisciplinary team. Despite the limitations, results from this multicenter, observational cohort study conducted by an Italian expert group, has confirmed that accurate management of BTcP from the baseline may improve several aspects of the HRQoL. Because of in cancer patients there is a high prevalence of BTcP and this severe acute pain has deleterious clinical consequences, this information can have an important clinical significance. In this population, more attention should be given to the treatment of sleep disturbances and the management of nausea and vomiting. Further studies are needed to verify the fascinating hypothesis that adequate BTcP treatment can probably reduce the number of episodes, also improving its response to therapy, and in turn, the HRQoL of these fragile individuals.

Author Contributions: Project administration, Arturo Cuomo; Conceptualization, Arturo Cuomo; formal analysis, C.A.F., G.E., S.D.S., A.C.; investigation, Arturo Cuomo, M.C., C.A.F., G.E., S.D.S., L.C., F.F., M.D., S.N., M.M., A.M., R.D.M., V.L., Sabrina Bimonte, Sandro Barni, G.P., and S.M.; methodology, Arturo Cuomo, S.M., S.N., G.E., A.C.; resources, S.D.S., A.M., and G.P.; supervision, Arturo Cuomo, and C.A.F.; validation, M.C., and F.F.; writing—original draft, M.C., and A.C; writing—review and editing, M.C., A.C., and Arturo Cuomo. All authors have read and agreed to the published version of the manuscript.

Funding: This research received no external funding.

Acknowledgments: This research was funded by TEVA and the APC was funded by IRCCS Pascale, Naples, Italy.

Conflicts of Interest: The authors declare no conflicts of interest.

References

1. Van den Beuken-van Everdingen, M.H.; Hochstenbach, L.M.; Joosten, E.A.; Tjan-Heijnen, V.C.; Janssen, D.J. Update on Prevalence of Pain in Patients With Cancer: Systematic Review and Meta-Analysis. *J. Pain Symptom Manag.* **2016**, *51*, 1070–1090. [CrossRef] [PubMed]
2. Scarborough, B.M.; Smith, C.B. Optimal pain management for patients with cancer in the modern era. *CA Cancer J. Clin.* **2018**, *68*, 182–196. [CrossRef] [PubMed]

3. Fallon, M.; Giusti, R.; Aielli, F.; Hoskin, P.; Rolke, R.; Sharma, M.; Ripamonti, C.I. ESMO Guidelines Committee. Management of cancer pain in adult patients: ESMO Clinical Practice Guidelines. *Ann. Oncol.* **2018**, *29*, iv166–iv191. [CrossRef] [PubMed]
4. Basch, E.; Deal, A.M.; Kris, M.G.; Scher, H.I.; Hudis, C.A.; Sabbatini, P.; Rogak, L.; Bennett, A.V.; Dueck, A.C.; Atkinson, T.M.; et al. Symptom monitoring with patient-reported outcomes during routine cancer treatment: A randomized controlled trial. *J. Clin. Oncol.* **2016**, *34*, 557–565. [CrossRef] [PubMed]
5. Mercadante, S.; Lazzari, M.; Reale, C.; Cuomo, A.; Fusco, F.; Marchetti, P.; Mediati, R.D.; Chiurazzi, B.; Ciuffedra, L.; Caraceni, A.; et al. Italian Oncological Pain Survey (IOPS): A multicentre Italian study of breakthrough pain performed in different settings. *Clin. J. Pain* **2015**, *31*, 214–221. [CrossRef]
6. Mercadante, S.; Marchetti, P.; Cuomo, A.; Caraceni, A.; Mediati, R.D.; Vellucci, R.; Mammucari, M.; Natoli, S.; Lazzari, M.; Dauri, M.; et al. IOPS-MS Study Group. Factors Influencing the Clinical Presentation of Breakthrough Pain in Cancer Patients. *Cancers* **2018**, *10*, 175. [CrossRef]
7. Camps Herrero, C.; Batista, N.; Díaz Fernández, N.; Escobar Álvarez, Y.; Gonzalo Gómez, A.; Isla Casado, D.; Salud, A.; Terrasa Pons, J.; Guillem Porta, V. Breakthrough cancer pain: Review and calls to action to improve its management. *Clin. Transl. Oncol.* **2020**. In press. [CrossRef]
8. Davies, A.N.; Patel, S.D.; Gregory, A.; Lee, B. Observational study of sleep disturbances in advanced cancer. *BMJ Support Palliat. Care* **2017**, *7*, 435–440. [CrossRef]
9. Vandenbroucke, J.P.; von Elm, E.; Altman, D.G.; Gøtzsche, P.C.; Mulrow, C.D.; Pocock, S.J.; Poole, C.; Schlesselman, J.J.; Egger, M.; STROBE Initiative. Strengthening the Reporting of Observational Studies in Epidemiology (STROBE): Explanation and elaboration. *Int. J. Surg.* **2014**, *12*, 1500–1524. [CrossRef]
10. Davies, A.; Zeppetella, G.; Andersen, S.; Damkier, A.; Vejlgaard, T.; Nauck, F.; Radbruch, L.; Sjolund, K.F.; Stenberg, M.; Buchanan, A. Multi-centre European study of breakthrough cancer pain: Characteristics and patient perceptions of current and potential management strategies. *Eur. J. Pain* **2011**, *15*, 756–763. [CrossRef]
11. Davies, A.; Buchanan, A.; Zeppetella, G.; Porta-Sales, J.; Likar, R.; Weismayr, W.; Slama, O.; Korhonen, T.; Filbet, M.; Poulain, P.; et al. Breakthrough cancer pain: An observational study of 1000 European oncology patients. *J. Pain Symptom Manag.* **2013**, *46*, 619–628. [CrossRef] [PubMed]
12. Groenvold, M.; Petersen, M.A.; Aaronson, N.K.; Arraras, J.I.; Blazeby, J.M.; Bottomley, A.; Fayers, P.M.; de Graeff, A.; Hammerlid, E.; Kaasa, S.; et al. The EORTC Quality of Life Group. The development of the EORTC QLQ-C15-PAL: A shortened questionnaire for cancer patients in palliative care. *Eur. J. Cancer* **2006**, *42*, 55–64. [CrossRef] [PubMed]
13. Moro, C.; Brunelli, C.; Miccinesi, G.; Fallai, M.; Morino, P.; Piazza, M.; Labianca, R.; Ripamonti, C. Edmonton symptom assessment scale: Italian validation in two palliative care settings. *Support Care Cancer* **2006**, *14*, 30–37. [CrossRef] [PubMed]
14. Buysse, D.J.; Reynolds, C.F., 3rd; Monk, T.H.; Berman, S.R.; Kupfer, D.J. The Pittsburgh Sleep Quality Index: A new instrument for psychiatric practice and research. *Psychiatry Res.* **1989**, *28*, 193–213. [CrossRef]
15. Osoba, D.; Rodrigues, G.; Myles, J.; Zee, B.; Pater, J. Interpreting the significance of changes in health-related quality-of-life scores. *J. Clin. Oncol.* **1998**, *16*, 139–144. [CrossRef]
16. Yen, T.Y.; Chiou, J.F.; Chiang, W.Y.; Su, W.H.; Huang, M.Y.; Hu, M.H.; Wu, S.C.; Lai, Y.L. Proportional dose of rapid-onset opioid in breakthrough cancer pain management: An open-label, multicenter study. *Medicine* **2018**, *97*, e11593. [CrossRef]
17. Jakobsen, G.; Engstrøm, M.; Fayers, P.; Hjermstad, M.J.; Kaasa, S.; Kloke, M.; Sabatowski, R.; Klepstad, P. Sleep quality with WHO Step III opioid use for cancer pain. *BMJ Support Palliat. Care* **2019**, *9*, 307–315. [CrossRef]
18. Cascella, M.; Thompson, N.S.; Muzio, M.R.; Forte, C.A.; Cuomo, A. The underestimated role of psychological and rehabilitation approaches for management of cancer pain. A brief commentary. *Recenti Prog. Med.* **2016**, *107*, 418–421.
19. Ahmed, Y.; Popovic, M.; Wan, B.A.; Lam, M.; Lam, H.; Ganesh, V.; Milakovic, M.; DeAngelis, C.; Malek, L.; Chow, E. Does gender affect self-perceived pain in cancer patients?—A meta-analysis. *Ann. Palliat. Med.* **2017**, *6* (Suppl. 2), S177–S184. [CrossRef]
20. Bodnar, R.J.; Kest, B. Sex difference in opioid analgesia, hyperalgesia, tolerance and withdrawal: Central mechanisms of action and roles of gonadal hormones. *Horm. Behav.* **2010**, *58*, 72–81. [CrossRef]

21. Doyle, H.H.; Eidson, L.N.; Sinkiewicz, D.M.; Murphy, A.Z. Sex Differences in Microglia Activity within the Periaqueductal Gray of the Rat: A Potential Mechanism Driving the Dimorphic Effects of Morphine. *J. Neurosci.* **2017**, *37*, 3202–3214. [CrossRef] [PubMed]
22. Cuomo, A.; Bimonte, S.; Forte, C.A.; Botti, G.; Cascella, M. Multimodal approaches and tailored therapies for pain management: The trolley analgesic model. *J. Pain Res.* **2019**, *12*, 711–714. [CrossRef] [PubMed]
23. Greco, M.T.; Corli, O.; Montanari, M.; Deandrea, S.; Zagonel, V.; Apolone, G. Epidemiology and Pattern of Care of Breakthrough Cancer Pain in a Longitudinal Sample of Cancer Patients: Results from the Cancer Pain Outcome Research Study Group. *Clin. J. Pain* **2011**, *27*, 9–18. [CrossRef] [PubMed]
24. Mercadante, S.; Costanzo, B.V.; Fusco, F.; Buttà, V.; Vitrano, V.; Casuccio, A. Breakthrough pain in advanced cancer patients followed at home: A longitudinal study. *J. Pain Symptom Manag.* **2009**, *38*, 554–560. [CrossRef] [PubMed]

4

Abuse of Licit and Illicit Psychoactive Substances in the Workplace: Medical, Toxicological and Forensic Aspects

Ricardo Jorge Dinis-Oliveira [1,2,3,*] and Teresa Magalhães [1,2,4,*]

1 IINFACTS—Institute of Research and Advanced Training in Health Sciences and Technologies, Department of Sciences, University Institute of Health Sciences (IUCS), CESPU, CRL, 4585-116 Gandra, Portugal
2 Department of Public Health and Forensic Sciences, and Medical Education, Faculty of Medicine, University of Porto, 4200-319 Porto, Portugal
3 UCIBIO-REQUIMTE, Laboratory of Toxicology, Department of Biological Sciences, Faculty of Pharmacy, University of Porto, 4050-313 Porto, Portugal
4 Fidelidade—Companhia de Seguros, SA, R. Direita de Campinas 324, 4100-207 Porto, Portugal
* Correspondence: ricardinis@med.up.pt (R.J.D.-O.); tmaga@med.up.pt (T.M.)

Abstract: About one-third of adult life is spent in the workplace. The use of psychoactive substances is a major preventable cause of morbidity and mortality. The consumption of psychoactive substances during or outside working hours greatly increases the frequency and severity of labor accidents, as well as the workers' poor general state of health and productivity, implying higher costs for enterprises. It is the responsibility of organizations to ensure the safety and health of their workers. These cannot be limited to traditional routine clinical exams, as other aspects also have an impact on health. Thus, prevention and intervention in the consumption of psychoactive substances (e.g., ethanol, opioids, central nervous system stimulants or depressants, hallucinogens, *Cannabis* derivatives, dissociative substances, and inhalants) in labor activity should be considered as an investment of organizations and not as a cost, in view of the professional, personal, and family advantages for workers and employers, with a potential impact on productivity, security, health, and quality of life at work. Despite the extensive literature on the subject, each article generally focuses on one or another aspect of a very specific nature, not tackling the problem in a holistic way by confronting clinical, safety, and legal issues. This article presents a reflection on the legal, laboratorial, clinical, ethical, forensic, and safety concerns related to the consumption of psychoactive substances in the workplace, and can be a cross-cutting contribution to occupational medicine, forensic medicine, and insurance medicine, as well as for entrepreneurs, lawyers, judges, workers, and technicians from the public and private sectors that develop projects in this area. This discussion is based on general principles established internationally and highlights the role of the occupational healthcare system and other decision-making actors in the prevention and supervision of workplace psychoactive consumption.

Keywords: occupational medicine; forensic medicine; insurance medicine; psychoactive substances; safety; clinical; forensic; law; ethics

---

1. Introduction

Workplaces reflect, to a certain extent, the widespread presence of ethanol and other psychoactive substances in society and the type of work, but sometimes both. There has been global growth in the use of workplace drug testing as a response to drug-related risks to safety and productivity [1,2]. Depending on the countries, the labor sectors, and the professions, statistics suggest high percentages of workers suffer from or are at risk of becoming dependent on ethanol [3]. Civil construction workers, transport workers, hotel staff, barmen, catering workers, farmers, and workers in the primary sectors are particularly affected by this problem, especially in terms of ethanol [3]. Additionally, ethanol-related indicators are often inversely proportional to the level of literacy, meaning that the higher this level is, the less likely workers are to become drunk [4]. However, in some countries, excessive ethanol or other substance consumption is clearly observed among some higher professional groups such as doctors and managers [5,6]. Regarding the consumption of other psychoactive substances in the workplace, the information is scarcer, with *Cannabis* being more prevalent among younger workers, whereas cocaine is more prevalent among highly skilled workers such as managers [7]. Indeed, because workplace drug testing is often performed on-site by occupational physicians, a global statistic spectrum is hard to obtain [8].

The consumption of psychoactive substances at work depends on the combination of multiple factors, some of them linked to individual characteristics and lifestyles, and others being of a professional nature, related for example to the typology of work, rhythms and cadences, shift work, and stress, among others [9,10].

It is obvious that the prevention and deterrence of problems associated with the use of psychoactive substances should be a global intervention involving the participation of all decision-making actors in the organization bodies, namely, occupational medicine, occupational safety and health, human resources, social action services, intermediate and direct leadership, workers' representatives, and workers themselves. Detection may or may not be part of the organization's health and safety policy procedures. In order to create a program that contemplates psychoactive substance testing, the underlying policy, objectives, and rights and responsibilities of all parties involved should be made explicit. Moreover, the analysis of results and the relationship with the worker must respect confidentiality, cooperation, mutual commitment, and capacity building. The final goals are beneficial both for employers and employees and include the increase of workplace productivity by reducing absenteeism, presenteeism, and workplace accidents, as well as raising awareness of the toxic effects of psychoactive substances and their consequences in workers' performance by adopting a more healthily behavior during and outside working hours [9,11,12].

This article presents a reflection on the legal, laboratorial, clinical, ethical, forensic, and safety concerns related to the consumption of psychoactive substances in the workplace, and can be a cross-cutting contribution to occupational medicine for businessmen, lawyers, juries, workers, and laboratory technicians that act in this area. We also aimed to discuss the best practices to be followed by laboratories providing workplace drug testing services.

2. Methods

A narrative review was performed by searching articles in English, French, Spanish, and Portuguese in PubMed, Scopus, Web of Science, and PsycINFO concerning legal, laboratorial, clinical, ethical, forensic, and safety concerns of workplace drug testing, without time limit. Besides these inclusion criteria, additional reports were obtained from the references of the articles identified in the original search. International reports from the World Health Organization; European Union; International Commission on Occupational Health; and legislation on psychoactive substance workplace consumption, testing, and prevention were also reviewed. Specifically, Portuguese legislation, under the European Union regulation, was used as a starting point and, regardless the jurisdiction, broad and transversal aspects general and useful for occupational medicine were discussed. The effects in workplace performance of ethanol, opioids, central nervous system stimulants or depressants, hallucinogens, *Cannabis* derivatives, dissociative substances, inhalants, and examples of new psychoactive substances were also reviewed. From this search, 192 documents were obtained and 105 were ultimately considered for the final version of the manuscript. The remaining documents were excluded if they focused on specific points of certain enterprises or on a very specific point of a country not considered useful for a broad discussion, or when those aspects do not fit well in the scope of occupational medicine, such as technical and analytical details of toxicological methods.

3. Psychoactive Substances and Occupational Risks

Psychoactive substances are those that act mainly on the central nervous system, where they alter brain function, resulting in temporary changes in perception, mood, consciousness, and behavior. The effect depends not only on the specific substance but also on the dose, previous consumption, tolerance, comorbidities, mixture with other substances, and route of administration, among other reasons. In a general overview, all psychoactive substances have, to a higher or lesser extent, a dysfunctional effect on work capability. Considering the clinical usefulness and their most important effects at the level of the central nervous systems at usual doses, psychoactive substances are classified into several groups, which are discussed below regarding their repercussions in terms of workplace performance.

Opioids are mainly used as analgesics and antitussives [13–17]. Physical work and high psychosocial work demands, excessive repetition of tasks, awkward postures, and heavy lifting are all known workplace risk factors for musculoskeletal pain and consequently lead to administration of opioids, according to prospective studies [18,19]. Interestingly, a recent randomized trial demonstrated that treatment with opioids was not better to treatment with nonopioid medications for improving pain-related function over 12 months in moderate to severe chronic back pain or hip or knee osteoarthritis pain [20]. Part of this group are natural compounds extracted from opium such as morphine, codeine, and thebaine; semisynthetic compounds such as heroin, oxycodone, hydrocodone, oxymorphone, etorphine, and hydromorphone; and the synthetics tramadol, tapentadol, meperidine (or pethidine), methadone, fentanyl, and pentazocine. Work-related injuries have been identified as a factor in the rise of opioid dependence and opioid-related overdoses [21,22]. Opioid use has also been associated with the risk of motor vehicle accidents in commercial drivers [23]. Indeed, several adverse effects are possible risk factors for workplace performance, namely, those mediated by μ-receptors, such as sedation, respiratory depression, suppression of cough reflex, sweating, euphoria, dysphoria, confusion, insomnia, agitation, fear, hallucinations, drowsiness, motor decoding and mood swings, miosis, and dependence [17,24,25].

Cocaine, amphetamines (i.e., *d*-amphetamine, *d*-methamphetamine, methylphenidate, 3,4-methylenedioxymethamphetamine), caffeine, nicotine, and ephedrine are **stimulants of the central nervous system** [26–28]. Xenobiotics belonging to this group exhibit, in general, a pronounced stimulating effect in the central nervous system. They reduce the feeling of mental (i.e., increased alertness) and physical fatigue (i.e., increased motor activity) and cause dependence [29,30]. Of these, the most consumed psychoactive substance is caffeine, which is present in coffee, tea, and chocolate, as well as in numerous foods, drugs, and beverages, as it increases energy and concentration, with no major negative labor effects having been reported [31], and it moreover has been linked to a reduced suicide risk [32]. In addition, considerable research suggests that nicotine enhances cognitive control-related processes (e.g., attention, memory) among nicotine-deprived smokers, both in terms of behavior and neural indices [33]. Indeed, smokers deprived of nicotine (e.g., 12 h smoking abstinence) exhibit reduced cognitive-attentional functioning [34]. Employees who tested positive for cocaine were four times more likely to be categorized as absentee employees and two times more likely to be terminated from employment than those who tested negative [35]. Comparing the consumers of amphetamines with those of other illicit psychoactive substances, it was found that they had higher absenteeism due to disease and/or accidents, as well as a higher incidence of behavioral risks. If consumption occurs outside working hours, the period of depression and asthenia and cognitive alterations may arise when they resume work activity. Low-to-moderate doses of stimulants (e.g., amphetamine, caffeine, modafinil) have been reported to be effective countermeasures for mood and performance decrements caused by sleep deprivation and fatigue [36,37].

More than 61 **cannabinoids** have been identified among more than 400 compounds documented in *Cannabis sativa* [16,38–40]. The most important forms are delta-9-tetrahydrocannabinol (Δ^9-THC; main psychoactive constituent), Δ^8-THC (almost as active as the previous one but at lower concentrations), cannabinol (low activity, but at high concentrations), and cannabidiol (not psychoactive, but in high concentrations). Δ^9-THC is the most widely abused illicit psychoactive substance and the potency of the derivative (e.g., marijuana, hashish, hashish oil) depends on the percentage of this xenobiotic [16,39–41]. Δ^9-THC produces euphoria followed by relaxation, distortion in space and time, hallucinations (in higher doses than those normally found clinically), changes in short-term memory, motor incoordination, behavioral disinhibition, concentration and learning issues, decreased appetite, and in high doses paranoid psychosis. It possesses a low risk of psychological dependence and its abstinence is typically characterized by insomnia [42]. Marijuana cigarettes containing low-to-moderate Δ^9-THC concentrations can decrease some night shift-related performance and mood disruptions [43,44]. Occupational medicine additional concerns come from the use of medicinal *Cannabis* [45–47]. Workers who have been authorized to use *Cannabis* should be required to report any change in product, dose, frequency, and timing of use or route of administration, and an occupational physician trained and knowledgeable on the impact and evaluation of potentially impairing substances in the workplace should be included [47]. Moreover, new psychoactive substances, such as synthetic cannabinoids, are now an additional concern to deal with [48]. Indeed, these compounds also bind to cannabinoid receptors and abuse can cause anxiety; confusion; hypertension; psychosis; hallucinations; tachycardia; seizures; and, in severe cases, it can lead to death [49–51].

Hallucinogens, such as the diethylamide of lysergic acid (LSD), mescaline, psilocybin, and psilocin, also have a pronounced effect on workplace performance [52,53]. Hallucinogens intensify sensory experiences and lead to behavioral alterations, delusions, as well as emotional lability at the time of and after consumption, confusional states, and *flashbacks* (i.e., reviving experiences). Chronic consumption can lead to depression, violent behavior, anxiety, and alteration in the perception of time, but the risk of dependence is absent.

The **central nervous system depressant** group mainly includes psychotropic drugs, notably the illicit use of anxiolytics, sedatives, and hypnotics, such as benzodiazepines; barbiturates; and non-benzodiazepine hypnotics such as zolpidem and ethanol [54,55]. Of all substances, ethanol is the one with the highest negative impact on work [9,56]. Globally, ethanol is the world's number one risk factor for ill-health and premature death amongst the 25- to 59-year-old age group, the core of the working-age population [57]. Moreover, in the USA, ethanol-induced impairment directly affects an estimated 15% of the workforce and causes more than 22% of the deaths as a result of injuries at work [58]. The main labor consequences of ethanol consumption are slow reaction time, motor incoordination, decreased visual acuity, emotional lability, reduced concentration, lower intellectual ability, behavioral changes, attendance/punctuality problems, lower productivity, absenteeism, presenteeism, workplace injuries, and higher employee turnover [59]. Several studies have shown that workers who drink the most are more often absent from work due to drinking [60], and they more often report alcohol-related presenteeism and inefficiency at work due to alcohol use [61]. Ethanol is anxiolytic/disinhibiting and has a high potential for abuse. Withdrawal leads to sweating, nausea, tremor, insomnia, decreased appetite, restlessness, aggression, anxiety, and eventually hallucinations. It is often used in conjunction with other substances to enhance the overall effect. Major international organizations such as the World Health Organization, the Council of the European Union, and the International Labor Office advertise the need as priority to actualize policies and programs focused on the issue of ethanol and work.

Among psychoactive drugs, benzodiazepines are the most prescribed drugs, especially as anxiolytic, sedative, or hypnotic drugs, and less often as antiepileptics and/or muscle relaxants [55]. Benzodiazepines have largely replaced barbiturates as they are safer drugs with fewer enzyme-inducing effects, and thus less severe interactions, less severe withdrawal symptoms, and a broad therapeutic margin [62]. However, persistent and longer than recommended use and self-medication is a reality. Benzodiazepines are distinguished between anxiolytic and hypnotic [24,55]. This distinction is somewhat artificial because all are anxiolytic, and all can change sleep as long as certain doses are reached [55,63]. What distinguishes them, however, is that so-called hypnotic benzodiazepines are potent drugs that can, therefore, modify sleep conditions at relatively low doses, whereas so-called anxiolytic benzodiazepines are less potent, allowing for a "therapeutic window" to exist where anxiolytic action can be obtained without significantly interfering with sleep [55]. All benzodiazepines may induce tolerance, dependence, and addiction, but to a lesser extent than barbiturates [62]. Short-acting benzodiazepines have the highest potential to induce dependence, and withdrawal syndrome may even occur when discontinuation is abrupt. The abuse of these drugs is generally higher in females and older workers. The toxic effects of benzodiazepines on quality of work are mostly related to the central nervous system depressant effects, particularly sleepiness, motor incoordination, and impaired thinking [64]. They have a significant impact on motor vehicle driving, workability, and interpersonal relationships, and thus their use should be taken into account in these circumstances [65]. They can also cause short-term memory impairment, that is, diminished ability to learn new information, leaving already learned information intact.

Among **dissociative drugs**, phencyclidine and ketamine were originally developed as dissociative general anesthetics, capable of promoting sensory loss and analgesia, amnesia, and paralysis, generating an intense sensation of dissociation of the environment but without real loss of consciousness and protective reflexes [66,67]. Only ketamine is still available in therapy due to the high frequency of delusions and hallucinations observed postoperatively with phencyclidine [67–70]. The most classic adverse effects of ketamine are delirium, hallucinations, tachycardia, mild respiratory depression, confusion, irrationality, violent or aggressive behavior, dizziness, ataxia, slurred speech, delayed reaction time, euphoria, altered body image, analgesia, amnesia, and coma [66,67].

4. Psychoactive Substances and Occupational Consequences

Employers, for their part, have a broad range of responsibilities, and it is the employer's obligation to ensure the individual and collective health of workers for the proper functioning of all work activities. Psychoactive substance abuse is a major preventable cause of morbidity and mortality and has direct impacts on workability [71]. Staying in the workplace under the influence of psychoactive substances depends on the combination of multiple factors, some linked to individual characteristics and lifestyles, and others of professional nature, such as work typology, rhythms and cadences, irregular working hours as occurs in shift work, stress, and psychological harassment, among others. The following are some of the consequences of the occupational psychoactive substance consumption and thus justify why employers aim for a "drug-free" workplace [72–74]: (i) increase in the rate of presenteeism (i.e., being present at workplace in an impaired state) and absenteeism that affects professional performance promoting errors, and hence the competitiveness and productivity of the enterprise, as well as the country's own wealth; (ii) creation of a negative image, leading to discrediting and despising of the organization; (iii) negative effect on the equipment integrity and therefore a potential cause of financial losses; (iv) negative effect on the workers' physical, psychosocial, and behavioral integrity; (v) risk of neglect and reduced decision-making and motor coordination, consequently leading to a higher number of errors and accidents and therefore costs (e.g., insurance premiums); (vi) workers being more often involved in conflict, violent behavior, and theft, and being more frequently the subject of complaint by coworkers who may also see their physical integrity or even their own lives affected as a result of lack of care or discernment, decreased alertness, or altered perceptions or judgements from others being under the influence of psychoactive substances; and (vii) workers tending to be non-punctual (arriving at work later and leaving early) than the rest of the working population, putting a greater strain on coworkers by introducing additional tasks that still need to be done.

5. Legal Aspects

Aiming at a legal interpretation of this theme, it is important to make clear what is an occupational accident and workplace. Although, these concepts may vary with the different legislation of each country or state, regardless the jurisdiction, these are broad concepts in most legislations. We used Portuguese legislation as a starting point for this approach.

The Portuguese Law no. 98/2009 of 4 September regulates the regime of compensation for occupational accidents and diseases, including occupational rehabilitation and reintegration, pursuant to article 284 of the Labor Code, approved by Law no. 7/2009 of 12 February. In accordance with Article 8, an ***occupational accident*** is one that occurs at the place and time of work and that directly or indirectly results in bodily injury, functional disturbance, or illness resulting in reduced working or earning capacity, or death. Therefore, it is an event that has a professional factor for its occurrence, including acts of violence that occurred within the scope of the workplace concept. Its major differences from the concept of occupational disease, in which occupational factors are also determinant, include (i) very short time (at most a few minutes), usually sudden and unexpected (acute); (ii) easy identification of the cause (professional); and (iii) easy identification of the lesion.

The concept of the ***workplace*** means any place where a worker is or should be by virtue of his/her work and that are directly or indirectly under the employer's control, including road accidents during work-related activities. The term "working time beyond the normal working period" is defined in Portuguese law as the time that (i) precedes its commencement, including preparatory acts; (ii) follows, including related acts; (iii) resulted from normal or forced interruptions of work. Article 9 extends the concept, and also considers a workplace accident as one that occurs (i) on the way to or from the workplace in the routes normally used and considering the period of time usually spent by the worker in those routes: between any of their workplaces if they have more than one job (the destination employer being the responsible for the accident), between his/her habitual or occasional residence and the workplace or the place of payment or the place where they will receive any kind of assistance or treatment by reason of a previous accident, or between the workplace and the place of meal and between the new place defined by the employer for a specific work and the usual workplace or his/her habitual or occasional residence. It is also considered a work accident when the normal route has been interrupted or changed in order to satisfy workers' needs, as well as due to force majeure or due to a fortuitous event (ii) while performing spontaneous services that may result in economic gain for the employer; (iii) at and outside the workplace while representing workers; (iv) at the workplace, when attending a training course, or outside the workplace, if the express permission from the employer for such attendance was obtained; (v) at the place of payment of remuneration and while staying there for that purpose; (vi) at the place where the worker should receive any form of assistance or treatment due to a previous accident and while staying there for that purpose; (vii) while job searching during the hours granted by law to workers with process of termination of the current work contract; and (viii) off-site or working time when verified in the performance of services determined by the employer or consented by him/her.

5.1. Workplace Drug Testing

The legislation applied to workplace drug testing also has some differences among countries [75]. Indeed, a multinational company may not be able to implement the same procedure in all its offices. In this work, we focused upon and discussed general consentaneous aspects that need to be followed in the application of a program for workplace drug testing; the Portuguese legislation was used as a platform for critical reflection. This approach is even more interesting because by adopting a radical step, in July 2001 Portugal became the first country in the world to decriminalize the possession for consumption of all illicit substances (Law no. 30/2000 of 20 November). Rather than being arrested, those caught with a personal supply are obliged to undergo rehabilitation treatment.

Although there are no specific propositions referring to psychoactive substance testing in the workplace, the Portuguese law appoints a set of very strict general rules regarding the worker's health. Indeed, the human life (Article 24); the moral and physical integrity of persons (Article 25); the right to preserve the intimacy of private life (Article 26); the right to the protection of personal data and the use of computers (Article 35); and the rights of all workers (regardless of age, sex, race, citizenship, territory of origin, religion, or political or ideological convictions) to have a job and work under conditions of hygiene, safety, and health, as well as the rights to have assistance and fair rehabilitation when they are victims of workplace accidents or occupational disease (Article 59) are rights constitutionally enshrined in the Constitution of the Portuguese Republic. Moreover, in Europe, any regulation must conform to the European Convention for the Protection of Human Rights and Fundamental Freedoms. The latter warranties for a person's right to privacy, which states that everyone has the right to his/her private and family life, his/her home, and his/her correspondence, and that public authorities must not interfere with the exercise of this right, except if the interests of national security, public safety, or the economic well-being of the country are at risk. On an international level, the matter might be covered by Universal Declaration of Human Rights (Article 12), which states that no one shall be subjected to arbitrary interference with his/her privacy.

The use of psychoactive substances in the workplace (or during working hours) is usually governed by health and safety laws that address the potential health and safety risks for themselves or co-workers [75–77]. Therefore, these laws usually legitimate the fact that the tests should be restricted to categories of workers whose activity may endanger their physical or third party integrity and make employers responsible for preventing psychoactive substance use in the workplace and impose them to carry out risk assessments and preventive measures [78]. The real question is how we can fulfil the purposes of the law, namely, the following Portuguese legislation: (i) Articles 15 (employer's general obligations), 16 (simultaneous or successive activities in the same workplace), and 17 (worker's obligations) of the legal regime promoting occupational safety and health (Law no. 102/2009 of 10 of September); (ii) Articles 19 (medical tests and examinations), 99 (internal company rules), 281 (general principles on safety and health at workplace), 282 (information, consultation, and training of workers), 283 (accidents at work and occupational diseases), and 284 (regulation of prevention and reparation) of the Labor Code (Law no. 7/2009 of 12 February); (iii) Decree-Law no. 4/2015 of 7 of January (Code of Administrative Procedure); and (iv) the General Data Protection Regulation 2016/679 of the European Parliament and of the Council of 27 of April of 2016. Besides these legislations, specific regulations of each enterprise should be also taking into account. The Portuguese State, through the Labor General Inspection, the Directorate-General of Health, and the National Protection Centre against Professional Risks, proceeds to inspections to see if the rules are followed.

5.1.1. The Legal Regime for the Promotion of Health and Safety at Work (Law no. 102/2009 of 10 September)

The legal regime for the promotion of health and safety at work (Law no. 102/2009 of 10 September) states that occupational safety and health must be based on a correct and permanent risk assessment and be developed according to principles, policies, standards, and programs, focusing on the promotion and monitoring of occupational health and the enhancement of technical and scientific research in the field of safety and health at the workplace, particularly the emergence of new risk factors (Article 5). In Portugal, the existence of in-house occupational safety and health services is mandatory in organizations with more than 400 workers or in those with more than 30 workers if they are exposed to high-risk activities. In cases where the enterprise does not have an internal occupational health and safety service, this must be assumed by the external entities that provide occupational health and safety services (Article 78).

There are several general obligations that the employer must continuously and permanently fulfil (Articles 15 and 18): (i) ensuring safety and health in the workplace, (ii) identifying all foreseeable risks in all activities of the organization, (iii) mitigating monotonous and repetitive work, and (iv) reducing psychosocial risks. These concerns should be balanced accordingly to the risks to which the workers are potentially exposed to and are recognized as causes for psychoactive substance use, which in turn is a risk factor for accidents and enhancer of work-related diseases. Nevertheless, it should be borne in mind that employers cannot legitimately invoke the obligation to carry out psychoactive substance screening tests to accomplish their duties of ensuring the health of workers (Article 108). Indeed, the obligation to perform clinical exams (i.e., for admission, periodic, or occasional) is duly specified in the legislation and its purpose is aimed at attesting and evaluating the physical and mental fitness of the worker to perform the activity, as well as possible repercussions. In other words, compulsory psychoactive substance testing undermines the rights, freedoms and personal guarantees enshrined in the Constitution of the Portuguese Republic, namely, the right to personal integrity (Article 25) and the right to privacy reserve (Article 26). This means that there will be no justification for drug testing in all (or random) workers in an organization, but only for those whose job requires high skills or involves considerable risk to themselves or other workers and in all who show manifested and serious signs of being influenced by psychoactive substances [79]. Moreover, it should be mentioned that the existence of an internal regulation that considers a program for workplace drug testing cannot be in itself a just cause for dismissal because it is not provided by law and violates the principle of job security and the fundamental right of workers accordingly the Article 53 of the Constitution of the Portuguese Republic.

On the other hand, it is also the worker's obligation to comply with the occupational safety and health requirements provided by legislation and collective labor regulation instruments, as well as for instructions determined for that purpose by the employer (Article 17).

5.1.2. The Labor Code (Law no. 7/2009 of 12 February)

Regarding the Portuguese Labor Code (Law no. 7/2009 of 12 February), the article 281 et seq. focuses on the prevention and reparation of accidents and occupational diseases in the workplace; workers have the right to provide work in safe and healthy conditions and should respect the occupational safety and health requirements laid down by law or collective labor regulation instruments, or those determined by the employer, and the employer should apply the necessary measures to provide such environments.

The carrying out of medical tests and examinations (Article 19) is within the scope of the organization of occupational safety and health services and must respect citizens' rights, freedoms, and guarantees. Regarding the detection of psychoactive substance use, this may or may not be part of the organization's health and safety policy. The most common procedure is to perform drug testing in those workers randomly nominated by the computer, as well as those appointed by the occupational physician, or to those who request according to the rules of procedure. As mentioned above, random drug testing has been prone to controversy because employers must ensure that every aspect of their policies is rooted in scientific evidence, linked rationally to the goal of workplace safety, and are ethically justifiable [79]. Some organizations also advocate testing following an accident of specific consequences (e.g., fatalities, injuries that require anyone to be removed from the scene for medical care, damage to vehicles or property above a specified monetary amount) in order to determine whether the abuse of psychoactive substances were a factor. Of course, a positive test for psychoactive substances cannot prove that this was the cause of the accident.

Considering the possibility of creating a program that includes toxicological analyses for detection of psychoactive substances, this must comply with the legal rules in force and be part of an internal regulation according to Article 99. This regulation should spell out the underlying policy, objectives, and rights and responsibilities of all parties involved, as well as issues regarding the protection of personal data, namely, assuring the right of the worker to privacy, the need for his/her consent to perform the tests, and the preventive and non-sanctioning character of the drug tests. These are important topics specially designed to increase the sensitivity of health and safety professionals to this problem and encourage them to raise awareness of them.

Screening tests for psychoactive substance use are restricted to the occupational physician or, under his/her guidance and control, to other health professionals obliged to professional secrecy (e.g., occupational nurses) and trained to use the kits for toxicological analysis. The same is true for the results of the tests because this represents health information. Therefore, clinical data can only be known to health professionals from the occupational medicine team, who are subject to confidentiality, and any hypothetic witnesses nominated by the worker.

In order to comply with professional secrecy and to guarantee the confidentiality of information resulting from medical examinations, the occupational physician must record results with "generic terms", namely, the worker (i) is fit (i.e., does not consume), (ii) is "fit with restrictions", or (iii) is temporarily unable (i.e., consumes) to perform his/her duties. According to no. 2 of Article 17 (on the protection of personal data) of the Labor Code, at no time should the physician report the test results to the employer. Only in this way is the adequacy of the preventive and deterrent measures ensured and it represents a very serious offence the disrespect of these directives. Accordingly to Article 195 of the Portuguese Penal Code, the disclosure of other people's secrets, known to someone on account of his/her state, job, employment, profession (e.g., physician), or arts, is punished by a term imprisonment of 1 year or fine until 240 days. Moreover, the physician also follows the Deontological Code of the Medical Association, which compels him/her to professional secrecy (Article 71).

It is also made clear by the Labor Code (Article 19), in addition to the situations provided in occupational safety and health legislation, that the employer cannot, for admission purposes or job maintenance, require the applicant or worker to perform or present tests or medical examinations of any nature (such as the results of psychoactive substance use tests), or prove physical or mental conditions and therefore health. An exception occurs when these examinations aim for the protection and safety of the worker or third parties, or when the demands inherent to the activity justify it. In these cases, the reasons must be provided in writing to the job seeker or worker. Therefore, conducting screening tests for psychoactive substance use will only be legitimate in exceptional cases where health, welfare, worker, employer, or third-party concerns are at stake. In cases of job admission, even if screening tests for psychoactive substance can be justifiably performed in candidates, the possibility of the job applicant stopping drug use several days before testing should be born in mind. However, the screening will no longer be legally acceptable on the principles of proportionality, appropriateness, and reasonableness when there are no objective grounds to perform them in order to assure safety to the workers, service users, or the wider community, or when, from this point of view, the risks are minimal.

It is also clear that a job applicant or worker who has provided personal information has the right to control his/her personal data, to be aware of its content and the intended purpose, and to ask for its correction and update.

6. Diagnosis of the Influence of Psychoactive Substances and Toxicological Analysis

It is fundamental to have the substances that will be monitored clearly defined in the rules of procedure. Suspicion of psychoactive substance consumption can be made at various levels, of a subjective and objective nature. The loss of productivity and decreased quality of work, lack of punctuality and absenteeism, indiscipline and inappropriate behaviors, and the increase in workplace accidents are warning signs that cannot be neglected. However, these signs of suspicion should be part of a broader clinical and laboratory evaluation under the responsibility of occupational medicine and, in some cases, with the contribution of insurance medicine as well as forensic medicine.

Occupational medicine is a medical specialty concerned with the maintenance of health in the workplace, including prevention and treatment of diseases and injuries. In other words, the aim of occupational medicine focuses on workers' health. Accordingly, the International Code of Ethics for Occupational Health Professionals published by the International Commission on Occupational Health (ICOH) states, "the aim of occupational health practice is to protect and promote workers' health, to sustain and improve their working capacity and ability, to contribute to the establishment and maintenance of a safe and healthy working environment for all, as well as to promote the adaptation of work to the capabilities of workers, taking into account their state of health" [80].

Many enterprises establish a drug policy with little or no structure for drug testing, namely, (i) quality control, (ii) systematic confirmation of positives, and (iii) procedures to accomplish the chain of custody. Indeed, procedures that ensure the chain of custody compliance are of utmost importance in toxicological analyses. Moreover, drug testing is usually performed on-site by occupational physicians, who are usually not familiarized with analytical toxicological aspects. In Europe, the European Guidelines for Workplace Drug Testing have been prepared and updated by the European Workplace Drug Testing Society (EWDTS) for different samples. These guidelines are designed to [81] (i) establish best practice and standard procedures whilst allowing individual countries to operate within the requirements of national customs and legislation, (ii) ensure that the entire drug testing process is conducted to give accurate and reliable information about a donor's drug use, (iii) maintain the legal defensibility and scrutiny either by an employment tribunal or a court of law, (iv) protect the dignity of the specimen donors and the validity of the specimen, (v) define common and critical quality control procedures for laboratories, and vi) help in the interpretation of the analytical results. Guidelines for collection of biological samples for toxicological analysis were recently published [82] and have largely conformed to the EWDTS guidelines, focusing on sample collection and testing in urine, hair, and oral fluid. Our work focused only on specific points relevant to the interpretation of workplace drug testing [75,81]. Trained personnel, who do not need to specifically be healthcare professionals, are required [81]. All samples must be kept for an agreed period or in respect of the national legislation of each country to allow rebuttal if any judicial sues are made regarding the obtained results. After the agreed time, the laboratory may discard the sample if the customer did not request the laboratory to retain the sample for an additional period. Samples must be retained within the secure laboratory area until the disposal date agreed with the customer [83].

6.1. Interpretation of Ethanol Results

The alcoholaemia is usually performed by quantitative breath analysis, using an alcohol meter (duly calibrated). In Portugal, there is a model certified by the Portuguese Institute of Quality that is based on the theoretical relationship defined in Law no. 18/2007 of 17 May, assuming that 1 mg/L in breath alcohol concentration (BrAC) is equal to 2.3 g/L of blood alcohol concentration (BAC) [65]. Counterproof should always be available to confirm results and should be provided by a referenced toxicology laboratory and by using a different technique and chemical principle from that of the screen test in order to ensure reliability and accuracy. Real BAC can be quantified by blood collection and further analysis by using gas chromatography with a flame ionization detector and a headspace system. The direct determination of ethanol itself in hair is not possible due to its volatility and its potential absorption from external sources [54]. Instead, the minor ethanol metabolites ethyl glucuronide (EtG) and/or fatty acid ethyl esters (FAEE) can be measured in hair by GC or LC coupled to MS/MS as a direct alcohol consumption marker [84].

There are no legally defined values for ethanol blood concentration in the workplace and it should be noted that the maximum limit established for the Portuguese Highway Code should not be generalized to all professions or tasks [65]. Nevertheless, several Portuguese organizations are governed by the values defined in the Highway Code. For instance, the Collective Bargaining Agreement for the Construction and Public Works Industry that has been in force since April 1, 2010, in clause no. 78 (on the prevention and control of alcoholaemia) considers that it is under the influence of alcohol the worker who, under examination by BrAC, reveals 0.5 g/L or more. For workers under the Highway Code, the BAC provided in that Code is applicable.

6.2. Interpretation of Other Psychoactive Substances Results

Regarding the analysis of other psychoactive substances, toxicological analysis can be performed in various biological samples, being more commonly analyzed in oral fluid [83–85] and urine [81,83] or in hair [86] and nails [87], given that, although analytically possible, the toxicological results are not relevant to allow for a quantitative interpretation [65]. Indeed, in most cases, only by using blood, serum, or plasma is it possible to truly document the impairment. Therefore, the most correct procedure will be to consider as positive the test that reveals the presence of illicit psychoactive substances above the defined concentrations cut-offs for screening and confirmation tests [88], regardless of the quantitative interpretation the test may provide [89]. Although urine is an important sample for toxicological screening, it is only useful if freshly voided and collection is witnessed and supervised to avoid adulteration. Indeed, the collection facilities should be arranged to prevent adulteration of the specimen as much as possible and adding coloring agents to toilet water has been recommended to reduce the risk [81]. Some authors suggest that all urine specimens taken for drug testing from both the workplace and court settings need to be tested for validity [90]. Nevertheless, urinating is a personal act and most people feel inhibited about being observed in such circumstances by close family members, medical staff, or even sexual partners, and the situation can never be less than humiliating. Furthermore, individuals may not want to disclose pregnancy or venereal diseases. A wide variety of collection devices are available in the market to collect oral fluid for toxicological analysis. A minimum validity test should be performed for oral fluid, such as visual inspection of the sample(s), measurement of oral fluid volume and testing on matrix authenticity through measurement of endogenous biomarkers such as salivary amylase and cortisol [83–85].

Hair samples have been gaining popularity. This is by far the most expensive method, but it is claimed to be more secure in the event of legal challenges, to provide conclusive evidence of rebuttal, and is an excellent indicator of addiction, as opposed to occasional use, which may be particularly suitable for pre-employment testing programs. Analysis of nail clippings may be a useful back-up for hair analysis when hair is unavailable [87,91,92]. Useful applications of nail analysis may be where contamination is highly unlikely (i.e., if the fingers do not become contaminated) as is the case during the consumption of tablets or capsules as medication or where the question of time or quantity of use rather than the fact of use is being investigated [92].

The most frequently analyzed substances are amphetamines and derivatives, cannabinoids, cocaine, opioids, and benzodiazepines. Regarding cocaine, immunoassays detect the metabolite benzoylecgonine quite accurately without much concern for false positive or negatives. Nevertheless, the metabolite is inactive and may be present up to 3 days after use, whereas most clinical effects of cocaine occur within 6 to 12 hours of use [26,27]. As for amphetamines, there are many false positives, including antihistamines, decongestants, antidepressants, or acid-blockers, and these may be detected 1 to 3 days after use. Indeed, methamphetamine only differs from pseudoephedrine in a single atom of oxygen. In fact, many methods flowed by clandestine laboratories use *l*-ephedrine (present in stimulant supplements and used for weight loss) or *d*-pseudoephedrine (present in several decongestants drugs) as starting reagents to produce *d*-methamphetamine [93].

Regarding cannabinoids, common over-the-counter analgesics such as ibuprofen and naproxen, as well as the increasing interest in the use of medical *Cannabis*, can increase the probability of cross-reaction with this assay, creating false positives. Many opioids can be missed during routine screening, generating significant false-negatives, and it has been reported that screening is also prone to many false-positive results in the presence of poppy seeds and quinolone antibiotics [13,94]. Indeed, poppy seed paste used in foods could lead to positive urine tests for opioids, even if increased cut-off levels are used and different biomarkers are considered for the differential diagnosis, such as the presence of thebaine to ensure justice for each individual [13,95]. Moreover, if an individual is currently taking a lawful medication containing codeine, the test can suggest that he/she has used heroin.

Nevertheless, it should be mentioned that there are several unscreened substances in existence, such as ketamine, chloral hydrate, gamma-hydroxybutyrate (GHB), psilocybin, mescaline, and cathinones. Moreover, qualitative or semi-quantitative immunoassays may cross-react with other substances, many of which are licit, namely, pharmaceutical drugs [89]. In this case, tests showing the presence of prescription drugs should not be considered positive.

On the basis of the technical limitation of the immunoassay analysis, whenever positive results (i.e., above a predefined cut-off level) emerge at the screening stage, confirmatory tests on the sample must be carried out by a referenced toxicology laboratory, normally by gas and liquid chromatography coupled with mass spectrometry. If the screen results are all negative, no further analysis is necessary. Results of confirmatory analysis are usually not readily available, and even if positive results are obtained, interpretation is required by skilled toxicological professionals in conjunction with a qualified occupation medicine physician [96].

Additionally, of note is that there are many other clinical situations with signs and symptoms similar to psychoactive substance poisoning, and thus definitive diagnosis is only possible through clinical examination. Therefore, a differential diagnosis is needed to find out whether the reason for the positive result can be explained by prescribed medication; some other acceptable reason; or whether it is, in fact, a question of drug abuse [97]. If an occupational physician is not present, the worker should be removed from activities that put his/her or others' safety at risk and should be properly referred to a health unit. It is underlined that in this case all labor rights, including remuneration, must be ensured for as long as the worker is away from work.

6.3. Worker's Refusal to Undergo Toxicological Analysis

Besides the health professional (or other) who is competent to carry out the sample collection for toxicological analysis, it should be made possible for the worker to request the assistance of a witness, having a defined time to do so, but the test cannot be stopped if the presentation of the witness was not feasible. Refusal to submit to screening tests for psychoactive substance use, although possible, does not imply that the worker is unsuitable for work. When unjustified, the worker may incur any disciplinary offence and, in some enterprises, the refusal leads to the assumption that the worker has a BAC of 0.5 g/L or higher and therefore the employee is unfit/inapt for work. Moreover, it should be highlighted that if a worker is declared unfit by the occupational medicine as a result of psychoactive substance use, it is not a just cause for dismissal or to affect career progression, as clinical results are confidential and as such cannot be made known to the hierarchical superiors or other entities outside the clinical sphere. Only the behavior that may result from the influenced state can be framed according to Article 351 (just cause for dismissal) of the Portuguese Labor Code and as such be subject to disciplinary sanction (and possibly dismissal) due to the unacceptable or breach of established rules.

As a precautionary measure, if a BAC of 0.5 g/L or greater is assumed or presumed, or if positive illicit psychoactive substances results are obtained, the worker will be immediately prevented from working during the remaining daily work period, with the consequent loss of remuneration for such period.

If the worker is found to abuse psychoactive substances in the workplace, it is possible and permissible to initiate disciplinary proceedings against the worker, especially in organizations with internal rules prohibiting the use of psychoactive substances in the workplace.

7. Conclusions and Future Perspectives

The use of psychoactive substances in the workplace is a public health problem that influences the safety and health of workers and extends beyond the workplace itself. It is a contentious issue that has moved up the human resources agenda in recent years, and different organizations take diverse approaches to psychoactive substance workplace testing, some of them following a zero-tolerance approach, whereas others have had to develop a more nuanced policy. Such cases may also have insurance and legal repercussions [98,99]. Indeed, workplace psychoactive substance testing is one of the latest components to be added to the discipline of forensic toxicology, which now comprises the triad fields of post-mortem, human performance, and workplace drug testing toxicology [88]. There are several studies that demonstrate that the psychic and motor disturbance due to the consumption of psychoactive substances is in the origin of several work accidents and related economic impacts [12,100,101]. Moreover, testing for psychoactive substances in the workplace, at random or by surprise, has a statistically significant preventive effect in overall professions [102]. Nevertheless, testing in the workplace is a complex topic because it is not often directly regulated by supranational or national law. Only a few countries report legislation that clearly and specifically address the issue of drug testing in the workplace [51].

The participation of workers and their representatives in the design of an occupational health promotion plan and in the definition of policies to be followed undoubtedly plays a decisive role in the implementation of prevention programs against the use of psychoactive substances in the workplace. Human resources policies aimed at promoting worker safety, health, and well-being that integrate worker assistance programs, information campaigns, and other interventions in this field reflect the level of organizational cultures that incorporate concepts and principles of corporate citizenship, encouraging entrepreneurs and managers to good practices, the production of deontological ethics, and codes that value the image of the company or organization and its end products. Workers should also be aware that the employer is committed to creating a work environment that promotes safety and health and that policies and related measures should be applied to all elements of the organizational system so that the individual and collective rights of society will be fully accomplished. Indeed, if on the one hand the use of illicit drugs in the workplace raises issues pertaining to prevention and safety and the responsibility of the various members of staff, on the other hand it also brings into question the interface between work and private life [103].

As a prerequisite to testing, the company must have an antidrug program aiming to ensure health and safety, including a written drug testing internal regulation. In this regulation, problems related to the use of psychoactive substances should be considered as health problems and consequently should be treated like other health problems in the workplace regarding temporary disability, sick pay, and other social benefits, especially during periods of rehabilitation treatment.

It is important to clarify that under the law, the screening, counterproof, or confirmatory analysis should not be charged to the worker because they are preventive health and safety activities of companies and the costs must always be supported by the employer. All these measures are stimulating and represent facilitating factors for recovery, although under treatment, the employer must also ensure that the workstation is maintained or transferred to other duties that do not pose a risk to the safety of himself or others without loss of rights or other benefits. Nevertheless, an employee's failure to successfully complete treatment requirements can eventually result in the termination of their employment.

Nowadays, we are witnessing a paradigm shift from an evolution centered on the treatment and rehabilitation of proven psychoactive substance dependents to a cross-cutting approach through the implementation of a specific regulation that includes (i) prevention of consumption through information actions on health consequences of the use of psychoactive substances; (ii) early detection; (iii) treatment at the enterprise (if it has the means), or through referral to other specialist physician, or to local or regional specialist services (e.g., integrated response centers or alcoholology units) to recover workers in compliance with personal freedom, and these treatments cannot be imposed by coercion; and (iv) socio-professional rehabilitation of the worker, aiming at relapse prevention.

For the full implementation of these objectives, the availability of skilled human resources specifically in occupational medicine with toxicological background and skilled toxicologists in clinical, forensic, and analytical aspects of psychoactive substances, to correctly interpret toxicological results, are needed. Given this reality, fulfilling the purposes of the law, namely, Article 19 of the Portuguese Labor Code, is an almost impossible task. There should be a balance between prevention and repression.

Finally, policies and educational interventions to reduce psychoactive substance consumption in the workplace are needed [104]. These should address awareness to workplace hazards, physician education to promote best practices for treatment, and overdose prevention. In addition, the phenomenon of the new psychoactive substances are also motifs of concern in the workplace that should not be disregarded [51]. Indeed, the consumption of new psychoactive substances poses a significant risk to public health and a challenge to national and international drug policies for occupational medicine, and only very recently have laboratories begun to offer screening and confirmation analysis for new psychoactive substances at lower costs [105].

Author Contributions: R.J.D.-O. created and designed the study, wrote the first draft of the manuscript, and analyzed and interpreted the literature. T.M. also analyzed and interpreted literature and wrote and revised the final version of the manuscript. All authors have read and agreed to the published version of the manuscript.

References

1. George, S. A snapshot of workplace drug testing in the UK. *Occup. Med. (Lond.)* **2005**, *55*, 69–71. [CrossRef] [PubMed]
2. Burke, R.J.; Richardsen, A.M. *Increasing Occupational Health and Safety in Workplaces: Individual, Workplaces*; Edward Elger Publishing: Cheltenham, UK, 2019.
3. World Health Organization. *Global Status Report on Alcohol and Health*; World Health Organization: Geneva, Switzerland, 2018.
4. Mackenbach, J.P.; Stirbu, I.; Roskam, A.-J.R.; Schaap, M.M.; Menvielle, G.; Leinsalu, M.; Kunst, A.E.; European Union Working Group on Socioeconomic Inequalities in Health. Socioeconomic inequalities in health in 22 European countries. *N. Engl. J. Med.* **2008**, *358*, 2468–2481. [CrossRef] [PubMed]
5. Cope, R.B. The potential for occupational exposure of veterinarians to ketamine resulting in positive drug tests. *Aust. Vet. J.* **2018**, *96*, 59–61. [CrossRef] [PubMed]
6. Airagnes, G.; Lemogne, C.; Renuy, A.; Goldberg, M.; Hoertel, N.; Roquelaure, Y.; Limosin, F.; Zins, M. Prevalence of prescribed benzodiazepine long-term use in the French general population according to sociodemographic and clinical factors: Findings from the CONSTANCES cohort. *BMC Public Health* **2019**, *19*, 566. [CrossRef] [PubMed]
7. Corral, A.; Durán, J.; Isusi, I. *Use of Alcohol and Drugs at the Workplace*; European Foundation for the Improvement of Living and Working Conditions: Dublin, Ireland, 2012.
8. Lillsunde, P.; Mukala, K.; Partinen, R.; Lamberg, M. Role of occupational health services in workplace drug testing. *Forensic Sci. Int.* **2008**, *174*, 103–106. [CrossRef] [PubMed]
9. Buvik, K.; Moan, I.S.; Halkjelsvik, T. Alcohol-related absence and presenteeism: Beyond productivity loss. *Int. J. Drug Policy* **2018**, *58*, 71–77. [CrossRef] [PubMed]
10. Ervasti, J.; Kivimäki, M.; Head, J.; Goldberg, M.; Airagnes, G.; Pentti, J.; Oksanen, T.; Salo, P.; Suominen, S.; Jokela, M.; et al. Sociodemographic differences between alcohol use and sickness absence: Pooled analysis of four cohort studies. *Alcohol Alcohol. (Oxf. Oxfs.)* **2018**, *53*, 95–103. [CrossRef]
11. Dams, J.; Buchholz, A.; Kraus, L.; Reimer, J.; Scherbaum, N.; Konnopka, A.; König, H.-H. Excess costs of alcohol-dependent patients in German psychiatric care compared with matched non-alcohol-dependent individuals from the general population: A secondary analysis of two datasets. *BMJ Open* **2018**, *8*, e020563. [CrossRef]
12. Sullivan, T.; Edgar, F.; McAndrew, I. The hidden costs of employee drinking: A quantitative analysis. *Drug Alcohol Rev.* **2019**, *38*, 543–553. [CrossRef]
13. Dinis-Oliveira, R.J. Metabolism and metabolomics of opiates: A long way of forensic implications to unravel. *J. Forensic Leg. Med.* **2019**, *61*, 128–140. [CrossRef]
14. Faria, J.; Barbosa, J.; Moreira, R.; Queirós, O.; Carvalho, F.; Dinis-Oliveira, R.J. Comparative pharmacology and toxicology of tramadol and tapentadol. *Eur. J. Pain (Lond. Engl.)* **2018**, *22*, 827–844. [CrossRef] [PubMed]
15. Ventura, L.; Carvalho, F.; Dinis-Oliveira, R.J. Opioids in the frame of new psychoactive substances network: A complex pharmacological and toxicological issue. *Curr. Mol. Pharmacol.* **2018**, *11*, 97–108. [CrossRef] [PubMed]
16. Dinis-Oliveira, R.J. Licit and ilicit uses of medicines. *Acta Med. Port.* **2014**, *27*, 755–766. [CrossRef] [PubMed]
17. Dinis-Oliveira, R.J.; Carvalho, F.; Moreira, R.; Duarte, J.A.; Proenca, J.B.; Santos, A.; Magalhaes, T. Clinical and forensic signs related to opioids abuse. *Curr. Drug Abus. Rev.* **2012**, *5*, 273–290. [CrossRef] [PubMed]
18. da Costa, B.R.; Vieira, E.R. Risk factors for work-related musculoskeletal disorders: A systematic review of recent longitudinal studies. *Am. J. Ind. Med.* **2010**, *53*, 285–323. [CrossRef]
19. Buttorff, C.; Trujillo, A.J.; Castillo, R.; Vecino-Ortiz, A.I.; Anderson, G.F. The impact of practice guidelines on opioid utilization for injured workers. *Am. J. Ind. Med.* **2017**, *60*, 1023–1030. [CrossRef]
20. Krebs, E.E.; Gravely, A.; Nugent, S.; Jensen, A.C.; DeRonne, B.; Goldsmith, E.S.; Kroenke, K.; Bair, M.J.; Noorbaloochi, S. Effect of opioid vs nonopioid medications on pain-related function in patients with chronic back pain or hip or knee osteoarthritis pain: The SPACE randomized clinical trial. *JAMA* **2018**, *319*, 872–882. [CrossRef]
21. Kowalski-McGraw, M.; Green-McKenzie, J.; Pandalai, S.P.; Schulte, P.A. Characterizing the interrelationships of prescription opioid and benzodiazepine drugs with worker health and workplace hazards. *J. Occup. Environ. Med.* **2017**, *59*, 1114–1126. [CrossRef]

22. Cheng, M.; Sauer, B.; Johnson, E.; Porucznik, C.; Hegmann, K. Comparison of opioid-related deaths by work-related injury. *Am. J. Ind. Med.* **2013**, *56*, 308–316. [CrossRef]
23. Howard, M.E.; Desai, A.V.; Grunstein, R.R.; Hukins, C.; Armstrong, J.G.; Joffe, D.; Swann, P.; Campbell, D.A.; Pierce, R.J. Sleepiness, sleep-disordered breathing, and accident risk factors in commercial vehicle drivers. *Am. J. Respir. Crit. Care Med.* **2004**, *170*, 1014–1021. [CrossRef]
24. Katzung, B.G. *Basic & Clinical Pharmacology*, 14th ed.; Katzung, B.G., Trevor, A.J., Eds.; McGraw-Hill: New York, NY, USA, 2018.
25. Negus, S.S.; Banks, M.L. Medications development for opioid abuse. *Cold Spring Harb. Perspect. Med.* **2013**, *3*, a012104. [CrossRef] [PubMed]
26. Dinis-Oliveira, R.J. Metabolomics of cocaine: Implications in toxicity. *Toxicol. Mech. Methods* **2015**, *25*, 494–500. [PubMed]
27. Oliveira, N.G.; Dinis-Oliveira, R.J. Drugs of abuse from a different toxicological perspective: An updated review of cocaine genotoxicity. *Arch. Toxicol.* **2018**, *92*, 2987–3006. [CrossRef] [PubMed]
28. Nóbrega, L.; Dinis-Oliveira, R.J. The synthetic cathinone α-pyrrolidinovalerophenone (α-PVP): Pharmacokinetic and pharmacodynamic clinical and forensic aspects. *Drug Metab. Rev.* **2018**, *50*, 125–139. [CrossRef] [PubMed]
29. Carvalho, M.; Carmo, H.; Costa, V.M.; Capela, J.P.; Pontes, H.; Remiao, F.; Carvalho, F.; Bastos Mde, L. Toxicity of amphetamines: An update. *Arch. Toxicol.* **2012**, *86*, 1167–1231. [CrossRef] [PubMed]
30. Lhermitte, M.; Frimat, P.; Labat, L.; Haguenoer, J.M. Use of illicit substances in the workplace. *Ann. Pharm. Fr.* **2012**, *70*, 3–14. [CrossRef]
31. McLellan, T.M.; Caldwell, J.A.; Lieberman, H.R. A review of caffeine's effects on cognitive, physical and occupational performance. *Neurosci. Biobehav. Rev.* **2016**, *71*, 294–312. [CrossRef]
32. Park, H.; Suh, B.S.; Lee, K. Relationship between daily coffee intake and suicidal ideation. *J. Affect. Disord.* **2019**, *256*, 468–472. [CrossRef]
33. Sutton, S.K.; Van Rensburg, K.J.; Jentink, K.G.; Drobes, D.J.; Evans, D.E. Nicotine-induced cortical activation among nonsmokers with moderation by trait cognitive control. *Psychopharmacology* **2016**, *233*, 2301–2308. [CrossRef]
34. Leventhal, A.M.; Waters, A.J.; Boyd, S.; Moolchan, E.T.; Lerman, C.; Pickworth, W.B. Gender differences in acute tobacco withdrawal: Effects on subjective, cognitive, and physiological measures. *Exp. Clin. Psychopharmacol.* **2007**, *15*, 21–36. [CrossRef]
35. Normand, J.; Salyards, S.D.; Mahoney, J.J. An evaluation of preemployment drug testing. *J. Appl. Psychol.* **1990**, *75*, 629–639. [CrossRef] [PubMed]
36. Hart, C.L.; Haney, M.; Vosburg, S.K.; Comer, S.D.; Gunderson, E.; Foltin, R.W. Modafinil attenuates disruptions in cognitive performance during simulated night-shift work. *Neuropsychopharmacol. Off. Publ. Am. Coll. Neuropsychopharmacol.* **2006**, *31*, 1526–1536. [CrossRef] [PubMed]
37. Hart, C.L.; Ward, A.S.; Haney, M.; Nasser, J.; Foltin, R.W. Methamphetamine attenuates disruptions in performance and mood during simulated night-shift work. *Psychopharmacology* **2003**, *169*, 42–51. [CrossRef] [PubMed]
38. Ross, S.A.; ElSohly, M.A.; Sultana, G.N.; Mehmedic, Z.; Hossain, C.F.; Chandra, S. Flavonoid glycosides and cannabinoids from the pollen of *Cannabis sativa* L. *Phytochem. Anal.* **2005**, *16*, 45–48. [CrossRef] [PubMed]
39. Dinis-Oliveira, R.J. Metabolomics of Delta9-tetrahydrocannabinol: Implications in toxicity. *Drug Metab. Rev.* **2016**, *48*, 80–87. [CrossRef] [PubMed]
40. Dinis-Oliveira, R.J. The Clinical Toxicology Perspective on the Therapeutic Use of Cannabis and Cannabinoids. *Acta Med. Port.* **2019**, *32*, 87–90. [CrossRef]
41. Sharma, P.; Murthy, P.; Bharath, M.M. Chemistry, metabolism, and toxicology of cannabis: Clinical implications. *Iran. J. Psychiatry* **2012**, *7*, 149–156.
42. Crane, N.A.; Schuster, R.M.; Fusar-Poli, P.; Gonzalez, R. Effects of cannabis on neurocognitive functioning: Recent advances, neurodevelopmental influences, and sex differences. *Neuropsychol. Rev.* **2013**, *23*, 117–137. [CrossRef]
43. Keith, D.R.; Gunderson, E.W.; Haney, M.; Foltin, R.W.; Hart, C.L. Smoked marijuana attenuates performance and mood disruptions during simulated night shift work. *Drug Alcohol Depend.* **2017**, *178*, 534–543. [CrossRef]
44. Dahlgren, M.K.; Sagar, K.A.; Smith, R.T.; Lambros, A.M.; Kuppe, M.K.; Gruber, S.A. Recreational cannabis use impairs driving performance in the absence of acute intoxication. *Drug Alcohol Depend.* **2020**. [CrossRef]

45. Anderson, D.M.; Rees, D.I.; Tekin, E. Medical marijuana laws and workplace fatalities in the United States. *Int. J. Drug Policy* **2018**, *60*, 33–39. [CrossRef] [PubMed]
46. Phillips, J.A.; Holland, M.G.; Baldwin, D.D.; Meuleveld, L.G.; Mueller, K.L.; Perkison, B.; Upfal, M.; Dreger, M. Marijuana in the workplace: Guidance for occupational health professionals and employers: Joint Guidance Statement of the American Association of Occupational Health Nurses and the American College of Occupational and Environmental Medicine. *J. Occup. Environ. Med.* **2015**, *57*, 459–475. [CrossRef] [PubMed]
47. Goldsmith, R.S.; Targino, M.C.; Fanciullo, G.J.; Martin, D.W.; Hartenbaum, N.P.; White, J.M.; Franklin, P. Medical marijuana in the workplace: Challenges and management options for occupational physicians. *J. Occup. Environ. Med.* **2015**, *57*, 518–525. [CrossRef] [PubMed]
48. Cho, B.; Cho, H.S.; Kim, J.; Sim, J.; Seol, I.; Baeck, S.K.; In, S.; Shin, D.H.; Kim, E. Simultaneous determination of synthetic cannabinoids and their metabolites in human hair using LC-MS/MS and application to human hair. *Forensic Sci. Int.* **2020**, *306*, 110058. [CrossRef]
49. Adamowicz, P.; Gieron, J.; Gil, D.; Lechowicz, W.; Skulska, A.; Tokarczyk, B. The effects of synthetic cannabinoid UR-144 on the human body-A review of 39 cases. *Forensic Sci. Int.* **2017**, *273*, e18–e21. [CrossRef]
50. Gounder, K.; Dunuwille, J.; Dunne, J.; Lee, J.; Silbert, P.; Lawn, N. The other side of the leaf: Seizures associated with synthetic cannabinoid use. *Epilepsy Behav.* **2020**, *104*, 106901. [CrossRef]
51. Salomone, A.; Palamar, J.J.; Vincenti, M. Should NPS be included in workplace drug testing? *Drug Test. Anal.* **2019**. [CrossRef]
52. Dinis-Oliveira, R.J.; Pereira, C.L.; da Silva, D.D. Pharmacokinetic and pharmacodynamic aspects of peyote and mescaline: Clinical and forensic repercussions. *Curr. Mol. Pharmacol.* **2019**, *12*, 184–194. [CrossRef]
53. Dinis-Oliveira, R.J. Metabolism of psilocybin and psilocin: Clinical and forensic toxicological relevance. *Drug Metab. Rev.* **2017**, *49*, 84–91. [CrossRef]
54. Dinis-Oliveira, R.J. Oxidative and Non-Oxidative Metabolomics of Ethanol. *Curr. Drug Metab.* **2016**, *17*, 327–335. [CrossRef]
55. Dinis-Oliveira, R.J. Metabolic profile of oxazepam and related benzodiazepines: Clinical and forensic aspects. *Drug Metab. Rev.* **2017**, *49*, 451–463. [CrossRef] [PubMed]
56. Gomez-Recasens, M.; Alfaro-Barrio, S.; Tarro, L.; Llaurado, E.; Sola, R. A workplace intervention to reduce alcohol and drug consumption: A nonrandomized single-group study. *BMC Public Health* **2018**, *18*, 1281. [CrossRef] [PubMed]
57. Griswold, M.; Fullman, N.; Hawley, C.; Arian, N.; Zimsen, S.R.M.; Tymeson, H.D.; Venkateswaran, V.; Tapp, A.D.; Forouzanfar, M.H.; Abate, K.H.; et al. Alcohol use and burden for 195 countries and territories, 1990–2016: A systematic analysis for the Global Burden of Disease Study 2016. *Lancet* **2018**, *392*, 1015–1035. [CrossRef]
58. Spicer, R.S.; Miller, T.R.; Smith, G.S. Worker substance use, workplace problems and the risk of occupational injury: A matched case-control study. *J. Stud. Alcohol* **2003**, *64*, 570–578. [CrossRef]
59. Bragazzi, N.L.; Dini, G.; Toletone, A.; Rahmani, A.; Montecucco, A.; Massa, E.; Manca, A.; Guglielmi, O.; Garbarino, S.; Debarbieri, N.; et al. Patterns of harmful alcohol consumption among truck drivers: Implications for occupational health and work safety from a systematic review and meta-analysis. *Int. J. Environ. Res. Public Health* **2018**, *15*, 1121. [CrossRef]
60. Edvardsen, H.M.; Moan, I.S.; Christophersen, A.S.; Gjerde, H. Use of alcohol and drugs by employees in selected business areas in Norway: A study using oral fluid testing and questionnaires. *J. Occup. Med. Toxicol.* **2015**, *10*, 46. [CrossRef]
61. Aas, R.W.; Haveraaen, L.; Sagvaag, H.; Thorrisen, M.M. The influence of alcohol consumption on sickness presenteeism and impaired daily activities. The WIRUS screening study. *PLoS ONE* **2017**, *12*, e0186503. [CrossRef]
62. Brunton, L.L.; Knollman, B.C.; Hilal-Dandan, R. *Goodman & Gilman's—The Pharmacological Basis of Therapeutics*, 13th ed.; McGraw-Hill—Medical Publishing Division: New York, NY, USA, 2017.
63. Dinis-Oliveira, R.J. Metabolic profile of flunitrazepam: Clinical and forensic toxicological aspects. *Drug Metab. Lett.* **2017**, *11*, 14–20. [CrossRef]
64. Hunt, D.L.; Artuso, R.D.; Kalia, N.; Leung, N.; Bernacki, E.J.; Tao, X.G. Association of opioid, anti-depressant, and benzodiazepines with workers' compensation cost: A cohort study. *J. Occup. Environ. Med.* **2019**, *61*, e206–e211. [CrossRef]

65. Dinis-Oliveira, R.J.; Nunes, R.; Carvalho, F.; Santos, A.; Teixeira, H.; Vieira, D.N.; Magalhaes, T. Ethical, technical and legal procedures of the medical doctor responsibility to accomplish the road enforcement law about driving under the influence of alcohol and psychotropic substances. *Acta Med. Port.* **2010**, *23*, 1059–1082.
66. Morgan, C.J.; Curran, H.V. Ketamine use: A review. *Addiction* **2012**, *107*, 27–38. [CrossRef] [PubMed]
67. Dinis-Oliveira, R.J. Metabolism and metabolomics of ketamine: A toxicological approach. *Forensic Sci. Res.* **2017**, *2*, 2–10. [CrossRef] [PubMed]
68. Orhurhu, V.J.; Claus, L.E.; Cohen, S.P. Ketamine toxicity. In *StatPearls*; StatPearls Publishing: Treasure Island, FL, USA, 2019.
69. Corriger, A.; Pickering, G. Ketamine and depression: A narrative review. *Drug Des. Dev. Ther.* **2019**, *13*, 3051–3067. [CrossRef] [PubMed]
70. Kintz, P.; Villain, M.; Dumestre, V.; Cirimele, V. Evidence of addiction by anesthesiologists as documented by hair analysis. *Forensic Sci. Int.* **2005**, *153*, 81–84. [CrossRef] [PubMed]
71. Cook, R.F.; Back, A.; Trudeau, J. Substance abuse prevention in the workplace: Recent findings and an expanded conceptual model. *J. Prim. Prev.* **1996**, *16*, 319–339. [CrossRef]
72. White, T. Drug testing at work: Issues and perspectives. *Subst. Use Misuse* **2003**, *38*, 1891–1902. [CrossRef] [PubMed]
73. Frone, M.R.; Trinidad, J.R. Perceived physical availability of alcohol at work and workplace alcohol use and impairment: Testing a structural model. *Psychol. Addict. Behav.* **2014**, *28*, 1271–1277. [CrossRef]
74. Takeshita, T. Prevention of alcohol-related health harm in the workplace. *Ind. Health* **2017**, *55*, 403–405. [CrossRef]
75. Pierce, A. Regulatory aspects of workplace drug testing in Europe. *Drug Test. Anal.* **2012**, *4*, 62–65. [CrossRef]
76. Rosso, G.L.; Montomoli, C.; Morini, L.; Candura, S.M. Seven years of workplace drug testing in Italy: A systematic review and meta-analysis. *Drug Test. Anal.* **2017**, *9*, 844–852. [CrossRef]
77. Ruehle, L. How to maintain a drug-free workplace and ensure audit success. *Occup. Health Saf.* **2016**, *85*, 76, 78, 80. [PubMed]
78. Waehrer, G.M.; Miller, T.R.; Hendrie, D.; Galvin, D.M. Employee assistance programs, drug testing, and workplace injury. *J. Saf. Res.* **2016**, *57*, 53–60. [CrossRef] [PubMed]
79. Christie, T. A discussion of the ethical implications of random drug testing in the workplace. *Healthc. Manag. Forum* **2015**, *28*, 172–174. [CrossRef] [PubMed]
80. International Commission on Occupational Health. *International Code of Ethics for Occupational Health Professionals*, 3rd ed.; International Commission on Occupational Health: Rome, Italy, 2014.
81. Taskinen, S.; Beck, O.; Bosch, T.; Brcak, M.; Carmichael, D.; Fucci, N.; George, C.; Piper, M.; Salomone, A.; Schielen, W.; et al. European guidelines for workplace drug testing in urine. *Drug Test. Anal.* **2017**, *9*, 853–865. [CrossRef] [PubMed]
82. Dinis-Oliveira, R.J.; Vieira, D.N.; Magalhaes, T. Guidelines for collection of biological samples for clinical and forensic toxicological analysis. *Forensic Sci. Res.* **2016**, *1*, 42–51. [CrossRef]
83. Brcak, M.; Beck, O.; Bosch, T.; Carmichael, D.; Fucci, N.; George, C.; Piper, M.; Salomone, A.; Schielen, W.; Steinmeyer, S.; et al. European guidelines for workplace drug testing in oral fluid. *Drug Test. Anal.* **2018**, *10*, 402–415. [CrossRef]
84. Moore, C. Oral fluid for workplace drug testing: Laboratory implementation. *Drug Test. Anal.* **2012**, *4*, 89–93. [CrossRef]
85. Desrosiers, N.A.; Huestis, M.A. Oral fluid drug testing: Analytical approaches, issues and interpretation of results. *J. Anal. Toxicol.* **2019**, *43*, 415–443. [CrossRef]
86. Salomone, A.; Tsanaclis, L.; Agius, R.; Kintz, P.; Baumgartner, M.R. European guidelines for workplace drug and alcohol testing in hair. *Drug Test. Anal* **2016**, *8*, 996–1004. [CrossRef]
87. Stowe, G.N.; Paulsen, R.B.; Hill, V.A.; Schaffer, M.I. A retrospective analysis of selected opioids in hair of workplace drug testing subjects. *J. Anal. Toxicol.* **2019**, *43*, 553–563. [CrossRef]
88. Karch, S.B. *Workplace Drug Testing*; CRC Press: Boca Raton, FL, USA, 2008.
89. Dinis-Oliveira, R.J. Heterogeneous and homogeneous immunoassays for drug analysis. *Bioanalysis* **2014**, *6*, 2877–2896. [CrossRef] [PubMed]
90. Lin, S.Y.; Lee, H.H.; Lee, J.F.; Chen, B.H. Urine specimen validity test for drug abuse testing in workplace and court settings. *J. Food Drug Anal.* **2018**, *26*, 380–384. [CrossRef] [PubMed]

91. Solimini, R.; Minutillo, A.; Kyriakou, C.; Pichini, S.; Pacifici, R.; Busardo, F.P. Nails in forensic toxicology: An update. *Curr. Pharm. Des.* **2017**, *23*, 5468–5479. [CrossRef] [PubMed]
92. Hill, V.A.; Stowe, G.N.; Paulsen, R.B.; Schaffer, M. Nail analysis for drugs: A role in workplace testing? *J. Anal. Toxicol.* **2018**, *42*, 425–436. [CrossRef] [PubMed]
93. Brzeczko, A.W.; Leech, R.; Stark, J.G. The advent of a new pseudoephedrine product to combat methamphetamine abuse. *Am. J. Drug Alcohol Abus.* **2013**, *39*, 284–290. [CrossRef]
94. Phan, H.M.; Yoshizuka, K.; Murry, D.J.; Perry, P.J. Drug testing in the workplace. *Pharmacotherapy* **2012**, *32*, 649–656. [CrossRef]
95. Ozbunar, E.; Aydogdu, M.; Doger, R.; Bostanci, H.I.; Koruyucu, M.; Akgur, S.A. Morphine Concentrations in Human Urine Following Poppy Seed Paste Consumption. *Forensic Sci. Int.* **2019**, *295*, 121–127. [CrossRef]
96. Dinis-Oliveira, R.J.; Carvalho, F.; Duarte, J.A.; Remiao, F.; Marques, A.; Santos, A.; Magalhaes, T. Collection of biological samples in forensic toxicology. *Toxicol. Mech. Methods* **2010**, *20*, 363–414. [CrossRef]
97. Verstraete, A.G.; Pierce, A. Workplace drug testing in Europe. *Forensic Sci. Int.* **2001**, *121*, 2–6. [CrossRef]
98. Smith, D.E.; Glatt, W.; Tucker, D.E.; Deutsch, R.; Seymour, R.B. Drug testing in the workplace: Integrating medical review officer duties into occupational medicine. *Occup. Med.* **2002**, *17*, 79–90.
99. Clark, H.W.; Johnson, B. Legal issues facing physicians: Substance abuse in the workplace. *Occup. Med.* **2002**, *17*, 119–135. [PubMed]
100. Ompad, D.C.; Gershon, R.R.; Sandh, S.; Acosta, P.; Palamar, J.J. Construction trade and extraction workers: A population at high risk for drug use in the United States, 2005–2014. *Drug Alcohol Depend.* **2019**, *205*, 107640. [CrossRef]
101. Carter, T.; Heaton, K.; Shirey, M.R. Should nursing institute random drug screening? *Workplace Health Saf.* **2019**, *67*, 604. [CrossRef]
102. Marques, P.H.; Jesus, V.; Olea, S.A.; Vairinhos, V.; Jacinto, C. The effect of alcohol and drug testing at the workplace on individual's occupational accident risk. *Saf. Sci.* **2014**, *68*, 108–120. [CrossRef]
103. Fantoni-Quinton, S.; Bossu, B.; Morgenroth, T.; Frimat, P. Illicit drugs, testing, prevention and work in France: Ethical and legal issues. *Med. Law* **2010**, *29*, 353–372. [PubMed]
104. Hawkins, D.; Roelofs, C.; Laing, J.; Davis, L. Opioid-related overdose deaths by industry and occupation-Massachusetts, 2011–2015. *Am. J. Ind. Med.* **2019**, *62*, 815–825. [CrossRef]
105. Kimble, A.N.; DeCaprio, A.P. Systematic analysis of novel psychoactive substances. II. Development of a screening/confirmatory LC-QqQ-MS/MS method for 800+ compounds and metabolites in urine. *Forensic Chem.* **2019**, *16*, 100189. [CrossRef]

5

Effect of an Electronic Medical Record-Based Screening System on a Rapid Response System: 8-Years' Experience of a Single Center Cohort

Se Hee Lee, Chae-Man Lim, Younsuck Koh, Sang-Bum Hong and Jin Won Huh *

Department of Pulmonary and Critical Care Medicine, Asan Medical Center, University of Ulsan College of Medicine, 88, Olympic-ro 43-gil, Songpa-gu, Seoul 05505, Korea; celestia7@gmail.com (S.H.L.); cmlim@amc.seoul.kr (C.-M.L.); yskoh@amc.seoul.kr (Y.K.); sbhong@amc.seoul.kr (S.-B.H.)

* Correspondence: jwhuh@amc.seoul.kr

Abstract: An electronic medical record (EMR)-based screening system has been developed as a trigger system for a rapid response team (RRT) that traditionally used direct calling. We compared event characteristics, intensive care unit (ICU) admission, and 28-day mortality following RRT activation of the two trigger systems. A total of 10,026 events were classified into four groups according to the activation time (i.e., daytime or on-call time) and the triggering type (i.e., calling or screening). Among surgical patients, the ICU admission was lowest for the on-call screening group (26.2%). Compared to the on-call screening group, the on-call calling group and daytime calling group showed higher ICU admission with an odds ratio (OR) of 2.07 (95% CI 1.50–2.84, $p < 0.001$) and OR of 2.68 (95% CI 1.91–3.77, $p < 0.001$), respectively. The 28-day mortality was lowest for the on-call screening group (8.7%). Compared to the on-call screening group, on-call calling (OR 1.88, 95% CI 1.20–2.95, $p = 0.006$) and daytime calling (OR 1.89, 95% CI 1.17–3.05, $p < 0.001$) showed higher 28-day mortality. The EMR-based screening system might be useful in detecting at-risk surgical patients, particularly during on-call time. The clinical usefulness of an EMR-based screening system can vary depending on patients' characteristics.

Keywords: clinical deterioration; early medical intervention; electronic health records; hospital rapid response team; intensive care units; medical records system; computerized

---

1. Introduction

Rapid response teams (RRT) were widely deployed in the early 2000s to promptly detect deteriorating patients outside critical care and to provide appropriate advanced critical care early on [1]. RRTs are activated by calls by medical staff based on the calling criteria and the clinical concern. Increasing the RRT dose could improve patient outcomes [2,3]. However, previous research indicates that only 30% of at-risk patients who satisfied the calling criteria received critical care from RRTs [1]. In addition, diurnal variation affects RRT activation and clinical outcomes. RRT calls frequently occur during the day. Diurnal variation in RRT utilization influences hospital mortality dependent upon the time of the call [4,5]. Delayed RRT activation occurs more frequently between midnight and 8:00 am and is associated with increased hospital mortality [6]. Infrequent activation during early morning hours is followed by a spike in mortality at 7:00 am [7]. These findings suggest a delay in recognition of at-risk patients and suboptimal RRT utilization by caregivers at night results in poor patient outcomes.

Abundant clinical data and conclusions derived from electronic medical records (EMR) can be utilized to improve not only health care quality but also point-of-care management by detecting clinical deterioration early. The 24-h accessibility of EMR is beneficial in that automatic EMR monitoring by RRTs tends to reinforce the screening of at-risk patients. Currently, vital signs and certain laboratory data in EMR are used as criteria parameters for detecting deteriorating patients working as an additional limb of RRT [8,9]. However, results of EMR-based RRT systems have been mixed [9–11]. In our hospital, an RRT with dual-triggering afferent limbs, which utilizes both direct calling from bedside doctors or nurses and 24-h based EMR screening criteria, was introduced in 2008. We adopted a single-parameter EMR screening system. Previous research that assessed clinical outcomes in the first two-year period after dual triggering system deployment reported that EMR screening resulted in lower intensive care unit (ICU) admission rates but only surgically ill patients had reduced 28-day mortality rates [12]. This study aimed to analyze the event characteristics and clinical outcomes of RRT activations according to the trigger-type and activation time using the 8-year-period RRT cohort.

2. Methods

2.1. Study Populations

The study protocol was approved by the Institutional Review Board (2016-0857) of Asan Medical Center. Due to the retrospective nature, informed consent was not required, and patients' data were used anonymously. This study was conducted at an academic tertiary care hospital with approximately 2400 adult beds. All adult patients in general wards who received treatment from the RRT were eligible. RRT operated for 24 h a day, 7 days a week during the study period. As the purpose of the study was to compare clinical characteristics and effectiveness of two triggering systems in early detection and management of at-risk patients, RRT events which were categorized as cardiopulmonary cerebral resuscitation (CPCR), post-CPCR care, educational purpose, procedure assistance, and counseling for end-of-life were excluded. Patients who requested to be listed as "do not resuscitate" (DNR) were also excluded. If the patient had more than one event in the same admission period, only the first event was included for analysis to eliminate redundancy.

Based on the duty hours of training residents, daytime for weekdays was defined as 7:00 am to 5:59 pm while on-call time was defined as 6:00 pm to 6:59 am on the following day. Daytime for weekends or holidays was defined as from 7:00 am to 11:59 am while on-call time was defined as from 12:00 pm to 6:59 am on the following day. Nursing staffs work in three shifts, day shift (6:30 am to 2:30 pm), evening shift (2:30 pm to 10:30 pm), and night shift (10:30 pm to 6:30 am on the following day), regardless of weekend or weekdays. We divided the type of activation events into four groups: calling vs. screening, based on trigger type, and daytime vs. on-call time, based on activation time.

At this hospital, the RRT not only provides advanced critical care but is also actively involved in monitoring and assessing at-risk patients throughout the day. Direct calling from ward physicians and nurses activates the RRT. Additionally, the EMR-based screening system is utilized, which automatically activates the RRT when the pre-defined criteria based on the vital signs and laboratory measurements of the patients' medical records are met. Details of the criteria are shown in Table S1.

2.2. Study Variables and Outcomes

Data were routinely collected for patients' demographics, illness-type (medical or surgical), RRT activation time and date (weekdays or weekend), trigger parameter for activation, therapeutic intervention during the event (e.g., intubation, ventilator, high flow nasal cannular (HFNC), bilevel positive airway pressure (BiPAP), advanced cardiovascular life support (ACLS), etc.), the outcome of the RRT intervention (e.g., ICU transfer vs. ward stay), and the 28-day mortality following the event. If the alarm was triggered by both calling and screening, the first trigger was recorded. Patients' vital signs (e.g., systolic/diastolic blood pressure (BP), pulse rate (PR), respiratory rate (RR), body temperature (BT), and mental status) at the time of the event were also collected to risk-stratify patients. We calculated a modified early warning score (MEWS), which was validated for both medical in-patients and surgical in-patients [13,14] and used this score for adjustment. MEWS is the sum of scores for five parameters: systolic BP, PR, RR, and mental status. Each parameter and detailed pre-assigned score are described in Table S2.

The number of RRT events per year and the number of RRT activations per clock hour were analyzed to identify the RRT activation pattern. RRT events per each clock hour were classified as per screening and calling which were further divided into doctor-calling, and nurse-calling. All events were categorized into four different groups: daytime calling, daytime screening, on-call calling, and on-call screening. The primary outcome considered was ICU admission after RRT activation. Twenty-eight day mortality following RRT activation was also assessed for the four groups.

2.3. Statistical Methods

Annual RRT activations and the number of RRT events for each clock hour are presented graphically. Differences between two groups (i.e., calling vs. screening in daytime, and calling vs. screening in on-call time) were tested using a Chi-square test for categorical variables, and the independent t-test for continuous variables. ICU admission and 28-day mortality were compared between the on-call screening group and the other three individual groups and presented as an odds ratio (OR) with a 95% confidence interval using a multivariate logistic regression model adjusting for age, sex, MEWS, weekend, and activation coding after univariate analysis. The risk factors for ICU admission and 28-day mortality were identified following univariate logistic analysis and statistically significant variables were further applied for the multivariate logistic regression. All statistical analyses were performed using SPSS software (version 24.0; IBM Corp., Armonk, NY).

3. Results

From 1 January 2009 to 31 December 2016, 15,641 RRT events were identified (Figure 1); of these, 10,026 events were included for analysis. All events were classified according to activation time and trigger type. A total of 6293 events occurred during on-call time and 54.3% (n = 3419) were activated by screening rather than calling. Figure 2 represents the number of RRT activation events per year over the 8-year period. The number of RRT triggers by calling did not vary significantly between each year but activation by screening increased steadily from 2009. This increase was more prominent during on-call time.

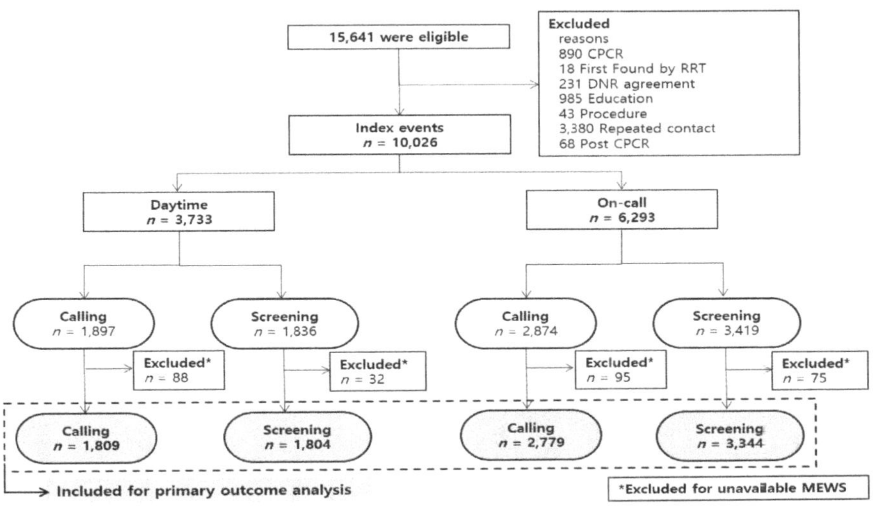

Figure 1. Schematic flow chart of the study Given that our rapid response team (RRT) performs a multifunctional role, only events related to early detection and management of at-risk patients were included for the study. Among 15,641 eligible events, 10,026 events were analyzed to describe the pattern of RRT activations. For clinical outcome analysis, 9736 events were included after excluding 290 events due to unavailable MEWS. Cardiopulmonary cerebral resuscitation (CPCR); Do not resuscitate (DNR); Rapid response team (RRT); Modified early weaning score (MEWS).

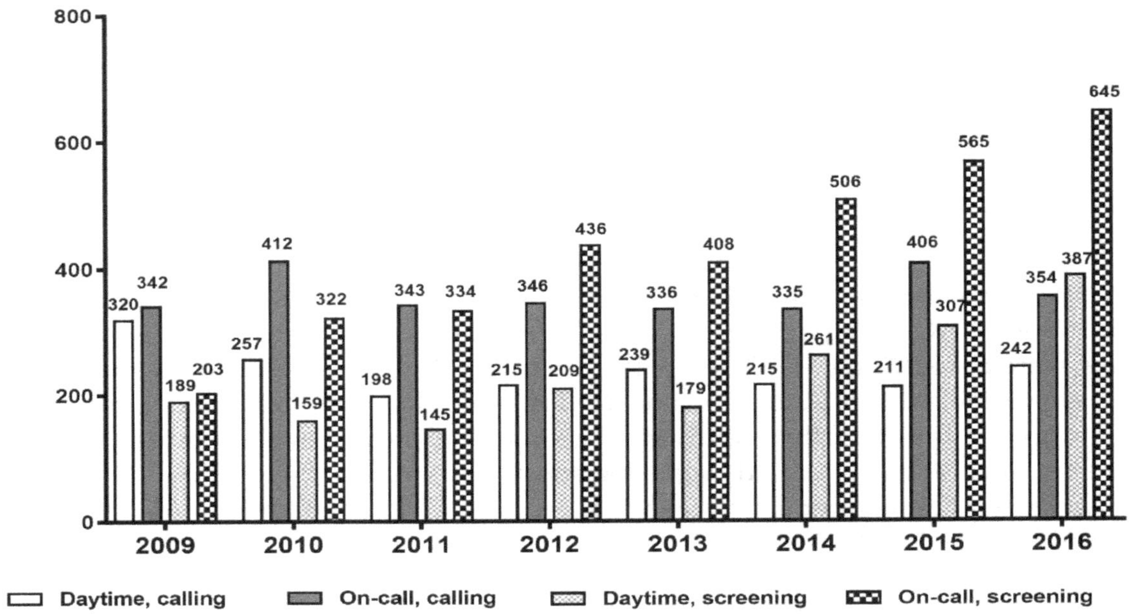

Figure 2. The number of RRT events per year since 2009. Overall RRT events increased from 1055 in 2009 to 1627 in 2016. The total number of RRT activations by screening in 2016 was 2.63-fold higher than that in 2009. Data are presented as number of events.

The number of events for each clock hour are illustrated in Figure 3. In total, 4771 events (47.6%) were call-triggered (doctor calling and nurse calling). The number of activations by nurse calling was relatively stable in each clock hour compared with the number of doctor calling. RRT contacts were most frequent from midnight to 00:59 am ($n = 952$, 9.5%). The proportions of activation by screening were higher during on-call time, particularly from midnight to 0:59 at which time the vital check is conducted by night duty nurses.

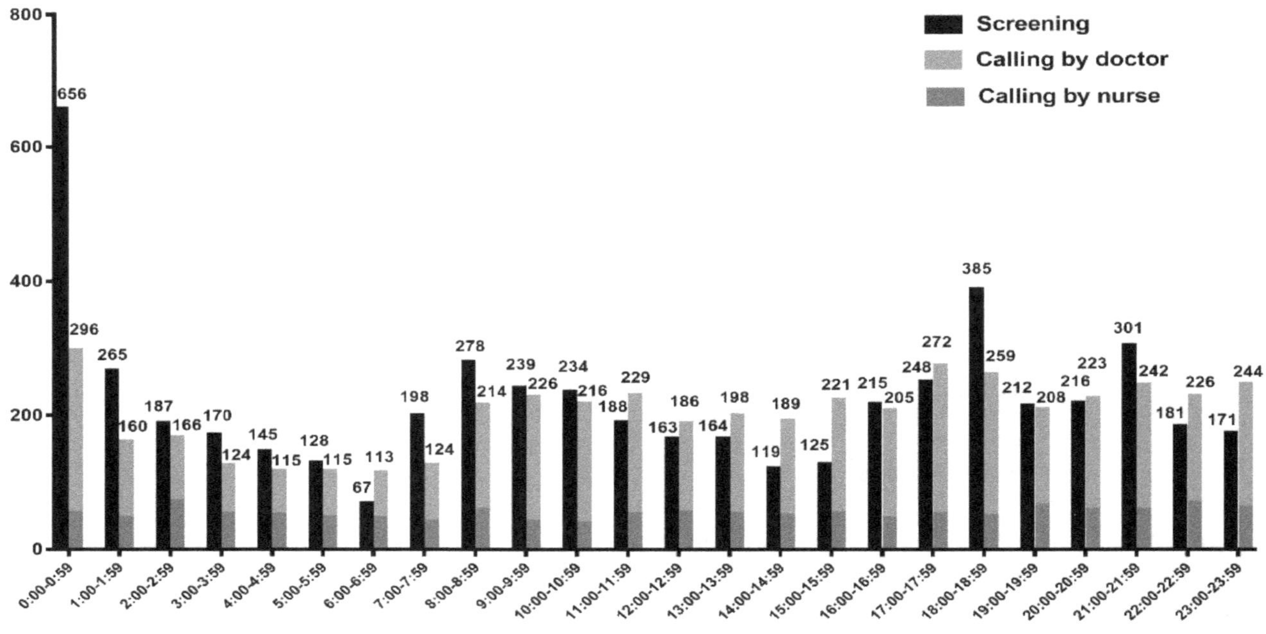

Figure 3. The RRT frequency according to each clock hour. Among 10,026 events, 4771 (47.6%) were triggered by calling and 5255 (52.4%) were triggered by screening. RRT contacts are most frequent at midnight to 00:59 am ($n = 952$, 9.5%). The total frequency was higher in order of 18:00 pm, 21:00 pm, and 8:00 am. Data are presented as number of events.

Patients' baseline characteristics, illness type, and MEWS are presented in Table 1. Approximately half of the patients in the screening group had solid malignancy (daytime 50.3% vs. 35.3%, $p < 0.001$; on-call time 50.2% vs. 41.5%, $p < 0.001$). Moreover, a greater number of patients had hematologic malignancy in the screening group than in the calling group (daytime 19.3% vs. 13.4%, $p < 0.001$; on-call time 16.7% vs. 11.6%, $p < 0.001$). In contrast, the proportion of patients with chronic lung disease, cardiovascular disease, or neurologic disease was higher in the calling group. Among surgical patients, a higher number of at-risk patients were activated by calling rather than screening (daytime 18.9% vs. 10.7%, $p < 0.001$: on-call time 19.6% vs. 12.9%, $p < 0.001$). MEWS was available in 9,736 events. MEWS was significantly higher in the calling group than in the screening group (daytime 4.54 vs. 4.30, $p = 0.031$; on-call 4.57 vs. 4.37, $p = 0.0017$). Activation coding and type of intervention are presented in Table S3.

Table 1. Baseline characteristics of included events.

	Daytime		**On-Call**	
	Calling	**Screening**	**Calling**	**Screening**
	***N* = 1897**	***N* = 1836**	***N* = 2874**	***N* = 3419**
Age	64 (52–73)	64 (53–72)	64 (53–73)	64 (53–72)
Sex				
Male—No. (%)	1165 (61.7)	1120 (61.0)	1768 (61.5)	2097 (61.3)
Underlying disease				
Solid malignancy	669 (35.3)	924 (50.3) ‡	1194 (41.5)	1717 (50.2) ‡
Hematologic malignancy	254 (13.4)	355 (19.3) ‡	334 (11.6)	571 (16.7) ‡
Chronic lung disease	277 (14.6) *	224 (12.2)	405 (14.1) *	375 (11.0)
Cardiovascular disease	839 (44.2) †	720 (39.2)	1327 (46.2) *	1483 (43.4)
Chronic liver disease	273 (14.4)	267 (14.5)	424 (14.8)	479 (14.0)
Gastrointestinal disease	7 (0.4)	6 (0.3)	16 (0.6)	14 (0.4)
Neurologic disease	262 (13.8) ‡	166 (9.0)	402 (14.0) ‡	322 (9.4)
Chronic kidney disease	158 (8.3) ‡	102 (5.6)	217 (7.6) *	203 (5.9)
Thyroid disease	95 (5.0) *	61 (3.3)	113 (3.9)	140 (4.1)
Diabetes mellitus	440 (23.2)	429 (23.4)	703 (24.5)	825 (24.1)
Solid organ transplant	70 (3.7)	58 (3.2)	86 (3.0)	93 (2.7)
Illness type				
Medical	1450 (78.7)	1627 (88.6) ‡	2251 (79.9)	2987 (87.4) ‡
Surgical	392 (21.3) ‡	209 (11.4)	567 (20.1) ‡	432 (12.6)
MEWS	4.54 ± 2.23 ‡	4.30 ± 2.02	4.57 ± 2.24 ‡	4.37 ± 2.01
Weekend	330 (17.4)	377 (20.5) *	1103 (38.4)	1347 (40.2)

Among continuous variables, age is presented as median (interquartile range) and MEWS are presented as mean ± SD. Categorical variables are presented as No. (%). MEWS was available in 9736 patients. * p-value < 0.05, † p-value < 0.01, ‡ p-value < 0.001. Chi-square test was done for the comparison between daytime calling and daytime screening. The same analytic technique was used for the comparison between on-call calling and on-call screening. MEWS = modified early weaning score.

The overall ICU admission was 28.9% and 28-day mortality was 30% among 9736 patients. As more patients in the screening group had a malignancy (Table 1), a subgroup analysis was conducted to compare the clinical outcomes between patients with cancer and those without cancer (Table 2). Among patients with an underlying malignancy, the overall ICU admission rate was 21.5% and the on-call screening group displayed the lowest ICU admission (14.9%). The overall 28-day mortality was 40.6% and mortality was lower for the on-call calling group compared to the on-call screening group (OR 0.84, 95% CI 0.72–0.98). Among patients without cancer, overall ICU admission and 28-day mortality were 36.1% and 21.4%, respectively. ICU admission was lowest for the on-call screening group (22.3%) as was 28-day mortality (18.6%). Similar to patients with cancer, the daytime screening group had higher mortality compared to on-call screening group (OR 1.48, 95% CI 1.14–1.93).

Table 2. Clinical outcomes among medical patients without cancer and with cancer.

		With Cancer ($N = 4980$)			Without Cancer ($N = 3256$)		
		OR	**95% CI**	***p*-Value**	**OR**	**95% CI**	***p*-Value**
ICU admission	On-call, screening	1			1		
	Daytime, screening	1.01	0.81–1.26	0.92	1.26	0.97–1.64	0.086
	On-call, calling	2.30	1.91–2.77	<0.001	2.42	1.98–2.97	<0.001
	Daytime, calling	3.85	3.11–4.77	<0.001	3.65	2.93–4.54	<0.001
28-day mortality	On-call, screening	1			1		
	Daytime, screening	1.16	0.99–1.35	0.063	1.48	1.14–1.93	0.004
	On-call, calling	0.84	0.72–0.98	0.026	1.10	0.88–1.38	0.417
	Daytime, calling	0.87	0.72–1.05	0.136	1.17	0.92–1.50	0.204

Data are presented as odds ratio (OR) with 95% confidence interval (CI). ICU admission and 28-day mortality were analyzed using a multivariate logistic regression model adjusting for age, sex, MEWS, weekend, and activation code. MEWS, weekend, and activation code were variables finally selected for the regression model for ICU admission in cancer patients. For 28-day mortality in cancer patients, sex, MEWS, weekend, and activation code were adopted variables for the regression model. Among patients without cancer, age, MEWS, and activation code were variables adopted for ICU admission and 28-day mortality. For patients with cancer: overall ($n = 4980$); on-call screening ($n = 1971$); daytime screening ($n = 1131$); on-call calling ($n = 1188$); daytime calling ($n = 690$). For patients without cancer: overall ($n = 3256$); On-call screening ($n = 961$); Daytime screening ($n = 472$); On-call calling ($n = 1063$); Daytime calling ($n = 760$).

Among patients with surgical illnesses (Table 3) overall ICU admission and 28-day mortality were 37.6% and 13.4%, respectively. The on-call screening group was significantly associated with lower ICU admission (26.2%); daytime screening had an ICU admission of 28.4% (OR 1.06, 95% CI 0.70–1.59, $p = 0.794$), on-call calling 42.4% (OR 2.07, 95% CI 1.50–2.84, $p < 0.001$), and daytime calling 46.1% (OR 2.68, 95% CI 1.91–3.77, $p < 0.001$). The on-call screening group was also associated with lower 28-day mortality (8.7%); the 28-day mortality for daytime screening was 12.9% (OR 1.44, 95% CI 0.82–2.51, $p = 0.203$), on-call calling 15.5% (OR 1.88, 95% CI 1.20–2.95, $p = 0.006$), and daytime calling 15.9% (OR 1.89, 95% CI 1.17–3.05, $p = 0.0009$).

Table 3. Clinical outcomes among patients with surgical illness.

		OR	**95% CI**	***p*-Value**
ICU admission	On-call, screening	1		
	Daytime, screening	1.06	0.70–1.59	0.794
	On-call, calling	2.07	1.50–2.84	<0.0001
	Daytime, calling	2.68	1.91–3.77	<0.0001
28-day mortality	On-call, screening	1		
	Daytime, screening	1.44	0.82–2.51	0.203
	On-call, calling	1.88	1.20–2.95	0.006
	Daytime, calling	1.89	1.17–3.05	0.009

Data are presented as odds ratio with 95% confidence interval (CI). ICU admission and 28-day mortality were analyzed using a multivariate logistic regression model adjusting for age, sex, MEWS, weekend, and activation code. Sex, MEWS, weekend, and activation code were variables finally selected for the regression model for ICU admission. For 28-day mortality, sex, MEWS, and activation code were adopted variables for the regression model. Overall ($n = 1500$); on-call screening ($n = 412$); daytime screening ($n = 201$); on-call calling ($n = 528$); daytime calling ($n = 359$).

The risk factors associated with ICU transfer and 28-day mortality following RRT activation are shown in Table S4. On-call time patients were less likely to be transferred to the ICU (OR 0.76, 95% CI: 0.68–0.84, $p < 0.001$) and had a lower mortality rate than daytime patients (OR 0.85, 95% CI: 0.78–0.94, $p < 0.001$). Compared to calling, the RRT activation by screening was associated with a lower ICU transfer rate, (OR 0.51, 95% CI: 0.46–0.57, $p < 0.001$) but a higher 28-day mortality rate (OR 1.19, 95% CI: 1.08–1.33).

4. Discussion

We evaluated the effects of an EMR-based screening system using the RRT cohort over an 8-year period following the employment of a dual triggering system. In addition to the calling system, the EMR-based screening system was implemented to aid in increasing the detection sensitivity of at-risk patients. Between 1 January 2009 and 31 December 2016, a total of 10,026 events were included. The number of RRT activations by screening system continually increased over the course of data collection. The higher proportion of screening group (especially on-call time) compared to the other study groups can be explained by two factors: (1) the experiences gained by the RRT over the study years might have led to an increase in the sensitivity of the screening system in detecting at-risk patients; (2) a small number of doctors on duty compared to daytime might result in a decrease in on-call calling, thus eventually increasing the burden of RRT work during on-call time.

Among the patients without cancer and surgical patients, the on-call screening group had lower ICU admission and lower 28-day mortality than other groups, possibly due to early detection using EMR screening during on-call time. However, this positive effect of the screening system was not observed among at-risk patients with cancer. Although more patients in the on-call calling group transferred to the ICU and had higher MEWS than the on-call screening group, 28-day mortality was significantly lower in the on-call calling group. The higher ICU admission rate in the calling group can be explained by the fact that activation by calling is (1) more likely to be associated with acute medical events and (2) more likely to reflect greater motivation on behalf of attending physicians to treat the patient. Alternatively, the daytime screening group had lower MEWS and lower ICU admission, but higher 28-day mortality. This result suggests that various factors affect mortality in medically ill at-risk patients. DNR agreement following RRT activation or consideration for end-of-life care might be closely related to 28-day mortality.

In many reports, the dose-response effect of the RRT was well described [15–17]. Increasing RRT dose was associated with dose-related reduction of cardiac arrest and cardiac arrests were most common overnight when RRT dose was the lowest. Because the trigger threshold by traditional calling criteria may vary depending on the experience or concern of ward physicians and nurses, the achievement of optimal RRT dose is important. Real-time monitoring by experienced RRT could increase the sensitivity of detecting clinical deterioration and improve clinical outcome. As our results indicate, triggering frequency itself is largely dependent on the interval of vital sign measurements. As vital sign check-ups at the ward are typically recorded by nurses at intervals of 8-h or 4-h, the activation frequency was higher during the regular vital sign check-up hours. Therefore, unless clinicians order frequent vital sign check-ups or laboratory tests for possible at-risk patients, the possibility of missing indicators of deteriorating patients will persist. Employment of automatic continuous monitoring could overcome this limitation [18].

We used single parameters including laboratory data, such as lactate levels and arterial blood gas analysis, as the triggers for the EMR-based system. Previous research indicates various degrees of sensitivity and the accuracy of multiple aggregate weighted scoring systems (AWSS) for predicting ICU transfer, cardiac arrest, and mortality [19,20]. However, the current AWSS depends mainly on vital signs, without assessing other characteristics of at-risk patients. Therefore, the development of a modified scoring system which includes vital signs, laboratory data, and characteristics of the patient population is necessary to increase the sensitivity and specificity of the screening system.

There are several limitations in this study. First, this is a single-center study and data were analyzed retrospectively. As our center is an academic tertiary hospital, the patients' disease severity is generally higher than in non-tertiary hospitals; thus, our results may not generalize well to non-teaching hospitals or hospitals with different patient populations. Nevertheless, the use of a screening system during on-call time seems to be associated with an improved 28-day mortality rate, particularly among surgically ill patients and patients without malignancy. As our hospital adopted a dual-triggering system at the time of the launch of RRT, for ethical and patient safety concerns, a prospective randomized trial comparing calling system and screening system based on the duty hours was not possible. A prospective multicenter study is required to evaluate the efficacy of the screening system more accurately. Second, the proportion of patients who agreed on a plan for end-of-life care following RRT activation was not considered. There are other factors affecting primary outcomes aside from the management of RRT, such as end-of-life care, spontaneous decisions by attending physicians, will of family caregivers, and the availability of ICU beds at the time of the RRT visit. Therefore, these results should be interpreted with careful consideration of multiple clinical factors, not by the RRT intervention alone.

5. Conclusions

Deployment of an EMR-based screening system offers additional improvement in detecting and managing at-risk patients, particularly during on-call time. However, the clinical effectiveness of this system can vary depending on patients' characteristics. The deployment of a modified screening system reflecting the physiologic parameters, laboratory measurements, and underlying diseases of the patient population at each hospital would maximize the beneficial role of the RRT in point of care management.

Author Contributions: S.H.L. contributed to analyzing data and writing of the manuscript. C.-M.L., Y.K., and S.-B.H. contributed in planning the study, clinical work, and approval of the submitted article. J.W.H. conceived the study; contributed in clinical work, integrity, and accuracy of data; preparation and approval of the submitted article. All authors have read and agreed to the published version of the manuscript.

Acknowledgments: The authors thank the nurses of rapid response team for their contribution to this work.

Abbreviations

ACLS: Advanced cardiovascular life support; AWSS: Aggregate weighted scoring systems; BiPAP: Bilevel positive airway pressure; CI: Confidence interval; CPCR: Cardiopulmonary cerebral resuscitation; DNR: Do not resuscitate; EMR: electronic medical record; HFNC: High flow nasal cannular; ICU: Intensive care unit; MEWS: Modified early warning score; RRT: Rapid response team

References

1. Hillman, K.; Chen, J.; Cretikos, M.; Bellomo, R.; Brown, D.; Doig, G.; Finfer, S.; Flabouris, A. Introduction of the medical emergency team (MET) system: A cluster-randomised controlled trial. *Lancet* **2005**, *365*, 2091–2097. [CrossRef] [PubMed]
2. Maharaj, R.; Raffaele, I.; Wendon, J. Rapid response systems: A systematic review and meta-analysis. *Crit. Care* **2015**, *19*, 254. [CrossRef] [PubMed]
3. Jones, D.; Bellomo, R.; DeVita, M.A. Effectiveness of the medical emergency team: The importance of dose. *Crit. Care* **2009**, *13*, 313. [CrossRef] [PubMed]
4. Galhotra, S.; DeVita, M.A.; Simmons, R.L.; Schmid, A. Impact of patient monitoring on the diurnal pattern of medical emergency team activation. *Crit. Care Med.* **2006**, *34*, 1700–1706. [CrossRef] [PubMed]
5. Sundararajan, K.; Flabouris, A.; Thompson, C. Diurnal variation in the performance of rapid response systems: The role of critical care services-a review article. *J. Intensive Care* **2016**, *4*, 15. [CrossRef] [PubMed]
6. Barwise, A.; Thongprayoon, C.; Gajic, O.; Jensen, J.; Herasevich, V.; Pickering, B.W. Delayed rapid response team activation is associated with increased hospital mortality, morbidity, and length of stay in a tertiary care institution. *Crit. Care Med.* **2016**, *44*, 54–63. [CrossRef] [PubMed]
7. Churpek, M.M.; Edelson, D.P.; Lee, J.Y.; Carey, K.; Snyder, A. Association between survival and time of day for rapid response team calls in a national registry. *Crit. Care Med.* **2017**, *45*, 1677–1682. [CrossRef] [PubMed]
8. Wong Lama, K.M.; DeVita, M.A. Trigger criteria: Big data. *Crit. Care Clin.* **2018**, *34*, 199–207. [CrossRef] [PubMed]
9. Kang, M.A.; Churpek, M.M.; Zadravecz, F.J.; Adhikari, R.; Twu, N.M.; Edelson, D.P. Real-time risk prediction on the wards: A feasibility study. *Crit. Care Med.* **2016**, *44*, 1468–1473. [CrossRef] [PubMed]
10. Green, M.; Lander, H.; Snyder, A.; Hudson, P.; Churpek, M.; Edelson, D. Comparison of the between the

flags calling criteria to the MEWS, NEWS and the electronic cardiac arrest risk triage (eCART) score for the identification of deteriorating ward patients. *Resuscitation* **2018**, *123*, 86–91. [CrossRef] [PubMed]

11. Kollef, M.H.; Chen, Y.; Heard, K.; LaRossa, G.N.; Lu, C.; Martin, N.R.; Martin, N.; Micek, S.T.; Bailey, T. A randomized trial of real-time automated clinical deterioration alerts sent to a rapid response team. *J. Hosp. Med.* **2014**, *9*, 424–429. [CrossRef] [PubMed]
12. Huh, J.W.; Lim, C.M.; Koh, Y.; Lee, J.; Jung, Y.K.; Seo, H.S.; Hong, S.B. Activation of a medical emergency team using an electronic medical recording-based screening system. *Crit. Care Med.* **2014**, *42*, 801–808. [CrossRef] [PubMed]
13. Subbe, C.P.; Kruger, M.; Rutherford, P.; Gemmel, L. Validation of a modified Early Warning Score in medical admissions. *Q J. Med.* **2001**, *94*, 521–526. [CrossRef] [PubMed]
14. Gardner-Thorpe, J.; Love, N.; Wrightson, J.; Walsh, S.; Keeling, N. The value of Modified Early Warning Score (MEWS) in surgical in-patients: A prospective observational study. *Ann. R Coll. Surg. Engl.* **2006**, *88*, 571–575. [CrossRef] [PubMed]
15. Foraida, M.I.; DeVita, M.A.; Braithwaite, R.S.; Stuart, S.A.; Brooks, M.M.; Simmons, R.L. Improving the utilization of medical crisis teams (Condition C) at an urban tertiary care hospital. *J. Crit. Care* **2003**, *18*, 87–94. [CrossRef] [PubMed]
16. Jones, D.; Bellomo, R.; Bates, S.; Warrillow, S.; Goldsmith, D.; Hart, G.; Opdam, H. Patient monitoring and the timing of cardiac arrests and medical emergency team calls in a teaching hospital. *Intensive Care Med.* **2006**, *32*, 1352–1356. [CrossRef] [PubMed]
17. Jones, D.; Bellomo, R.; Bates, S.; Warrillow, S.; Goldsmith, D.; Hart, G.; Opdam, H.; Gutteridge, G. Long term effect of a medical emergency team on cardiac arrests in a teaching hospital. *Crit. Care* **2005**, *9*, R808–R815. [CrossRef] [PubMed]
18. Bellomo, R.; Ackerman, M.; Bailey, M.; Beale, R.; Clancy, G.; Danesh, V.; Hvarfner, A.; Jimenez, E.; Konrad, D.; Lecardo, M.; et al. A controlled trial of electronic automated advisory vital signs monitoring in general hospital wards. *Crit. Care Med.* **2012**, *40*, 2349–2361. [CrossRef] [PubMed]
19. Jansen, J.O.; Cuthbertson, B.H. Detecting critical illness outside the ICU: The role of track and trigger systems. *Curr. Opin. Crit. Care* **2010**, *16*, 184–190. [CrossRef] [PubMed]
20. Churpek, M.M.; Yuen, T.C.; Edelson, D.P. Risk stratification of hospitalized patients on the wards. *Chest* **2013**, *143*, 1758–1765. [CrossRef] [PubMed]

6

Role of Nutrition and Exercise Programs in Reducing Blood Pressure

Roman Jurik and Petr Stastny *

Department of Sport, Faculty of Physical Education and Sport, Charles University, 162 52 Prague, Czech Republic; rjurik@centrum.cz

* Correspondence: stastny@ftvs.cuni.cz

Abstract: The combined effect of diet and strength training (ST) on blood pressure (BP) seems to be very important for the treatment of prehypertension and hypertension (HT). Therefore, the aim of this study was to determine whether ST alone or combined with nutrition or supplementation has an impact on the arterial pressure reduction in normotensive and hypertensive populations. A systematic computerized literature search was performed according to the PRISMA guidelines using PubMed, Scopus and Google Scholar; only English language studies published from 1999 until 2018 were included. This systematic search identified the results of 303 individuals from nine studies. The ST program alone had a similar effectiveness as the nutrition program (NP) alone; however, their combination did not result in increased effectiveness in terms of a high BP reduction. The consumption of L-citrulline had a similar effect as ST on lowering BP; on the other hand, caffeine led to an increase in BP during the ST session. Our data suggest that a combination of ST 2–3 times a week at moderate intensity and a NP seems to be equally effective in terms of lowering BP (systolic and diastolic) as ST and NP alone.

Keywords: resistance training; hypertension; arterial pressure; disease prevention; caffeine

---

1. Introduction

The nonpharmacological approach to hypertension (HT) reduction is based on lifestyle changes using nutritional and exercise strategies; different training interventions [1–7] or nutritional plans [8–10] have been shown to decrease arterial pressure values. Previous reviews have summarized the approaches of aerobic training [11–13], anaerobic training [14–17] and nutrition [18–21], and those strategies were effective for HT reduction with expected decreases of 5 mmHg in systolic blood pressure (SBP) and 3 mmHg in diastolic pressure (DBP) [22] after three months. However, nonpharmacological strategies do not contraindicate each other, and their combination has been shown to be effective for other health improvements, such as bodyweight reduction [10,23–27]. Therefore, there is a question as to what kind of intervention or their combination has an improved effect on the HT decrease.

One of the well-documented interventions that has been shown to reduce arterial pressure is strength training (ST), which has already been reviewed to set optimal training loads, such as the number of sets [28–31], repetitions [32–35] and rest intervals during training sessions [32–34,36–38]. One of the ST effects is eliciting high muscle protein degradation followed by protein synthesis, which increases basal metabolism and is therefore usually accompanied by changes in nutritional requirements. In clinical practice, it is typical that ST is prescribed along with a low carb diet [39–41], specific protein intake [42–49] or another strategy that might support and magnify the arterial pressure decrease. However, there is currently no recommendation regarding whether the ST program should be accompanied by specific nutritional support that could result in a greater effect of HT reduction.

Numerous studies have shown that different nutritional programs (NP) and strategies might lead to nonpharmacological decreases in arterial pressure [50–55], while many strategies place a high demand on patients to make changes in their eating habits. One way to easily change food intake might be accomplished by using food supplements, which have a synergistic effect with the application of ST. Some food supplements have been shown to decrease arterial pressure when used with aerobic training [56–59] or alone. On the other hand, some food supplements might have a positive effect alone but when used simultaneously with exercise might cause side effects, such as post-exercise hypotension [60–66].

In the current literature, there is no current overview of whether ST or nutritional strategies have a stronger effect on HT reduction. Therefore, the aim of this study was to determine whether ST alone or ST combined with nutrition or a supplement has the greatest impact on arterial pressure reduction in normotensive and hypertensive populations. Additionally, this review aimed to summarize what kind of combined ST and NP might be effective for HT reduction without side effects. The main hypothesis of this article is that the biggest effect on HT should be observed when strength training is combined with energy intake restriction. Based on this result, practitioners can establish nonpharmacological treatment for the individuals with increased blood pressure (BP).

2. Methods

This systematic review is reported in accordance with recommendations as presented in the Preferred Reporting Items for Systematic Reviews and Meta-Analysis (PRISMA) statement [67]. The protocol for this systematic review was published on PROSPERO under registration number CRD42019130631.

2.1. Search Strategy

A systematic computerized literature search was performed using PubMed, and Scopus and included studies published in English from 1966 until November 2018. The search formula included the following terms: Blood pressure AND hypertension OR cardiovascular disease OR hypotension AND resistance training OR strength training OR weightlifting OR bodybuilding OR exercise. The search was limited by article types, species, subjects, language, age, and text availability. A manual search was performed using the identified reviews, reference lists of the selected articles and Google Scholar.

2.2. Types of Studies

The review considered cohort studies, analytical cross-sectional studies, randomized control trials, nonrandomized control trials, intervention studies, case-control studies and others that included BP and HR measurements as well as data on NP and ST in all adult populations. The review studies were used for manual searches of their reference list. Dissertations, theses, conference proceedings, conference monographies, and other reviews were not included. Retrospective studies were not included because the area of interest requires performing experiments. The qualitative component also considered the type of ST and NP and methodological designs. All titles and abstracts were screened according to the above-mentioned inclusion criteria after removing the duplicates. Full texts of eligible articles were retrieved and assessed by two reviewers (R. J. and P.S.). Any discrepancies between the two reviewers were managed by a consensus discussion.

2.3. Types of Outcomes

The review considered studies that included the following outcome measures: Acute SBP and DBP variability before, during, and after exercise or a nutritional treatment; the HR variability before, during, and after exercise or treatment; and a mean arterial pressure before, during, and after exercise. The exclusion criteria were as follows: Full text was not available in English, the study did not contain an appropriate description of measurement devices and procedures, the study did not include a proper exercise or nutrition task, or the study did not report how raw data were processed.

2.4. *Data Extraction and Evaluation*

Data extraction included aspects of the study population, such as the average age and sex, specific aspects of the NP and ST intervention (sample size, type of exercise performed, presence of supervision, frequency, and, duration of each session, type of diet, type of supplements), outcome measures and results presented, and the values of BP or HR (Tables S1–S3); however, the studies were not rejected if any part were missing. The Physiotherapy Evidence Database (PEDro) scale was used to assess the methodological quality of a study based on general criteria, such as concealed allocation, intention-to-treat analysis, and adequacy of follow-up. These characteristics make the PEDro scale a useful tool to assess methodological quality [68]. Extraction was performed by two reviewers (R. J. and P.S.). The lack of clarity during the extraction process was resolved by the reviewer's discussion. The PEDro scale based on a Delphi list [69] was used for all articles even if the trials had already been rated by trained evaluators of the PEDro database (http://www.pedro.fhs.usyd.edu.au/).

3. Results

3.1. *Study Characteristics*

The systematic literature search through database searching identified 15,302 records. However, after duplicates were removed, 11,558 records were screened based on the title and abstract. The title and abstract screening resulted in 144 records for full-text eligibility. From these records, nine studies satisfied the quality and exclusion criteria and were selected for this systematic review after full-text screening (Figure 1).

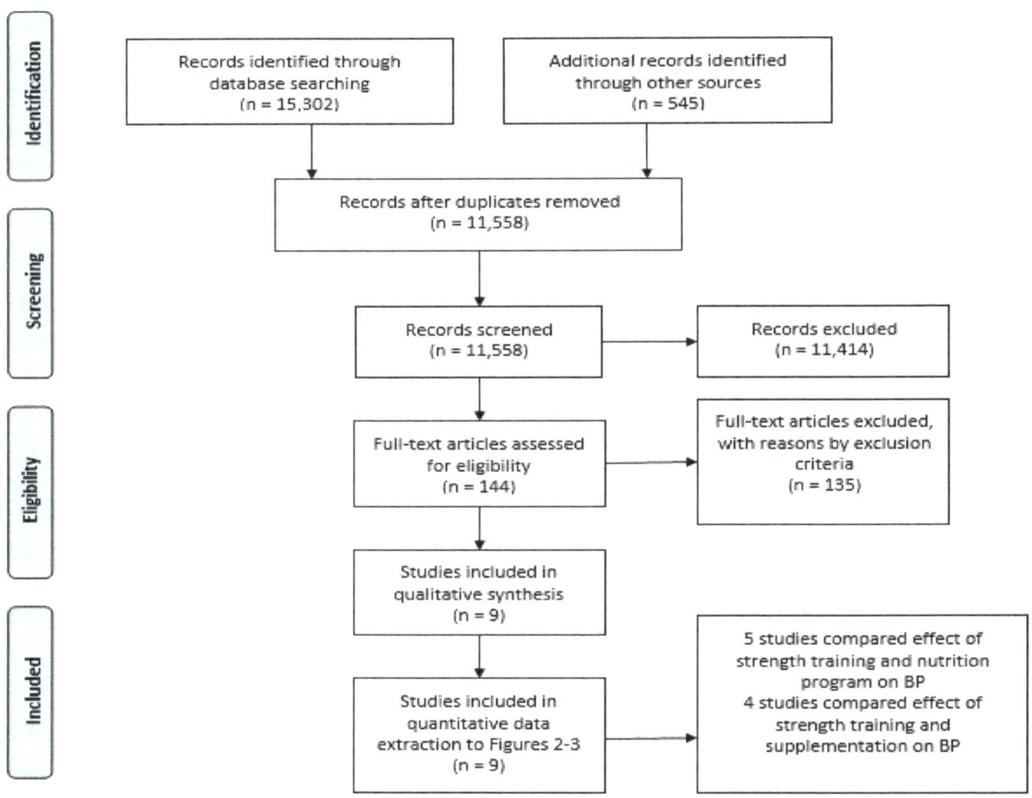

Figure 1. Flowchart of the selection process. BP = blood pressure.

Table 1 provides a general description of each study, sample, and intervention characteristics. Only two studies included seniors [70] and [71]. One study included only men [72], and three included a mixed sample of men and women [70,71,73]. Five studies included only women [74–78]. In total, five studies compared the effect of ST with the NP intervention effect on BP [70,73–76]. Another three studies compared the effect of ST and supplementation intervention on BP [71,72,78,79] and one study analysed the effect of ST and supplementation sesion in cross sectional design [71].

Based on the study results compilation, it can be stated that ST alone has a positive effect on the BP values (Figure 2A,B). However, the effect did not depend on the type of ST (resistance training, bodyweight training or training on vibration platforms, etc. Table 2). An important prerequisite for effective ST is the selection of suitable parameters and methods; otherwise, there is a risk of injury or side effects. All studies used training parameters (Table 2) in accordance with recommendations established by The American College of Sport Medicine (ACSM) and the Canadian Hypertension Education Program, according to Pescatello et al. [80]. However, each study chose different training parameters based on the performance and health state of their subjects.

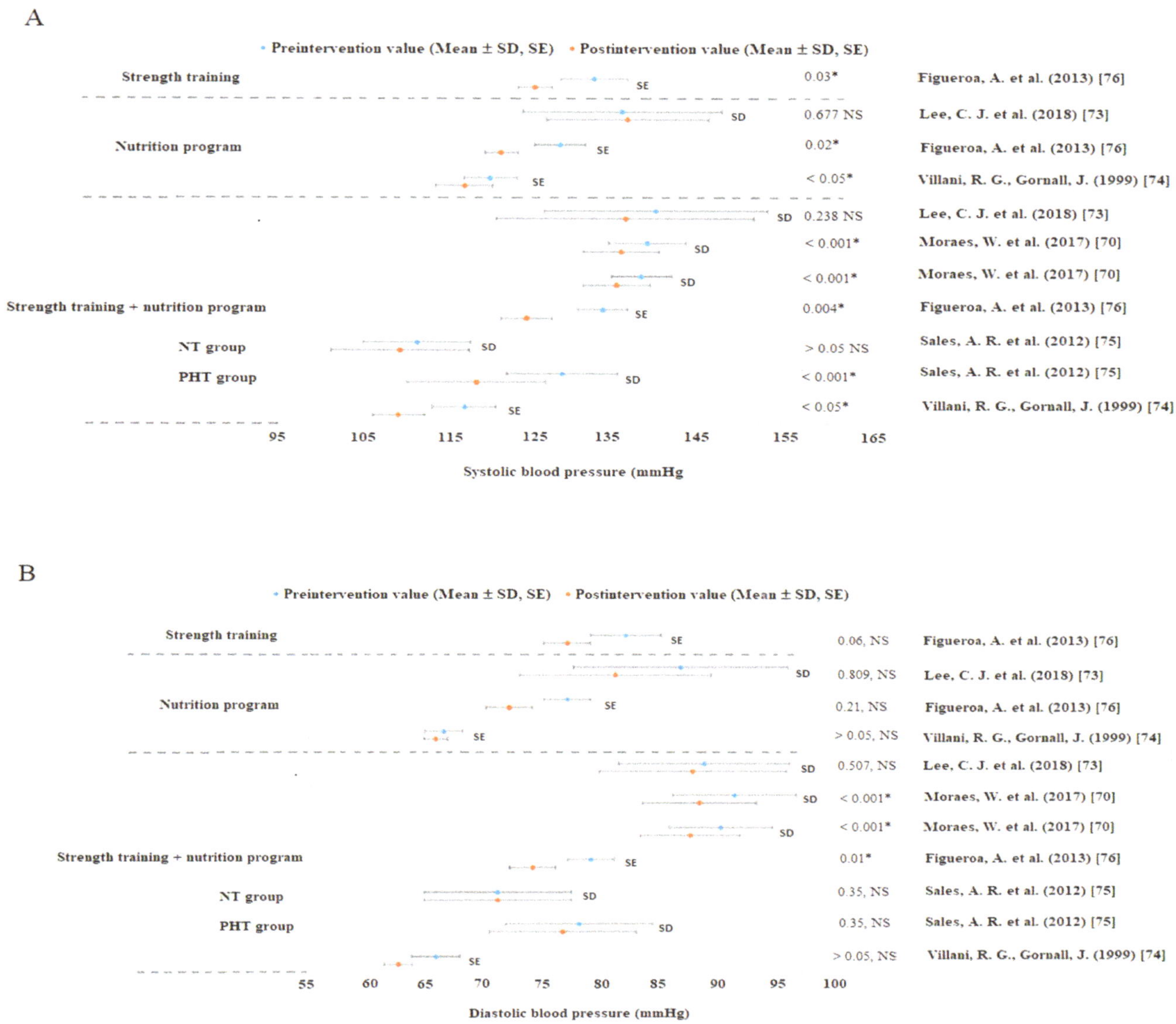

Figure 2. Changes in systolic (**A**) and diastolic (**B**) blood pressure (mmHg) in nutrition and strength training program studies. Abbreviations: NP = nutrition program, NT = normotension group, PHT = prehypertension group, SD = standard deviation, SE = standard error, ST = strength training, NS = not significant change—no change; * significant difference on reported p value.

Table 1. General description of each study, sample, and intervention characteristics.

Authors	Subjects	Aim	Results
Villani and Gornall (1999) [74]	Premenopausal women NP-only group: n = 10, mean age (y) = 33, weight (kg) = 75.78 ± 3.2 NP + Strength training group: n = 10, mean age (y) = 33, weight (kg) = 79.50 ± 2.86	The aim of the study was to investigate the combined influences of very-low-kilojoule diets and strength training on BP.	Resistance exercise did not significantly alter the BP reduction observed with short-term severe dieting.
Sales et al. (2012) [75]	Women with prehypertension: n = 10, age (y) = 39 ± 6, weight (kg) = 71.5 ± 10.7 Women with normotension n = 10, age (y) = 35 ± 11, weight (kg) = 66.5 ± 6.8	The aim of the study was to investigate the effect of diet and exercise training on BP and autonomic modulation in women with prehypertension.	Diet and exercise training reduced SBP in women with prehypertension, and this was associated with parasympathetic augmentation and probably reduction in sympathetic cardiac modulation.
Astorino and Martin (2013) [72]	Hypertensive men: n = 7, age (y) = 23.9 ± 4.6, height (m) = 1.8 ± 0.1, mass (kg) = 89 ± 16.2 Normotensive men: n = 7, age (y) = 22.4 ± 4.0, height (m) = 1.8 ± 0.1, weight (kg) = 77.9 ± 6.4	The primary aim of the study was to compare changes in BP in normotensive and prehypertensive men completing resistance exercise following caffeine ingestion.	Post-exercise hypotension did not occur in either treatment, suggesting that intense resistance training with or without caffeine intake may mitigate the BP-lowering effect of resistance exercise.
Figueroa et al. (2013) [76]	Postmenopausal women LIRET: n = 14, age (y) = 54 ± 1, height (m) = 1.66 ± 0.02, weight (kg) = 88.4 ± 4.6 Postmenopausal women NP: n = 13, age (y) = 54 ± 1, height (m) = 1.62 ± 0.02, weight (kg) = 89.0 ± 4.4 Postmenopausal women NP + LIRET: n = 14, age (y) = 54 ± 1, height (m) = 1.63 ± 0.02, weight (kg) = 86.7 ± 2.7	The aim of the study was to evaluate the independent and combined effects of a hypocaloric diet and LIRET with slow movement on PWV and body composition.	A hypocaloric diet decreases baPWV mainly by reducing legPWV, and this reduction was related to the loss of truncal fat. Although LIRET alone does not affect PWV or body composition, LIRET combined with diet improves baPWV and muscle strength while preventing loss of lean body mass in obese postmenopausal women.
Arazi et al. (2014) [77]	Middle-aged women: n = 24, age (y) = 46.4 ± 6.3, height (m) = 1.66 ± 4.2, weight (kg) = 66.6 ± 9.2 kg	The aim of the study was to investigate the effects of green tea extract on BP, HR, and RPP responses to low-intensity resistance exercise in hypertensive women.	Three weeks of green tea extract ingestion did not influence SBP, DBP or HR but may be have a favorable effect on MAP and RPP responses to an acute resistance exercise during a 1-h exercise recovery.

Table 1. *Cont.*

Authors	Subjects	Aim	Results
Wong et al. (2016) [78]	Postmenopausal women whole-body vibration training + Placebo: n = 14, age (y) = 58 ± 4.0, height (m) = 1.6 ± 0.06, weight (kg) = 89.5 ± 10.6 Postmenopausal women L-citrulline: n = 14, age (y) = 58 ± 4.0, height (m) = 1.6 ± 0.05, weight (kg) = 83.8 ± 8.4 Postmenopausal women WBVT + L-citrulline: n = 13, age (y) = 58 ± 3.0, height (m) = 1.62 ± 0.05, weight (kg) = 88.3 ± 3.9	The aim of the study was to examine the combined and independent effects of whole-body vibration training and L-citrulline supplementation on aortic hemodynamics and plasma nitric oxide metabolites in postmenopausal women.	This study supports the effectiveness of whole-body vibration training + L-citrulline as a potential intervention for the prevention of hypertension-related cardiac diseases in obese postmenopausal women.
Moraes et al. (2017) [70]	Low milk intake group: n = 16, age (y) = 70.2 ± 4.9 and weight (kg) = 70.1 ± 7.6 High milk intake group: n = 12, age (y) = 70.3 ± 5.0, weight (kg) = 68.6 ± 7.7	The aim of the study was to investigate whether the maintenance of exercise training benefits are associated with adequate milk and dairy product intake in elderly hypertensive subjects after detraining.	Maintenance of exercise training benefits related to pressure levels, lower extremity strength and aerobic capacity is associated with adequate milk and dairy product intake in hypertensive elderly subjects following six weeks of detraining.
Romero et al. (2017) [71]	Adults (men and women): n = 9, age (y) = 68 ± 5, height (m) = 1.65 ± 5, weight (kg) = 70 ± 8	The purpose of this study was to test the hypothesis that folic acid ingestion improves skeletal muscle blood flow in aged adults performing graded handgrip and plantar flexion exercise via increased vascular conductance.	Folic acid ingestion increases blood flow to active skeletal muscle primarily via improved local vasodilation in aged adults.
Lee et al. (2018) [73]	Adults (men and women) Advice-only comparison group: n = 28, age (y) = 43.4 ± 14.5, weight (kg) = 69.9 ± 9.2 Diet education group: n = 30, age (y) = 43.0 ± 13.5, weight (kg) = 72.8 ± 15.2 Diet and exercise education group: n = 27, age (y) 49.1 ± 10.1, weight (kg) = 76.6 ± 10.7	The aim of this study was to evaluate the effectiveness of a home-based lifestyle modification intervention on BP management.	Lifestyle modification emphasizing both diet and exercise was effective for lowering BP and should be favored over diet-only modifications.

baPWV, brachial–ankle pulse-wave velocity; BP, blood pressure; DBP, diastolic blood pressure; HR, heart rate; LIRET, low-intensity resistance exercise training, PWV, pulse-wave velocity; MAP, mean arterial pressure; RPP, rate pressure product; SBP, systolic blood pressure; y, year.

Table 2. Strength training parameters and methods in each study.

Authors	Sets	Rest Between Sets	Repetitions	Intensity	Frequency	Strength Training Methods	Number of Exercises
Villani and Gornall (1999) [74]	3	1–2 min	10	10 RM	3x per week	Resistance training	6
Sales et al. (2012) [75]	3	-	10	45–85% 1RM	3x per week	Resistance + aerobic training	10
Astorino and Martin (2013) [72]	4	2 min	As much as possible	70–80% 1RM	2 measurements	Resistance free weight training	4
Figueroa et al. (2013) [76]	2–3	-	18–22x	-	3x per week	Resistance machine training	4
Arazi et al. (2014) [77]	2	2 min	6–10	50% 1 RM	1 measurement	Resistance training	6
Wong et al. (2016) [78]	1–5	0.5–1 min	0.5–1 min	25–40 Hz	3x per week	Bodyweight training	8
Moraes et al. (2017) [70]	-	-	-	-	2x per week	Resistance + endurance + flexibility + stability training	-
Romero et al. (2017) [71]	2	20 min	1	3, 6, 9 kg	2 measurements	Isometric training	2
Lee et al. (2018) [73]	3	-	-	Mild–moderate intensity	Every day	Circuit training	5–7

RM = repetition maximum.

3.2. Strength Training Intervention

In studies by Figueroa et al. [76], Arazi et al. [77], Wong et al. [78] and Astorino et al. [72], a reduction in SBP after ST alone was detected in prehypertensive individuals. Only Astorino et al. [72] observed a negligible improvement in the BP values in normotensive individuals. Figueroa et al. [76] also detected a reduction in DBP after ST. It seems that ST is one of the initiators of post-exercise hypotension in adults, regardless of the type of ST (see in Figure 2A,B, Figure 3 and Tables S1–S3).

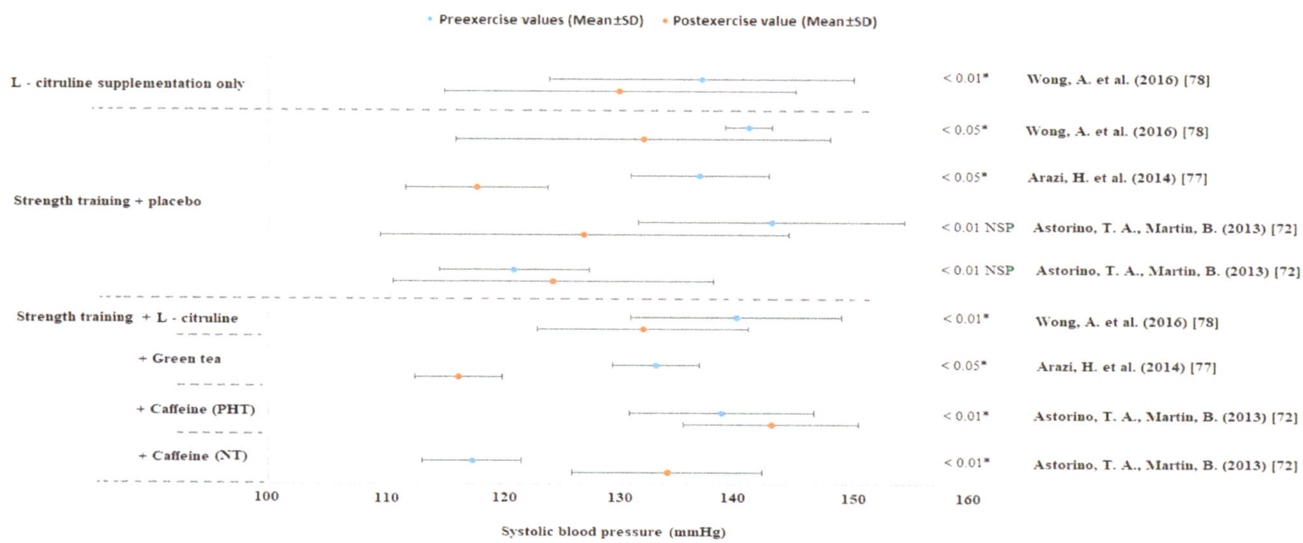

Figure 3. Changes in systolic blood pressure (mmHg) in supplement studies. Abbreviations: SD = standard deviation, * significant difference on reported "p" value. NSP = not significant according to the post hoc test.

Body composition and strength parameters have been improved by ST alone in the study by Figueroa et al. [76]. This confirmed the assumption that ST has a generally positive effect on health status because it might reduce body fat and increase muscle mass and other conditioning values. Strength abilities were improved in participants of studies combining ST and nutrition, and these findings have been reported by Sales et al. [75], Figueroa et al. [76], Moraes et al. [70], and Lee et al. [73]. Strength abilities worsened in the nontraining group (only NP) in the study by Figueroa et al. [76]. In contrast, the Dietary Approaches to Stop Hypertension (DASH) diet group had no negative effect on strength according to Lee et al. [73]. A comparison of the effect of ST alone or ST and NP on absolute and relative strength bring very similar results as those shown by Figueroa et al. [76]. The aerobic parameters were improved in the ST group with NP in the studies by Moraes et al. [70] and Lee et al. [73], and the VO2max was improved in the study by Sales et al. [75].

3.3. Nutrition Program

Figure 2A,B show that SBP and DBP decreased after a nutrition program [74,76]. Only a study by Lee et al. [73] reported a negligible increase in SBP after eight weeks of a NP in individuals with prehypertension (PHT) and HT. Moraes et al. [70] showed that a higher intake of dairy products together with combined aerobic and anaerobic training can lead to a slightly larger drop in BP than that associated with a lower intake of dairy products. Moreover, the higher intake of dairy products resulted in a smaller increase in BP (i.e., return of BP to the initial values) after six weeks of nontraining [70]. It appears that the inclusion of more dairy products in the NP together with combined aerobic and anaerobic training has a positive effect on the reductions in the SBP and DBP values.

A study by Villani, Gornall [74], Figueroa et al. [76], and Lee et al. [73] revealed that a training program combined with a NP leads to a significant drop in BP. Moreover, one study showed that ST alone had similar effectiveness as that of the NP [76].

3.4. *The Effectivity of Food Supplements*

Caffeine is a very popular pre-workout stimulant among athletes. Astorino et al. [72] found that caffeine intake immediately before training increases SBP ($p < 0.05$). However, the effect on HR ($p = 0.16$) and DBP ($p = 0.10$) was similar for the caffeine and placebo. Values of a HR and BP were significantly higher in men with PHT than in normotensive men ($p < 0.05$).

A study by Arazi et al. [77] performed on middle-aged women with HT revealed practically the same reduction in BP after resistance training with or without green tea supplementation (Figure 3). There was no significant difference between the placebo and green tea intake groups (500 mg daily = 245 mg polyphenol, 75 mg epigallocatechin gallate, 25 mg caffeine) or placebo (490 mg maltodextrin). The participants performed circuit training consisting of two sets with a resistance of 50% one repetition maximum (1RM). BP was measured at zero, 15, 30, 45, and 60 min after training.

Wong et al. [78] observed the BP changes in postmenopausal obese women with a BMI ≥ 25 kg/m^2. There was a similar decrease in the brachial and arterial BP in all groups ($p < 0.05$). Vibration training in combination with the placebo, vibration training with L-citrulline or L-citrulline alone can be used as effective ways to lower BP (Figure 3). However, there was no improvement in body composition between the study groups.

Romero et al. [71] observed the effects of folic acid supplementation for six weeks among seniors. The authors found that the folic acid intake immediately before training reduces HR but not mean arterial pressure. At the end of the six-week experiment, the HR values and mean arterial pressure were higher than the baseline values ($p = 0.05$ compared to acute folic acid ingestion). A significant positive feature is the fact that folic acid increases the blood flow to active skeletal muscles, mainly due to better local vasodilation.

4. Discussion

The present study is the first systematic review to analyze the evidence for the effectiveness of ST combined with the NP or supplementation on the BP values. This systematic research analyzed the results of 303 individuals from nine studies. Studies by Moraes et al. [70], Villani, Gornall [74], Sales et al. [75], Figueroa et al. [76], and Lee et al. [73] compared the effects of ST combined with a NP on BP. All of these studies used different methods and parameters for the ST protocol and the NP. A common feature of these five studies was the reductions in SBP and DBP or mean arterial pressure in all experimental groups, regardless of the type of training or diet. Only four studies with supplements met the criteria for inclusion in the systematic review: Astorino et al. [72], Arazi et al. [77], Wong et al. [78] and Romero et al. [71]. The effects of caffeine, L-citrulline, folic acid, and green tea were investigated. Only two supplements had a positive impact on BP: L-citrulline and green tea. On the other hand, caffeine and folic acid did not decrease BP, and caffeine has even been reported to increase BP.

In general, the issue of ST and diet or supplementation has been considered as completely different disciplines, which should be examined separately. However, in the case of treatment of PHT and HT, their combination may appear to be the most effective method. Although this study was not able to conclude whether ST alone or ST combined with the NP has the greatest impact on arterial pressure reduction, it successfully summarized current studies comparing different ST and NP interventions.

4.1. *Blood Pressure Reduced by Strength Training Alone*

It is generally known that ST increases strength, muscle mass, and bone mass and simultaneously helps reduce the symptoms of various chronic diseases, such as heart disease [81–85]. In 2005, the AHA (American Heart Association) started to recommended ST for lowering BP [2] because ST induces a post-exercise BP decrease, as supported by many reviews [14–16,86]. One of the first long-term ongoing studies conducted on cardiovascular disease was the Framingham Heart Study [24], where one of the findings reported was that a 2 mmHg reduction in DBP was associated with an estimated 17%

decrease in the prevalence of HT. However, unsuitable training parameters such as the work load, reps per set, rest interval, etc., can increase BP [87] above the recommended values, i.e., 220/105 mmHg [1]. This study summarize that ST alone can decrease SBP from 132 ± 4 mmHg to 125 ± 2 mmHg [76] or from 141 ± 2 mmHg to 132 ± 16 mmHg [78], and can decrease DBP from 82 ± 3 mmHg to 77 ± 2 mmHg [76], which is much more than the smallest significant values of 2 mmHg. The one-time effect of ST induced a SBP decrease (from 136.88 ± 5.9 mmHg to 117.82 ± 6.09 mmHg) in the study by Arazi et al. [77] and in the prehypertensive group of the study by Astorino et al. [72] (from 143 ± 11.4 mmHg to 131.7 ± 16.6 mmHg). However, in a study by Arazi et al. [77], the biggest BP reduction was not observed immediately after training but after 1 h. There is great diversity between the training sessions in this systematic review. None of the included studies was identical in terms of the training parameters, methods, or exercises (Table 2), but all included studies set up the ST intervention according to the recommended parameters and methods published by Pescatello et al. [80]. Moreover, no study reported a dangerous increase of BP over 220/105 mmHg (according to the ACSM) or substantial post-exercise hypotension. According to the results of this review, ST alone can be recommended as an effective nonpharmacological intervention and prevention method for people with HT or PHT.

4.2. Blood Pressure was Reduced by the Nutrition Program

Nutrition-based approaches are recommended as a first-line therapy for the prevention of HT [72], where the AHA recommends a specific program called the DASH diet to treat and prevent HT. However, some food components such as alcohol, sodium, simple sugar, and saturated fat, have been shown to increase BP [9,51,88]. It has also been found that for HT reduction, weight loss is essential, which has been shown to reduce BP in overweight hypertensive and prehypertensive individuals [10,89–92]. This systematic review included only one study that used the DASH diet. The Korean variation of the DASH diet in a study by Lee et al. [73] improved SBP and DBP only in conjunction with ST (from 139.3 ± 13.2 mmHg to 135.7 ± 15.3 mmHg). Diet alone increased SBP (from 135.3 ± 11.8 mmHg to 135 ± 9.6 mmHg), but decreased DBP (from 86.7 ± 9.2 mmHg to 81.1 ± 8.2 mmHg [73]. Conversely, Villani, Gornall [74], Sales et al. [75] and Figueroa et al. [76] included hypocaloric diets, which led to a reduction in BP in both groups (ST group and NP alone). Moreover, it emerged that ST alone had similar effectiveness as the NP alone [76]. Based on this review result, we recommend a NP that takes into account the individual components of the food and that also leads to a drop in BP. Moraes et al. [70] showed that the inclusion of more dairy products in the NP, together with training, can have a positive effect on the lowering of the SBP (from 138.3 ± 4.6 mmHg to 135.2 ± 4.5 mmHg) and DBP (from 91.3 ± 5.3 mmHg to 88.3 ± 4.9 mmHg) values. The same higher intake of dairy products resulted in a smaller increase in BP (i.e., return of BP to the initial values) after six weeks of nontraining. It seems that a higher intake of dairy products prolongs training hypotension. Therefore, multiple effects of ST and a NP should not be expected for the BP lowering. Although their combination is not more effective, their combination might result in more health benefits (such as weight loss) than ST and NP alone.

4.3. Effect of Supplements on Blood Pressure

Caffeine is a central nervous stimulant whose physiological effects for increasing sport performance are extensive, but sometimes conflicting or contradicting [93,94]. Caffeine supplementation has been shown to decrease feelings of fatigue and promote mood and perceptual responses during any exercise, including ST [94–96]. It has been found that SBP and DBP increase after caffeine ingestion due to the vasoconstrictive effects of caffeine [93]. However, some studies have reported mixed results regarding caffeine intake and BP. In randomized controlled trials (RCTs), short-term caffeine intake caused an acute increase in SBP and DBP by 2/1 mmHg, respectively, compared with the effects of decaffeinated coffee or abstinence [8,97]. Caffeine supplementation, according to the results of Astorino et al. [72], cannot be recommended in individuals with HT or PHT because it not only increases the resting BP but also maintains the BP at a high level after the end of the workout. Therefore, the hypotensive effect of ST is completely lost [72]. For that reason, we cannot recommend caffeine to individuals with HT or PHT although caffeine reduces body fat, increases sport performance, and delays fatigue [94–96].

L-citrulline is a precursor of L-arginine, a substrate for nitric oxide synthase, in the production of nitric oxide. Deficiencies in the L-arginine supply have been strongly implicated in cardiovascular diseases, including HT, atherosclerosis, diabetic vascular disease, hyperhomocysteinemia, heart failure, etc. [98–100]. In a study by Wong et al. [78], L-citrulline decreased BP in individuals performing ST or not performing ST. Both combinations led to a reduction, but slightly better results were achieved in the group that performed the ST alone. Here, again, this study confirmed that ST plays a primary role in the entire process of hypotension. The main and indisputable advantage of L-citrulline is that it reduces BP alone but also in combination with NP or ST. However, more studies are needed to explore this supplement.

A link between green tea and BP reduction has been explored for decades in Chinese populations [101]. However, there are few studies regarding the long-term effects of tea drinking on the risk of HT, and the results of the few studies investigating the relationship between tea consumption and BP were opposing. In epidemiological studies, a higher consumption of black tea in Norwegian individuals was associated with a lower SBP [102], while the green tea intake in Japanese self-defense officials was unrelated to BP [103]. Long-term effects of green tea consumption do not reduce the values of SBP or DBP after training in comparison with the effects of training alone. In contrast, a significant difference between the two groups was observed in the increase in HR after the end of the training. The green tea group performing RT showed a smaller increase in HR than the training group alone. These positive effects can be attributed, at least in part, to the antioxidant properties and vasodilating effects of the catechins in green tea [104]. Unlike caffeine, green tea is not dangerous for individuals with a high BP because it does not increase BP. For this reason, it can be included for its stimulating effects as a preworkout drink. A very significant drop in the systolic blood pressure was measured in the study by Arazi et al. [77], where blood pressure dropped from preintervention values from 133.12 mmHg (± 3.7) to 116.25 mmHg (± 3.71) in the group that combine ST and green tea. According to this information, green tea can be recommended as a suitable food supplement for the treatment of HT. However, supplementation with green tea together with ST does not lead to a bigger reduction in BP in comparison with the effects of the ST alone.

The primary risk factor for a stroke, is HT as stated by Meschia et al. [105]. For this reason, the effect of folic acid on the frequency of infarcts was investigated. Most of the relevant randomized trials were designed for secondary prevention and have not shown a beneficial effect of folic acid for cardiovascular disease prevention [106–109]. Based on this study result, folic acid had an effect on the HR and mean arterial pressure [71]. The acute folate intake before exercise induced a reduction in HR but not a long-term decrease. Even the long-term intake did not lead to reduction. For all measurements, a similar increase in HR and mean arterial pressure during isometric exercises was observed with the acute and long-term intake of folic acid [71]. Based on this study, folic acid supplementation in elderly individuals does not lead to a significant decrease in the mean arterial BP or HR during exercise compared to the measurements of the control subjects [71]. Similar results were observed in studies by Huo et al. [63] and Hernández-Díaz et al. [110]. According to these findings, we cannot recommend folic acid alone for lowering BP.

4.4. *Combined Effect of Strength Training, Nutrition Program and Supplementation on Blood Pressure*

Although BP lowering is effective using ST alone [76–78], NP alone [74,76] and some food supplements alone [77,78], the combination of ST, NP, and supplementation did not have additional systolic BP lowering effectivity (Supplemetary Table S1). On the other hand, the combination of ST and NP seems to be necessary to decrease the diastolic BP [70,78] (Supplemetary Table S2). Moreover, the combination of ST with green tea or L-citrulline decreased the systolic BP on a higher significance or effect size (Supplemetary Table S3) than the ST alone, although the significant difference between the ST and ST with supplementation has not been directly reported. This findings supports the notion that total behavioral modification such as lifestyle modifications, rather than focusing on modifying a single behavioral target, is more important. Therefore, a combination of ST with the energy intake restriction NP, which include food supplement stimulants green tea and L-citrulline should be used for BP lowering and additional health benefits such as body composition changes.

4.5. Changes in Body Composition

Body composition improvements have been shown as a result of ST and NPs in studies by Villani et al. [74], Sales et al. [75], Figueroa et al. [76], Moraes et al. [70], and Lee et al. [73]. Slightly better results, in terms of improved body composition, were achieved by a NP alone in the studies by Villani et al. [74] and Figueroa et al. [76]. On the other hand, better results were not achieved by the DASH alone compared with the DASH diet and a training program in the latest study by Lee et al. [73]. Only a small improvement in the body composition was recorded by Figueroa et al. [76] in the ST group. Furthermore, Figueroa et al. [76] found that a hypocaloric diet decreased the brachial–ankle pulse-wave velocity mainly by reducing the leg pulse-wave velocity, and this reduction was related to fat loss. Although ST alone does not affect the pulse-wave velocity or body composition, ST combined with NP improves the brachial–ankle pulse-wave velocity and muscle strength while preventing the loss of lean body mass in obese postmenopausal women. The results of the pulse-wave velocity are considered an independent predictor of systolic hypertension [111].

In this case, a NP appears to be important for body composition transformation. However, the advantages of ST cannot be overlooked, and their combination seems to be the optimal variant. This systematic review reported some important findings concerning the different effects of various training, nutrition, and supplementary strategies on HT. Individuals with a high BP can improve their BP values, not only by using medication but also by utilizing a nonpharmacological method, which will not only have a positive impact on BP but also on other health components, such as body composition, muscle strength, and bone density. Future studies should more closely examine the effect of specific training, nutrition, and supplementation programs on individuals with HT, normotension, and PHT. Additionally, future studies should explore mechanisms of how different nutrition programs and supplements lower BP.

5. Conclusions

Presented data suggest that a combination of ST and NP seems to be an effective solution for lowering BP (systolic and diastolic). This method can be recommended for individuals with PHT or HT. However, an essential role can be attributed to the strength training program alone. In both aerobic and anaerobic forms, exercise causes post-exercise hypotension, but the effect depends on the selected training parameters. A NP based on the restriction of energy intake positively affects BP and body fat. However, this study cannot recommend caffeine supplementation because it increases BP during ST, while a more suitable stimulant is green tea or L-citrulline, which lower BP. For BP lowering in clinical practice, it is recommended to prescribe a combination of ST with the energy intake restriction NP, which include food supplements stimulants green tea and L-citrulline.

Author Contributions: Conceptualization, R.J. and P.S.; Methodology, R.J. and P.S.; Writing—original draft preparation, R.J. and P.S.; Writing—review and editing, R.J. and P.S.

Acknowledgments: This study was supported by Charles University grant no. UNCE/HUM/032, SVV 2017-2019 260466 and GACR GA19-12150S.

References

1. American College of Sports Medicine. American College of Sports Medicine position stand. Progression models in resistance training for healthy adults. *Med. Sci. Sports Exerc.* **2009**, *41*, 687. [CrossRef] [PubMed]
2. Pickering, T.G.; Hall, J.E.; Appel, L.J.; Falkner, B.E.; Graves, J.W.; Hill, M.N.; Jones, D.W.; Kurtz, T.; Sheps, S.G.; Roccella, E.J. Recommendations for blood pressure measurement in humans: An AHA scientific statement from the council on high blood pressure research professional and public education subcommittee. *J. Clin. Hypertens.* **2005**, *7*, 102–109. [CrossRef]
3. Chobanian, A.V.; Bakris, G.L.; Black, H.R.; Cushman, W.C.; Green, L.A.; Izzo, J.L., Jr.; Jones, D.W.; Materson, B.J.; Oparil, S.; Wright, J.T., Jr.; et al. Seventh Report of the Joint National Committee on Prevention, Detection, Evaluation, and Treatment of High Blood Pressure. *Hypertension* **2003**, *42*, 1206–1252. [CrossRef] [PubMed]
4. Lamotte, M.; Niset, G.; Van De Borne, P. The effect of different intensity modalities of resistance training on beat-to-beat blood pressure in cardiac patients. *Eur. J. Cardiovasc. Prev. Rehabil.* **2005**, *12*, 12–17. [CrossRef]
5. Meyer, K. Resistance exercise in chronic heart failure—Landmark studies and implications for practice. *Clin. Investig. Med.* **2006**, *29*, 166–169.
6. Pescatello, L.S.; Franklin, B.A.; Fagard, R.; Farquhar, W.B.; Kelley, G.A.; Ray, C.A. American College of Sports Medicine position stand. Exercise and hypertension. *Med. Sci. Sports Exerc.* **2004**, *36*, 533–553. [CrossRef] [PubMed]
7. Thompson, P.D.; Arena, R.; Riebe, D.; Pescatello, L.S.; American College of Sports Medicine. ACSM's new preparticipation health screening recommendations from ACSM's guidelines for exercise testing and prescription, ninth edition. *Curr. Sports Med. Rep.* **2013**, *12*, 215–217. [CrossRef]
8. Hamer, M. The anti-hypertensive effects of exercise: Integrating acute and chronic mechanisms. *Sports Med.* **2006**, *36*, 109–116. [CrossRef] [PubMed]
9. Sacks, F.M.; Svetkey, L.P.; Vollmer, W.M.; Appel, L.J.; Bray, G.A.; Harsha, D.; Obarzanek, E.; Conlin, P.R.; Miller, E.R.; Simons-Morton, D.G.; et al. Effects on Blood Pressure of Reduced Dietary Sodium and the Dietary Approaches to Stop Hypertension (DASH) Diet. *N. Engl. J. Med.* **2001**, *344*, 3–10. [CrossRef]
10. Stevens, V.J.; Obarzanek, E.; Cook, N.R.; Lee, I.M.; Appel, L.J.; West, D.S.; Milas, N.C.; Mattfeldt-Beman, M.; Belden, L.; Bragg, C.; et al. Long-term weight loss and changes in blood pressure: Results of the trials of hypertension prevention, phase II. *Ann. Intern. Med.* **2001**, *134*, 1–11. [CrossRef]
11. LaMonte, M.J.; Yanowitz, F.G. Aerobic exercise for lowering blood pressure: A metaanalysis. *Clin. J. Sport Med.* **2002**, *12*, 407. [PubMed]
12. Pescatello, L.S.; Kulikowich, J.M. The aftereffects of dynamic exercise on ambulatory blood pressure. *Med. Sci. Sports Exerc.* **2001**, *33*, 1855–1861. [CrossRef] [PubMed]
13. Whelton, S.P.; Chin, A.; Xin, X.; He, J. Effect of aerobic exercise on blood pressure: A meta-analysis of randomized, controlled trials. *Ann. Intern. Med.* **2002**, *136*, 493–503. [CrossRef] [PubMed]
14. da Rocha, P.E.C.P.; da Silva, V.S.; Camacho, L.A.B.; Vasconcelos, A.G.G. Effects of long-term resistance training on blood pressure: A systematic review. *Revista Brasileira de Cineantropometria Desempenho Humano* **2017**, *19*, 730–742.
15. Inder, J.D.; Carlson, D.J.; Dieberg, G.; McFarlane, J.R.; Hess, N.C.; Smart, N.A. Isometric exercise training for blood pressure management: A systematic review and meta-analysis to optimize benefit. *Hypertens. Res.* **2016**, *39*, 88–94. [CrossRef]
16. Lemes, I.R.; Ferreira, P.H.; Linares, S.N.; MacHado, A.F.; Pastre, C.M.; Netto, J. Resistance training reduces systolic blood pressure in metabolic syndrome: A systematic review and meta-analysis of randomised controlled trials. *Br. J. Sports Med.* **2016**, *50*, 1438–1442. [CrossRef] [PubMed]
17. Wewege, M.A.; Thom, J.M.; Rye, K.A.; Parmenter, B.J. Aerobic, resistance or combined training: A systematic review and meta-analysis of exercise to reduce cardiovascular risk in adults with metabolic syndrome. *Atherosclerosis* **2018**, *274*, 162–171. [CrossRef]
18. Hovell, M.F. The experimental evidence for weight-loss treatment of essential hypertension: A critical review. *Am. J. Public Health* **1982**, *72*, 359–368. [CrossRef]
19. Ndanuko, R.N.; Tapsell, L.C.; Charlton, K.E.; Neale, E.P.; Batterham, M.J. Dietary Patterns and Blood Pressure in Adults: A Systematic Review and Meta-Analysis of Randomized Controlled Trials. *Adv. Nutr.* **2016**, *7*, 76–89. [CrossRef]

20. Saneei, P.; Salehi-Abargouei, A.; Esmaillzadeh, A.; Azadbakht, L. Influence of Dietary Approaches to Stop Hypertension (DASH) diet on blood pressure: A systematic review and meta-analysis on randomized controlled trials. *Nutr. Metab. Cardiovasc. Dis.* **2014**, *24*, 1253–1261. [CrossRef]
21. Schwingshackl, L.; Chaimani, A.; Schwedhelm, C.; Toledo, E.; Pünsch, M.; Hoffmann, G.; Boeing, H. Comparative effects of different dietary approaches on blood pressure in hypertensive and pre-hypertensive patients: A systematic review and network meta-analysis. *Crit. Rev. Food Sci Nutr.* **2018**. [CrossRef] [PubMed]
22. Herrod, P.J.J.; Doleman, B.; Blackwell, J.E.M.; O'Boyle, F.; Williams, J.P.; Lund, J.N.; Phillips, B.E. Exercise and other nonpharmacological strategies to reduce blood pressure in older adults: A systematic review and meta-analysis. *J. Am. Soc. Hypertens.* **2018**, *12*, 248–267. [CrossRef] [PubMed]
23. Aucott, L.; Poobalan, A.; Smith, W.C.S.; Avenell, A.; Jung, R.; Broom, J. Effects of weight loss in overweight/obese individuals and long-term hypertension outcomes: A systematic review. *Hypertension* **2005**, *45*, 1035–1041. [CrossRef] [PubMed]
24. Moore, L.L.; Visioni, A.J.; Qureshi, M.M.; Bradlee, M.L.; Ellison, R.C.; D'Agostino, R. Weight loss in overweight adults and the long-term risk of hypertension the framingham study. *Arch. Intern. Med.* **2005**, *165*, 1298–1303. [CrossRef] [PubMed]
25. Mulrow, C.D.; Chiquette, E.; Angel, L.; Cornell, J.; Summerbell, C.; Anagnostelis, B.; Grimm, R., Jr.; Brand, M.B. Dieting to reduce body weight for controlling hypertension in adults. *Cochrane Database Syst. Rev.* **2000**, *2*, CD000484.
26. Sjostrom, M.; Karlsson, A.B.; Kaati, G.; Yngve, A.; Green, L.W.; Bygren, L.O. A four week residential program for primary health care patients to control obesity and related heart risk factors: Effective application of principles of learning and lifestyle change. *Eur J. Clin. Nutr* **1999**, *53* (Suppl. 2), S72–S77. [CrossRef]
27. Stevens, V.J.; Corrigan, S.A.; Obarzanek, E.; Bernauer, E.; Cook, N.R.; Hebert, P.; Mattfeldt-Beman, M.; Oberman, A.; Sugars, C.; Dalcin, A.T.; et al. Weight loss intervention in phase 1 of the Trials of Hypertension Prevention. The TOHP Collaborative Research Group. *Arch. Intern. Med.* **1993**, *153*, 849–858. [CrossRef]
28. Figueiredo, T.; Rhea, M.R.; Peterson, M.; Miranda, H.; Bentes, C.M.; dos Reis, V.M.; Simao, R. Influence of number of sets on blood pressure and heart rate variability after a strength training session. *J. Strength Cond. Res.* **2015**, *29*, 1556–1563. [CrossRef]
29. Moraes, M.R.; Bacurau, R.F.; Simoes, H.G.; Campbell, C.S.; Pudo, M.A.; Wasinski, F.; Pesquero, J.B.; Wurtele, M.; Araujo, R.C. Effect of 12 weeks of resistance exercise on post-exercise hypotension in stage 1 hypertensive individuals. *J. Hum. Hypertens.* **2012**, *26*, 533–539. [CrossRef]
30. Scher, L.M.; Ferriolli, E.; Moriguti, J.C.; Scher, R.; Lima, N.K. The effect of different volumes of acute resistance exercise on elderly individuals with treated hypertension. *J. Strength Cond. Res.* **2011**, *25*, 1016–1023. [CrossRef]
31. Tokmakidis, S.P.; Kalapotharakos, V.I.; Smilios, I.; Parlavantzas, A. Effects of detraining on muscle strength and mass after high or moderate intensity of resistance training in older adults. *Clin. Physiol. Funct. Imaging* **2009**, *29*, 316–319. [CrossRef] [PubMed]
32. Baum, K.; Rüther, T.; Essfeld, D. Reduction of blood pressure response during strength training through intermittent muscle relaxations. *Int. J. Sports Med.* **2003**, *24*, 441–445. [PubMed]
33. Gjovaag, T.; Hjelmeland, A.K.; Øygard, J.B.; Vikne, H.; Mirtaheri, P. Acute hemodynamic and cardiovascular responses following resistance exercise to voluntary exhaustion. Effects of different loadings and exercise durations. *J. Sports Med. Phys. Fit.* **2016**, *56*, 616–623.
34. Gjøvaag, T.; Hjelmeland, A.K.; Øygard, J.B.; Vikne, H.; Mirtaheri, P. Resistance exercise and acute blood pressure responses. *J. Sports Med. Phys. Fit.* **2016**, *56*, 616–623.
35. Nascimento Dda, C.; Tibana, R.A.; Benik, F.M.; Fontana, K.E.; Ribeiro Neto, F.; Santana, F.S.; Santos-Neto, L.; Silva, R.A.; Silva, A.O.; Farias, D.L.; et al. Sustained effect of resistance training on blood pressure and hand grip strength following a detraining period in elderly hypertensive women: A pilot study. *Clin. Interv. Aging* **2014**, *9*, 219–225. [CrossRef] [PubMed]
36. Lamotte, M.; Fleury, F.; Pirard, M.; Jamon, A.; van de Borne, P. Acute cardiovascular response to resistance training during cardiac rehabilitation: Effect of repetition speed and rest periods. *Eur. J. Prev. Cardiol.* **2010**, *17*, 329–336. [CrossRef] [PubMed]
37. Paulo, A.C.; Tricoli, V.; Queiroz, A.C.C.; Laurentino, G.; Forjaz, C.L.M. Blood Pressure Response During Resistance Training of Different Work-to-Rest Ratio. *J. Strength Cond. Res.* **2019**, *33*, 399–407. [CrossRef]

38. Veloso, J.; Polito, M.D.; Riera, T.; Celes, R.; Vidal, J.C.; Bottaro, M. Effects of rest interval between exercise sets on blood pressure after resistance exercises. *Arquivos Brasileiros de Cardiologia* **2010**, *94*, 482–487.
39. Boden, G.; Sargrad, K.; Homko, C.; Mozzoli, M.; Stein, T.P. Effect of a low-carbohydrate diet on appetite, blood glucose levels, and insulin resistance in obese patients with type 2 diabetes. *Ann. Intern. Med.* **2005**, *142*, 403–411. [CrossRef]
40. Yancy, W.S., Jr.; Foy, M.; Chalecki, A.M.; Vernon, M.C.; Westman, E.C. A low-carbohydrate, ketogenic diet to treat type 2 diabetes. *Nutr. Metab.* **2005**, 2. [CrossRef]
41. Yancy, W.S., Jr.; Westman, E.C.; McDuffie, J.R.; Grambow, S.C.; Jeffreys, A.S.; Bolton, J.; Chalecki, A.; Oddone, E.Z. A randomized trial of a low-carbohydrate diet vs orlistat plus a low-fat diet for weight loss. *Arch. Intern. Med.* **2010**, *170*, 136–145. [CrossRef]
42. Burke, V.; Hodgson, J.M.; Beilin, L.J.; Giangiulioi, N.; Rogers, P.; Puddey, I.B. Dietary protein and soluble fiber reduce ambulatory blood pressure in treated hypertensives. *Hypertension* **2001**, *38*, 821–826. [CrossRef]
43. Attina, D.A.; Cupelli, V.; Milicia, R.; Catalano, G.; Scavelli, A. Effects of physical exercise of different duration in hypertensive elderly subjects. *Int. J. Sports Cardiol.* **1996**, *5*, 67–70.
44. Fekete, A.A.; Giromini, C.; Chatzidiakou, Y.; Givens, D.I.; Lovegrove, J.A. Whey protein lowers blood pressure and improves endothelial function and lipid biomarkers in adults with prehypertension and mild hypertension: Results from the chronic Whey2Go randomized controlled trial. *Am. J. Clin. Nutr.* **2016**, *104*, 1534–1544. [CrossRef]
45. Fekete, Á.A.; Giromini, C.; Chatzidiakou, Y.; Givens, D.I.; Lovegrove, J.A. Whey protein lowers systolic blood pressure and Ca-caseinate reduces serum TAG after a high-fat meal in mildly hypertensive adults. *Sci. Rep.* **2018**, 8. [CrossRef]
46. Fekete, Á.A.; Ian Givens, D.; Lovegrove, J.A. Casein-derived lactotripeptides reduce systolic and diastolic blood pressure in a meta-analysis of randomised clinical trials. *Nutrients* **2015**, *7*, 659–681. [CrossRef]
47. He, J.; Gu, D.; Wu, X.; Chen, J.; Duan, X.; Chen, J.; Whelton, P.K. Effect of soybean protein on blood pressure: A randomized, controlled trial. *Ann. Intern. Med.* **2005**, *143*, 1–9. [CrossRef]
48. Pal, S.; Ellis, V. The chronic effects of whey proteins on blood pressure, vascular function, and inflammatory markers in overweight individuals. *Obesity* **2010**, *18*, 1354–1359. [CrossRef]
49. Rebholz, C.M.; Friedman, E.E.; Powers, L.J.; Arroyave, W.D.; He, J.; Kelly, T.N. Dietary protein intake and blood pressure: A meta-analysis of randomized controlled trials. *Am. J. Epidemiol.* **2012**, *176*, S27–S43. [CrossRef]
50. Al-Solaiman, Y.; Jesri, A.; Mountford, W.K.; Lackland, D.T.; Zhao, Y.; Egan, B.M. DASH lowers blood pressure in obese hypertensives beyond potassium, magnesium and fibre. *J. Hum. Hypertens.* **2010**, *24*, 237–246. [CrossRef]
51. Appel, L.J.; Moore, T.J.; Obarzanek, E.; Vollmer, W.M.; Svetkey, L.P.; Sacks, F.M.; Bray, G.A.; Vogt, T.M.; Cutler, J.A.; Windhauser, M.M.; et al. A clinical trial of the effects of dietary patterns on blood pressure. *N. Engl. J. Med.* **1997**, *336*, 1117–1124. [CrossRef]
52. Bazzano, L.A.; Green, T.; Harrison, T.N.; Reynolds, K. Dietary approaches to prevent hypertension. *Curr. Hypertens. Rep.* **2013**, *15*, 694–702. [CrossRef]
53. Estruch, R.; Martínez-González, M.A.; Corella, D.; Salas-Salvadó, J.; Ruiz-Gutiérrez, V.; Covas, M.I.; Fiol, M.; Gómez-Gracia, E.; López-Sabater, M.C.; Vinyoles, E.; et al. Effects of a Mediterranean-Style Diet on Cardiovascular Risk Factors a Randomized Trial. *Ann. Intern. Med.* **2006**, *145*, 1–11. [CrossRef]
54. Rees, K.; Hartley, L.; Flowers, N.; Clarke, A.; Hooper, L.; Thorogood, M.; Stranges, S. 'Mediterranean' dietary pattern for the primary prevention of cardiovascular disease. *Cochrane Database Syst. Rev.* **2013**, *2013*. [CrossRef]
55. Svetkey, L.P.; Simons-Morton, D.; Vollmer, W.M.; Appel, L.J.; Conlin, P.R.; Ryan, D.H.; Ard, J.; Kennedy, B.M. Effects of dietary patterns on blood pressure: Subgroup analysis of the Dietary Approaches to Stop Hypertension (DASH) randomized clinical trial. *Arch. Intern. Med.* **1999**, *159*, 285–293. [CrossRef]
56. Barbeau, P.A.; Holloway, T.M.; Whitfield, J.; Baechler, B.L.; Quadrilatero, J.; van Loon, L.J.C.; Chabowski, A.; Holloway, G.P. α-Linolenic acid and exercise training independently, and additively, decrease blood pressure and prevent diastolic dysfunction in obese Zucker rats. *J. Physiol.* **2017**, *595*, 4351–4364. [CrossRef]
57. Moradi, H.; Nikbakht, H.; Ebrahim, P.R.; Abed-Natanzi, H. The effects of 8 weeks of aerobic training and grape seed extract on some cardiovascular functional indexes in non-active men. *J. Isfahan Med. Sch.* **2017**, *34*, 1439–1444.

58. Neto, M.M.; da Silva, T.F.; de Lima, F.F.; Siqueira, T.M.Q.; Toscano, L.T.; de Moura, S.; Silva, A.S. Whole Red Grape Juice Reduces Blood Pressure at Rest and Increases Post-exercise Hypotension. *J. Am. Coll. Nutr.* **2017**, *36*, 533–540. [CrossRef] [PubMed]
59. Puga, G.M.; De, P.; Novais, I.; Katsanos, C.S.; Zanesco, A. Combined effects of aerobic exercise and l-arginine ingestion on blood pressure in normotensive postmenopausal women: A crossover study. *Life Sci.* **2016**, *151*, 323–329. [CrossRef]
60. Digiesi, V.; Cantini, F.; Brodbeck, B. Effect of coenzyme Q10 on essential arterial hypertension. *Curr. Ther. Res.* **1990**, *47*, 841–845.
61. Digiesi, V.; Cantini, F.; Bisi, G.; Guarino, G.; Oradei, A.; Littarru, G. Mechanism of action of coenzyme Q10 in essential hypertension. *Curr. Ther. Res.* **1992**, *51*, 668–672.
62. Dyckner, T.; Wester, P.O. Effect of magnesium on blood pressure. *Br. Med. J.* **1983**, *286*, 1847–1849. [CrossRef]
63. Huo, Y.; Li, J.; Qin, X.; Huang, Y.; Wang, X.; Gottesman, R.F.; Tang, G.; Wang, B.; Chen, D.; He, M.; et al. Efficacy of folic acid therapy in primary prevention of stroke among adults with hypertension in China: The CSPPT randomized clinical trial. *JAMA* **2015**, *313*, 1325–1335. [CrossRef] [PubMed]
64. Mente, A.; O'Donnell, M.J.; Rangarajan, S.; McQueen, M.J.; Poirier, P.; Wielgosz, A.; Morrison, H.; Li, W.; Wang, X.; Di, C.; et al. Association of urinary sodium and potassium excretion with blood pressure. *N. Engl. J. Med.* **2014**, *371*, 601–611. [PubMed]
65. Simopoulos, A.P. Omega-3 fatty acids in health and disease and in growth and development. *Am. J. Clin. Nutr.* **1991**, *54*, 438–463. [CrossRef] [PubMed]
66. Xiong, X.J.; Wang, P.Q.; Li, S.J.; Li, X.K.; Zhang, Y.Q.; Wang, J. Garlic for hypertension: A systematic review and meta-analysis of randomized controlled trials. *Phytomedicine* **2015**, *22*, 352–361. [CrossRef] [PubMed]
67. Moher, D.; Liberati, A.; Tetzlaff, J.; Altman, D.G.; The, P.G. Preferred Reporting Items for Systematic Reviews and Meta-Analyses: The PRISMA Statement. *PLOS Med.* **2009**, *6*, e1000097. [CrossRef] [PubMed]
68. Maher, C.G.; Sherrington, C.; Herbert, R.D.; Moseley, A.M.; Elkins, M. Reliability of the PEDro scale for rating quality of randomized controlled trials. *Phys. Ther.* **2003**, *83*, 713–721. [PubMed]
69. Verhagen, A.P.; de Vet, H.C.; de Bie, R.A.; Kessels, A.G.; Boers, M.; Bouter, L.M.; Knipschild, P.G. The Delphi List: A criteria list for quality assessment of randomized clinical trials for conducting systematic reviews developed by delphi consensus. *J. Clin. Epidemiol.* **1999**, *51*, 1235–1241. [CrossRef]
70. Moraes, W.; Santos, N.S.D.; Aguiar, L.P.; Sousa, L.G.O. Maintenance of exercise training benefits is associated with adequate milk and dairy products intake in elderly hypertensive subjects following detraining. *Einstein* **2017**, *15*, 289–294. [CrossRef] [PubMed]
71. Romero, S.A.; Gagnon, D.; Adams, A.N.; Moralez, G.; Kouda, K.; Jaffery, M.F.; Cramer, M.N.; Crandall, C.G. Folic acid ingestion improves skeletal muscle blood flow during graded handgrip and plantar flexion exercise in aged humans. *Am. J. Physiol.-Heart Circ. Physiol.* **2017**, *313*, H658–H666. [CrossRef] [PubMed]
72. Astorino, T.A.; Martin, B.J.; Schachtsiek, L.; Wong, K. Caffeine ingestion and intense resistance training minimize postexercise hypotension in normotensive and prehypertensive men. *Res. Sports Med.* **2013**, *21*, 52–65. [CrossRef] [PubMed]
73. Lee, C.J.; Kim, J.Y.; Shim, E.; Hong, S.H.; Lee, M.; Jeon, J.Y.; Park, S. The effects of diet alone or in combination with exercise in patients with prehypertension and hypertension: A randomized controlled trial. *Korean Circ. J.* **2018**, *48*, 637–651. [CrossRef] [PubMed]
74. Villani, R.G.; Gornall, J. Short-Term resistance exercise does not alter the hypotensive effect of low-energy dieting. *J. Strength Cond. Res.* **1999**, *13*, 286–288.
75. Sales, A.R.; Silva, B.M.; Neves, F.J.; Rocha, N.G.; Medeiros, R.F.; Castro, R.R.; Nobrega, A.C. Diet and exercise training reduce blood pressure and improve autonomic modulation in women with prehypertension. *Eur. J. Appl. Physiol.* **2012**, *112*, 3369–3378. [CrossRef] [PubMed]
76. Figueroa, A.; Vicil, F.; Sanchez-Gonzalez, M.A.; Wong, A.; Ormsbee, M.J.; Hooshmand, S.; Daggy, B. Effects of diet and/or low-intensity resistance exercise training on arterial stiffness, adiposity, and lean mass in obese postmenopausal women. *Am. J. Hypertens.* **2013**, *26*, 416–423. [CrossRef] [PubMed]
77. Arazi, H.; Samami, N.; Kheirkhah, J.; Taati, B. The effect of three weeks green tea extract consumption on blood pressure, heart rate responses to a single bout resistance exercise in hypertensive women. *High Blood Press. Cardiovasc. Prev.* **2014**, *21*, 213–219. [CrossRef] [PubMed]

78. Wong, A.; Alvarez-Alvarado, S.; Jaime, S.J.; Kinsey, A.W.; Spicer, M.T.; Madzima, T.A.; Figueroa, A. Combined whole-body vibration training and l-citrulline supplementation improves pressure wave reflection in obese postmenopausal women. *Appl. Physiol. Nutr. Metab.* **2016**, *41*, 292–297. [CrossRef] [PubMed]
79. Arazi, H.; Ghiasi, A.; Asgharpoor, S. A comparative study of cardiovascular responses to two rest intervals between circuit resistance exercises in normotensive woman. *Revista Brasileira de Medicina do Esporte* **2013**, *19*, 176–180. [CrossRef]
80. Pescatello, L.S.; MacDonald, H.V.; Lamberti, L.; Johnson, B.T. Exercise for Hypertension: A Prescription Update Integrating Existing Recommendations with Emerging Research. *Curr. Hypertens. Rep.* **2015**, *17*, 87. [CrossRef]
81. Castaneda, C.; Gordon, P.L.; Uhlin, K.L.; Levey, A.S.; Kehayias, J.J.; Dwyer, J.T.; Fielding, R.A.; Roubenoff, R.; Singh, M.F. Resistance Training To Counteract the Catabolism of a Low-Protein Diet in Patients with Chronic Renal Insufficiency: A Randomized, Controlled Trial. *Ann. Intern. Med.* **2001**, *135*, 965–976. [CrossRef] [PubMed]
82. Kannel, W.B. Blood Pressure as a Cardiovascular Risk Factor: Prevention and Treatment. *JAMA* **1996**, *275*, 1571–1576. [CrossRef] [PubMed]
83. Nelson, M.E.; Fiatarone, M.A.; Morganti, C.M.; Trice, I.; Greenberg, R.A.; Evans, W.J. Effects of high-intensity strength training on multiple risk factors for osteoporotic fractures: A randomized controlled trial. *JAMA* **1994**, *272*, 1909–1914. [CrossRef] [PubMed]
84. Skelton, D.A.; Young, A.; Greig, C.A.; Malbut, K.E. Effects of Resistance Training on Strength, Power, and Selected Functional Abilities of Women Aged 75 and Older. *J. Am. Geriatr. Soc.* **1995**, *43*, 1081–1087. [CrossRef] [PubMed]
85. Singh, N.A.; Clements, K.M.; Fiatarone, M.A. A randomized controlled trial of progressive resistance training in depressed elders. *J. Gerontol. Ser. A Biol. Sci. Med. Sci.* **1997**, *52*, M27–M35. [CrossRef] [PubMed]
86. Cornelissen, V.A.; Fagard, R.H.; Coeckelberghs, E.; Vanhees, L. Impact of resistance training on blood pressure and other cardiovascular risk factors: A meta-analysis of randomized, controlled trials. *Hypertension* **2011**, *58*, 950–958. [CrossRef]
87. MacDougall, J.D.; Tuxen, D.; Sale, D.G.; Moroz, J.R.; Sutton, J.R. Arterial blood pressure response to heavy resistance exercise. *J. Appl. Physiol.* **1985**, *58*, 785–790. [CrossRef]
88. Joint National Committee on Prevention, Detection, Evaluation, and Treatment of High Blood Pressure. The Sixth Report of the Joint National Committee on Prevention, Detection, Evaluation, and Treatment of High Blood Pressure. *Arch. Intern. Med.* **1997**, *157*, 2413–2446. [CrossRef]
89. Reisin, E.; Frohlich, E.D.; Messerli, F.H.; Dreslinski, G.R.; Dunn, F.G.; Jones, M.M.; Batson, H.M. Cardiovascular changes after weight reduction in obesity hypertension. *Ann. Intern. Med.* **1983**, *98*, 315–319. [CrossRef]
90. Langford, H.G.; Blaufox, M.D.; Oberman, A.; Hawkins, C.M.; Curb, J.D.; Cutter, G.R.; Wassertheil-Smoller, S.; Pressel, S.; Babcock, C.; Abernethy, J.D. Dietary therapy slows the return of hypertension after stopping prolonged medication. *JAMA* **1985**, *253*, 657–664. [CrossRef]
91. Stamler, R.; Stamler, J.; Gosch, F.C.; Civinelli, J.; Fishman, J.; McKeever, P.; McDonald, A.; Dyer, A.R. Primary prevention of hypertension by nutritional-hygienic means: Final report of a randomized, controlled trial. *JAMA* **1989**, *262*, 1801–1807. [CrossRef] [PubMed]
92. Stamler, R.; Stamler, J.; Grimm, R.; Gosch, F.C.; Elmer, P.; Dyer, A.; Berman, R.; Fishman, J.; Van Heel, N.; Civinelli, J. Nutritional therapy for high blood pressure: Final report of a four-year randomized controlled trial—the Hypertension Control Program. *JAMA* **1987**, *257*, 1484–1491. [CrossRef] [PubMed]
93. Happonen, P.; Voutilainen, S.; Salonen, J.T. Coffee drinking is dose-dependently related to the risk of acute coronary events in middle-aged men. *J. Nutr.* **2004**, *134*, 2381–2386. [CrossRef] [PubMed]
94. Grgic, J.; Grgic, I.; Pickering, C.; Schoenfeld, B.J.; Bishop, D.J.; Pedisic, Z. Wake up and smell the coffee: Caffeine supplementation and exercise performance—an umbrella review of 21 published meta-analyses. *Br. J. Sports Med.* **2019**. [CrossRef] [PubMed]
95. Glade, M.J. Caffeine—not just a stimulant. *Nutrition* **2010**, *26*, 932–938. [CrossRef]
96. Ali, A.; O'Donnell, J.; Foskett, A.; Rutherfurd-Markwick, K. The influence of caffeine ingestion on strength and power performance in female team-sport players. *J. Int. Soc. Sports Nutr.* **2016**, *13*, 46. [CrossRef] [PubMed]
97. Jee, S.H.; He, J.; Whelton, P.K.; Suh, I.; Klag, M.J. The Effect of Chronic Coffee Drinking on Blood Pressure. *Hypertension* **1999**, *33*, 647–652. [CrossRef]

98. Creager, M.A.; Cooke, J.P.; Mendelsohn, M.E.; Gallagher, S.J.; Coleman, S.M.; Loscalzo, J.; Dzau, V.J. Impaired vasodilation of forearm resistance vessels in hypercholesterolemic humans. *J. Clin. Investig.* **1990**, *86*, 228–234. [CrossRef]
99. Mayhan, W.G. Role of nitric oxide in disruption of the blood-brain barrier during acute hypertension. *Brain Res.* **1995**, *686*, 99–103. [CrossRef]
100. Rector, T.S.; Bank, A.J.; Mullen, K.A.; Tschumperlin, L.K.; Sih, R.; Pillai, K.; Kubo, S.H. Randomized, double-blind, placebo-controlled study of supplemental oral L-arginine in patients with heart failure. *Circulation* **1996**, *93*, 2135–2141. [CrossRef]
101. Yang, Y.-C.; Lu, F.-H.; Wu, J.-S.; Wu, C.-H.; Chang, C.-J. The protective effect of habitual tea consumption on hypertension. *Arch. Intern. Med.* **2004**, *164*, 1534–1540. [CrossRef]
102. Stensvold, I.; Tverdal, A.; Solvoll, K.; Foss, O.P. Tea consumption. Relationship to cholesterol, blood pressure, and coronary and total mortality. *Prev. Med.* **1992**, *21*, 546–553. [CrossRef]
103. Wakabayashi, K.; Kono, S.; Shinchi, K.; Honjo, S.; Todoroki, I.; Sakurai, Y.; Umeda, T.; Imanishi, K.; Yoshizawa, N. Habitual coffee consumption and blood pressure: A study of self-defense officials in Japan. *Eur. J. Epidemiol.* **1998**, *14*, 669–673. [CrossRef] [PubMed]
104. Álvarez, E.; Campos-Toimil, M.; Justiniano-Basaran, H.; Lugnier, C.; Orallo, F. Study of the mechanisms involved in the vasorelaxation induced by (−)-epigallocatechin-3-gallate in rat aorta. *Br. J. Pharmacol.* **2006**, *147*, 269–280. [CrossRef]
105. Meschia, J.F.; Bushnell, C.; Boden-Albala, B.; Braun, L.T.; Bravata, D.M.; Chaturvedi, S.; Creager, M.A.; Eckel, R.H.; Elkind, M.S.V.; Fornage, M.; et al. Guidelines for the primary prevention of stroke: A statement for healthcare professionals from the American Heart Association/American Stroke Association. *Stroke* **2014**, *45*, 3754–3832. [CrossRef] [PubMed]
106. Armitage, J.M.; Bowman, L.; Clarke, R.J.; Wallendszus, K.; Bulbulia, R.; Rahimi, K.; Haynes, R.; Parish, S.; Sleight, P.; Peto, R. Effects of homocysteine-lowering with folic acid plus vitamin B12 vs placebo on mortality and major morbidity in myocardial infarction survivors: A randomized trial. *JAMA* **2010**, *303*, 2486–2494.
107. Lonn, E. Heart Outcomes Prevention Evaluation (HOPE) 2 Investigators. Homocysteine lowering with folic acid and B vitamins in vascular disease. *Nat. Clin. Pract. Cardiovasc. Med.* **2006**, *3*, 414–415.
108. Toole, J.F.; Malinow, M.R.; Chambless, L.E.; Spence, J.D.; Pettigrew, L.C.; Howard, V.J.; Sides, E.G.; Wang, C.-H.; Stampfer, M. Lowering homocysteine in patients with ischemic stroke to prevent recurrent stroke, myocardial infarction, and death: The Vitamin Intervention for Stroke Prevention (VISP) randomized controlled trial. *JAMA* **2004**, *291*, 565–575. [CrossRef]
109. Bønaa, K.H.; Njølstad, I.; Ueland, P.M.; Schirmer, H.; Tverdal, A.; Steigen, T.; Wang, H.; Nordrehaug, J.E.; Arnesen, E.; Rasmussen, K. Homocysteine lowering and cardiovascular events after acute myocardial infarction. *N. Engl. J. Med.* **2006**, *354*, 1578–1588. [CrossRef]
110. Hernández-Díaz, S.; Werler, M.M.; Louik, C.; Mitchell, A.A. Risk of gestational hypertension in relation to folic acid supplementation during pregnancy. *Am. J. Epidemiol.* **2002**, *156*, 806–812. [CrossRef]
111. Najjar, S.S.; Scuteri, A.; Shetty, V.; Wright, J.G.; Muller, D.C.; Fleg, J.L.; Spurgeon, H.P.; Ferrucci, L.; Lakatta, E.G. Pulse wave velocity is an independent predictor of the longitudinal increase in systolic blood pressure and of incident hypertension in the Baltimore Longitudinal Study of Aging. *J. Am. Coll. Cardiol.* **2008**, *51*, 1377–1383. [CrossRef] [PubMed]

7

Ensemble Learning to Improve the Prediction of Fetal Macrosomia and Large-for-Gestational Age

Shangyuan Ye [1], Hui Zhang [2], Fuyan Shi [3], Jing Guo [4], Suzhen Wang [3,*] and Bo Zhang [5,*]

1 Department of Population Medicine, Harvard Pilgrim Health Care Institute and Harvard Medical School, Boston, MA 02115, USA; shangyuan_ye@harvardpilgrim.org
2 Division of Biostatistics, Department of Prevention Medicine, Northwestern University Feinberg School of Medicine, Chicago, IL 60611, USA.; hzhang@northwestern.edu
3 School of Public Health and Management, Weifang Medical University, Weifang, Shandong 261053, China; shifuyan@wfmc.edu.cn
4 School of Public Health, Peking University, Beijing 100191, China; jing624218@bjmu.edu.cn
5 Department of Neurology and ICCTR Biostatistics and Research Design Center, Boston Children's Hospital and Harvard Medical School, Boston, MA 02115, USA
* Correspondence: wangsz@wfmc.edu.cn (S.W.); bo.zhang@childrens.harvard.edu (B.Z.)

Abstract: Background: The objective of this study was to investigate the use of ensemble methods to improve the prediction of fetal macrosomia and large for gestational age from prenatal ultrasound imaging measurements. Methods: We evaluated and compared the prediction accuracies of nonlinear and quadratic mixed-effects models coupled with 26 different empirical formulas for estimating fetal weights in predicting large fetuses at birth. The data for the investigation were taken from the Successive Small-for-Gestational-Age-Births study. Ensemble methods, a class of machine learning techniques, were used to improve the prediction accuracies by combining the individual models and empirical formulas. Results: The prediction accuracy of individual statistical models and empirical formulas varied considerably in predicting macrosomia but varied less in predicting large for gestational age. Two ensemble methods, voting and stacking, with model selection, can combine the strengths of individual models and formulas and can improve the prediction accuracy. Conclusions: Ensemble learning can improve the prediction of fetal macrosomia and large for gestational age and have the potential to assist obstetricians in clinical decisions.

Keywords: macrosomia; large for gestational age; machine learning; ensemble methods; prediction; sensitivity; specificity

1. Introduction

Excessive fetal growth poses risks to maternal and infant well-being [1]. The term "macrosomia" is used to describe the condition of a fetus with a birth weight of more than 4000 g, regardless of gestational age [1,2]. Macrosomia is sometimes confused with "large for gestational age" (LGA), which describes an infant with a 90th percentile or higher birthweight for gestational age [1]. It has been shown that the infants with either macrosomia or LGA pose a large risk of perinatal morbidity and mortality to their mothers [2,3]. Therefore, accurately predicting and diagnosing these conditions has been a major goal of obstetric investigators, for purposes of conducting early intervention or targeted perinatal medical care to reduce the risks.

Measurements taken from prenatal ultrasound imaging are the primary quantitative resources for predicting birth weights and diagnosing macrosomia or LGA. Zhang et al. [4] took the empirical formula given by Hadlock et al. [5] for estimating fetal weights and implemented a joint mixed-effects model to predict macrosomia and LGA. This procedure of predicting macrosomia or LGA from prenatal ultrasound measurements was a two-step supervised learning process. In the first step, an empirical formula was chosen to derive the estimated fetal weights (EFWs) from sonographic ultrasound measurements at each of the gestational time points when the ultrasound measurements were taken and recorded. In the second step, a joint mixed-effects model with latent subject-specific random effects was fitted. One component of the joint model was a quadratic mixed-effects model to derive the predicted birth weights (PBWs). Another component was a probit mixed-effects model, from which the classification of macrosomia or LGA was determined from the PBWs by comparing the PBWs with a pre-specified threshold [6]. However, previous literature has noted that there were 26 candidate empirical formulas for estimating fetal weights [7–9]. In addition, some literature also argued that nonlinear mixed-effects models should be more appropriate in modeling growth curves than linear or quadratic mixed-effects models [10]. Selecting a particular EFW empirical formula and a quadratic mixed-effects model, as in Zhang et al. [4], increases the uncertainties in predicting macrosomia or LGA, because these empirical formulas and the statistical models function diversely.

In this article, we investigate the use of ensemble methods to aggregate prediction results given by different EFW empirical formulas and the statistical models. The goal of this practice is to improve the prediction in macrosomia or LGA. With ensemble methods, it is not required to select any specific statistical model or empirical formulas. Instead, the prediction capability of each combination of the empirical formulas and statistical models is combined and aggregated to generate a learning procedure that gives the best prediction performance.

2. Methods

2.1. Data

The Successive Small-for-Gestational-Age Births study (SGA study) was funded by the National Institute of Child Health and Human Development (NICHD), in the National Institutes of Health of the USA in 1983. The study was conducted concurrently by the University of Bergen in Norway, the University of Uppsala in Sweden, and the University of Alabama, USA, from 1984 to 1985 [11]. The initial goal of the SGA study was to characterize the different types of intra-uterine growth restriction and to assess the associated risk factors.

To demonstrate the strengths of ensemble methods in predicting fetal macrosomia or LGA, we took the Scandinavian data in the SGA study that were collected in Norway and Sweden. The Scandinavia SGA data were collected from January 1st, 1986, through March 31st, 1988 from nulliparous (parity 1) and primiparous (parity 2) Caucasian pregnant women prior to the 20th gestational week who had a singleton pregnancy and spoke one of the Scandinavian languages. A total of 6354 women were recruited to the study, and 632 of them were excluded from the study, according to the exclusion criteria (n = 432) or due to absence of first prenatal visit (n = 200). The remaining 5722 patients were split into three subgroups. A random sample of 561 patients was first selected. Then, a "high-risk" group of 1384 patients was identified out of the random sample of 561 patients on the basis of five small-for-gestational-age (SGA) risk factors: giving birth to an infant with birthweight below 2750 g in the past, maternal cigarette smoking at conception, pre-pregnancy weight lower than 50 kg, a previous perinatal death, and the presence of chronic maternal disease (chronic renal disease, hypertension, or heart disease). The remaining 3777 patients were considered as the "low-risk" group. The patients from the random sample and "high-risk" group were eligible to participate in a detailed follow-up study, during which the women were examined at approximately 17th, 25th, 33rd, and 37th weeks of gestation. For each visit, ultrasound examination was performed, and demographic and medical information were collected. At the end of the Scandinavia SGA study, only 1945 were able to complete the follow-up study.

In our study, we restricted the study data to the 1115 women in the Scandinavia SGA study who had all four ultrasound examinations and complete covariate information (maternal age, pre-pregnancy body weight and height, previous diseases history, and smoking history) in the Scandinavia SGA study. In the ultrasound examination records in the Scandinavia SGA study, there were three fetal measurements: biparietal diameter (BPD), middle abdominal diameter (MAD), and femur length (FL).

2.2. An Ensemble Learning Procedure of Predicting Macrosomia and LGA

Here, we developed a four-step ensemble learning procedure to predict macrosomia or LGA from prenatal ultrasound measurements. The output of the learning procedure is the binary classification of either macrosomia or LGA. The prediction of macrosomia and LGA is conducted based upon a set of input features. The primary input features are the sonographic measurements BPDs, MADs, and FLs collected from 17th, 25th, 33rd, and 37th weeks of gestation, as well as gestational age at delivery, in the Scandinavia SGA study. Other features also include maternal age, pre-pregnancy body mass index, parity, smoking status, existing diabetes, and gestational diabetes. Figure 1 shows a diagram that delineates the four steps in the ensemble learning procedure, to predict macrosomia or LGA. Step 1 is to take the sonographic measurements for each of the gestational weeks and each of the empirical formulas in Table A2, to obtain EFWs at each gestational time point. Step 2 is to fit either a nonlinear mixed-effects model or a quadratic mixed-effects model to predict the corresponding PBWs at birth from the EFWs obtained in Step 1. Step 3 is to use the PBWs to derive the classification of macrosomia or LGA by using a specified threshold. Step 4 is the ensemble learning step, in which prediction output from various empirical formulas and the nonlinear and quadratic mixed-effects models are combined to generate the ensemble learning prediction results.

2.3. Estimated Fetal Weights with 26 Empirical Formulas

In the ultrasound examination records in the Scandinavia SGA study, there were three fetal measurements BPD, MAD, and FL. Melamed et al. [7] summarized 26 different empirical sonographic formulas (see Appendix A Table A1) that can be taken to estimate fetal weights from sonographic ultrasound measures. In our ensemble learning procedure, we considered all the 26 models in our analysis. Abdominal circumference (AC) in the empirical sonographic formulas can be calculated by $3.1416 \times$ MAD, and head circumference (HC) can be derived by the formula introduced in [12].

2.4. Mixed-Effects Models for Predicting PBWs and Deriving the Classification of Macrosomia or LGA

We built a nonlinear three-parameter mixed-effects logistic model with latent random effects to predict PBWs and derive the classification of macrosomia or LGA [10,13]. The three-parameter mixed-effects logistic model for the ith fetus ($i = 1, \cdots, n$ indexing the study subjects) at gestational time t_{ij} ($j = 1, 2, 3, 4$ indexing the time when the gestational ultrasound measurements were recorded, $j = 5$ indexing the time of birth) is as follows:

$$y_{ij} = \frac{\phi_{1i}}{1 + \exp\left[-\left(t_{ij} - \phi_{2i}\right)/\phi_{3i}\right]} + \epsilon_{ij},$$

where y_{ij} is the EFW obtained from one of the 26 formulas in Table A1 at gestational time t_{ij}, $j = 1, 2, 3$, and 4, and y_{ij} is the birth weight when $j = 5$, $\phi_i = (\phi_{1i}, \phi_{2i}, \phi_{3i})$ are model parameters in which ϕ_{1i} indicates amplitude, ϕ_{2i} indicates the smoothness, ϕ_{3i} indicates stretch, and ϵ_{ij} are within-subject random errors. For the nonlinear mixed-effects model, each parameter ϕ_{ki} ($k = 1, 2, 3$ indexing the parameter), can be further modeled by a linear representation:

$$\phi_{ki} = X'_{ij}\beta_k + b_{ki},$$

where X_{ij} is a vector of fixed-effects the covariates of maternal age, pre-pregnancy body mass index, previous disease history, including diabetes, cardiac disease, high blood pressure, renal disorders, and other diseases, and smoking during pregnancy; and β_k denotes the corresponding regression parameters. The first element in X_{ij} equals 1 for the interception. In our learning procedure, the covariates were included in the linear term $\phi_{1i} = X'_{ij}\beta_1 + b_{1i}$, and ϕ_{2i} and ϕ_{3i} were specified as $\phi_{2i} = \beta_2 + b_{2i}$ and $\phi_{3i} = \beta_3 + b_{3i}$. We also considered the nonlinear three-parameter mixed-effects logistic model without any covariates in ϕ_{1i} such that $\phi_{1i} = \beta_1 + b_{1i}$. The random effects $b_i = (b_{1i}, b_{2i}, b_{3i})'$ represent the latent individual variations that are not explained by the covariates. We assumed the random effects, b_i, independently follow a multivariate normal distribution, with a vector of mean 0 and a variance-covariance matrix Σ, where Σ was assumed to be positive, definite, and unstructured. Further, we assumed the following heteroscedastic model [10] for the within-subject random errors ϵ_{ij}:

$$\epsilon_{ij} \sim N\left(0, \left|\frac{\phi_{1i}}{1+\exp\left[-\left(t_{ij}-\phi_{2i}\right)/\phi_{3i}\right]}\right|^{2\delta}\right).$$

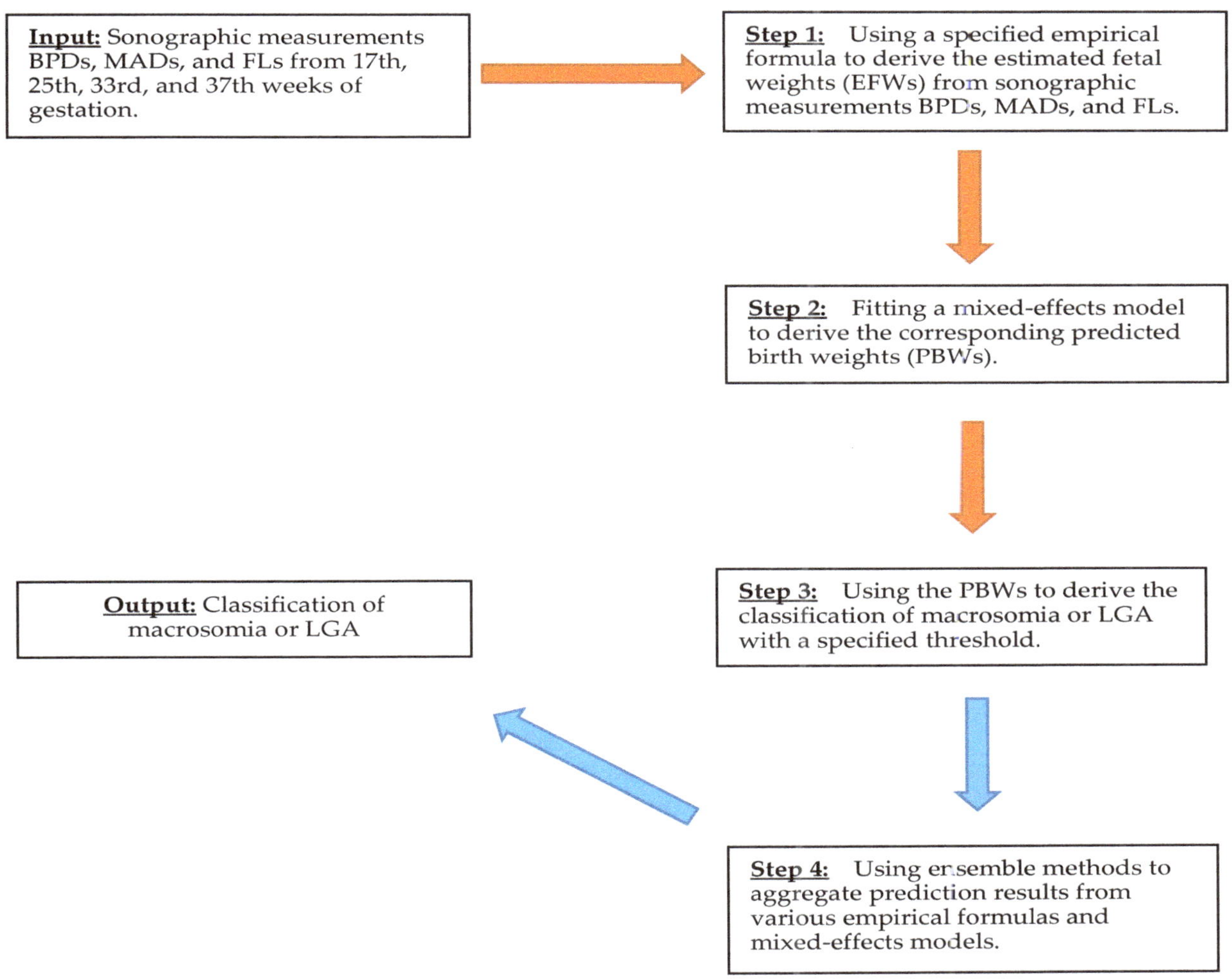

Figure 1. An ensemble learning procedure to predict macrosomia or LGA from prenatal ultrasound measurements.

We compared the above nonlinear mixed-effects models with the following quadratic mixed-effects model implemented in Zhang et al. [4].

$$y_{ij} = X'_{ij}\beta + \theta_1 t_{ij} + \theta_2 t_{ij}^2 + b_{i0} + b_{i1} t_{ij} + b_{i2} t_{ij}^2 + \epsilon_{ij}.$$

The configuration of X_{ij}, β, b_i, and ϵ_{ij} is identical to those in the nonlinear mixed-effects model, and $\theta = (\theta_1, \theta_2)$ are the parameters of time fixed-effects t_{ij} and t_{ij}^2. For the quadratic mixed-effects model, we also considered the one without any covariates for predicting the birth weights and deriving the classification of macrosomia or LGA.

2.5. Ensemble Learning Methods

Here, we propose to apply ensemble methods [14], to combine the prediction results generated from 26 individual EFW empirical formulas and from nonlinear and linear mixed-effects models. One appealing property for ensemble methods is that they combine the classification strengths of individual models but do not overfit the data. Two types of ensemble algorithms, majority voting and stacking, are considered. Majority voting is one of the most fundamental ensemble methods for classification [14]. For a binary classification problem, the final classification of majority voting is the class that receives more than half of the votes from the individual learning models. Because the individual learning models can be correlated, it is necessary to select among individual learning models that are combined in majority voting [15–17]. Here, we implemented least absolute shrinkage and selection operator (LASSO) [18], smoothed clipped absolute deviation (SCAD) [19], and minimax penalized likelihood (MCP) [20] to select individual learning models.

The stacking method [21,22] is one of the most known meta-learning methods. It combines the prediction results from several different individual learning models, called "first-level learners", by another learning model, named "second-level learner" or "meta-learner". Van der Laan et al. [23] proposed to train the meta-learner by a unified cross-validation algorithm or super learner and proved its oracle properties. The unified cross-validation algorithm is summarized as follows. For a K-fold cross-validation procedure ($K = 10$ is set here), the training dataset was split into K equal-sized groups, stratified by the response variable. Then, let the k-th group be the validation data, take the remaining data to train the first-level learners, and collect the prediction values from the validation data as the covariates of the meta-leaner. By repeating the above procedure on every fold of data, along with the original response variable, a complete dataset, called the "leave-one data", is generated for training the meta-learner. Several reports [21,22,24] proposed using the logistic regression with positive constraint on the regression coefficients as the meta-learner for classification, whereas Van der Laan et al. [23] used linear regression as the meta-learner for regression models. Debray et al. [24] suggested performing model selection on the meta-learner, so we applied LASSO, SCAD, and MCP to conduct model selection on the meta-learner.

2.6. Evaluation of Prediction Performance

In our investigation, the original dataset was randomly divided into a training dataset (70%, n = 781) and a testing dataset (30%, n = 334), stratified by the presence of macrosomia or LGA. For an individual mixed-effects model with a particular EFW empirical formula, the entire training dataset, along with the ultrasound measures and demographic information in the testing dataset, was used to fit the model. The birth time, birthweight, and the true macrosomia or LGA status in the testing dataset were used to evaluate the prediction performance. For ensemble methods, the ensemble learner was trained by the training dataset and tested by the testing dataset.

The prediction accuracy of each individual mixed-effects model with a particular EFW empirical formula, as well as the ensemble learner, was assessed by the areas under the receiver operating characteristic curve (AUC), sensitivity, specificity, positive predictive value (+PV), negative predictive value (−PV), positive likelihood ratio (+LR), negative likelihood ratio (−LR), and Youden's index (sensitivity + specificity − 1) for predicting both macrosomia and LGA.

3. Results

Table 1 shows the baseline characteristics of our study subjects (n = 1115). The mean maternal age of the study subjects was 28 years (standard deviation or SD: 4 years), and the average height and weight before pregnancy were 166 centimeters (SD: 6 centimeters) and 59 kg (SD: 10 kg), respectively. Twenty-one percent of women had a history of SGA births, and about half of them smoked at enrollment. Only a few had high blood pressure, cardiac disease, diabetes, or renal disorder, but 15% had other types of diseases. The mean gestational age at birth was 280 days (SD: 8 days), and the mean birthweight was 3562 g (SD: 478 g). Seventeen percent of infants had macrosomia, 11% had LGA at birth, and, among the LGA infants, 9 of them (7%) were not macrosomia infants. The current study sample was used as the reference of LGA [11].

Table 1. Baseline characteristics of study subjects.

Demographic Characteristic	**Mean (Standard Deviation) n = 1115**
Maternal age (years)	28.32 (4.12)
Birthweight (grams)	3562 (478)
Gestational age (days)	279.99 (8.34)
Maternal height (centimeters)	165.96 (5.99)
Maternal weight (kilograms)	59.20 (10.00)
Health History	**Number of Subjects (Percentage)**
High blood pressure	20 (1.8)
Cardiac disease	10 (0.9)
Diabetes	3 (0.3)
Renal disorders	11 (1.0)
Other diseases	172 (15.4)
Small for gestational age	235 (21.1)
Large for gestational age	124 (11.1)
Macrosomia	195 (17.5)
Smoking at enrollment (cigarettes/day)	
0	436 (49.1)
1–9	180 (16.1)
10–19	397 (35.6)
20+	102 (9.2)

3.1. Prediction Performance of Individual Models and Empirical Formulas in Macrosomia

We predicted macrosomia or LGA with the nonlinear and quadratic mixed-effects models described above, and also considered those models with or without the covariates. Thus, four mixed-effects models combined with 26 empirical formulas for EFWs, totally 104 learning models, were fitted. The prediction performance of individual learning models in predicting macrosomia is reported in Appendix A Tables A2–A5. For the three-parameter mixed-effects logistic models, their prediction performance varied with different EFW empirical formulas, and adding covariates into the models did not improve their prediction performance (see Appendix A Tables A2 and A3). The three-parameter mixed-effects logistic models, either with or without covariates, predicted all birth weights to be under 4000 g when combined with empirical formula 3 in Table A1. The two nonlinear mixed-effects models combined with empirical formula 11 in Table A1 gave the highest value of Youden's index of 0.670, and the lowest value of Youden's index of 0.050 was obtained by empirical formula 18 in Table A1 without covariates. The best sensitivities of 0.857 and 0.839 were obtained from the two models with or without covariates, respectively, when coupled with empirical formula 7 in Table A1. The AUCs for these models ranged from 0.871 to 0.910. The prediction performance of the quadratic mixed-effects models also varied among different empirical formulas, and adding covariates did not improve their prediction performance either (see Appendix A Tables A4 and A5). The quadratic mixed-effects models combined with empirical formula 12 in Table A1 gave the highest value of Youden's index of 0.663, whereas the lowest value of Youden's index of 0.310 was obtained by empirical formula 3, in Table A1, without covariates. The best sensitivity of 0.982 was obtained from the two models with or without covariates when coupled with empirical formulas 7 and 11 in Table A1. The AUCs for these models ranged from 0.857 to 0.905.

3.2. Prediction Performance of Individual Models and Empirical Formulas in LGA

LGA is defined as a newborn with a birthweight greater than the 90th percentile for gestational age. Here, given the input of sonographic ultrasound measures, both the nonlinear and quadratic mixed-effects models can generate PBWs for each of fetuses at any time point, regardless of its actual birth time. A newborn was classified as LGA if his or her PBW was above the 90th percentile of PBWs of all other fetuses, when the fetuses were assumed to be born at the identical birth time as that newborn. The prediction performance of the nonlinear and quadratic mixed-effects models is reported in Appendix A Tables A6–A9. The prediction performance showed small variation among different EFWs empirical formulas and among these models. The Youden's indexes ranged from 0.354 to 0.526, the sensitivities ranged from 0.424 to 0.576, the specificities ranged from 0.930 to 0.950, and the AUCs ranged from 0.863 to 0.894.

3.3. Prediction Performance of Ensemble Methods

Two ensemble methods, voting and stacking methods, were applied to combine the 104 learning models for the prediction of macrosomia. The voting method was implemented by using two approaches: voting from all learning models without selection and voting from the selected learning models. To select among the learning models, a penalized logistic regression was run with either a LASSO, SCAD, or MCP penalty. When the stacking method was implemented, we fit a linear regression model as our meta-learner, either without variable selection or with three variable selection methods, LASSO, SCAD, and MCP. The prediction performance of the ensemble methods for the prediction of macrosomia is summarized in Table 2. The voting and stacking methods with the SCAD selection yielded the best Youden's indexes of 0.681 and 0.688, respectively, which were higher than the Youden's indexes generated by any other individual learning models in Tables A2–A5. The voting method with the SCAD and MCP selection and the stacking method with the LASSO, SCAD, and MCP selection outperformed most of the individual learning models listed in Tables A2–A5. The voting method with the SCAD or MCP model selection generated an AUC of 0.932 and 0.924, respectively, higher than the AUCs generated by any other individual learning models in Tables A2–A5.

We also applied the voting and stacking methods for the prediction of LGA, to combine the 104 learning models. The voting method was implemented as described in the prediction of macrosomia. When the stacking method was implemented, we fit a logistic regression with positive constraints [22], without further selection on first-level learners, and a logistic regression with the LASSO, SCAD, and MCP selection on first-level learners as our meta-learner. The results are summarized in Table 3. These results showed that the best prediction results were supplied by the voting method with the MCP selection with a Youden's index of 0.537 and a sensitivity of 0.636, both higher than any of the individual learning models in Tables A6–A9.

Table 2. Prediction performance of macrosomia by the ensemble methods.

Method	AUC (95% CI)	Sensitivity (95% CI)	Specificity (95% CI)	+LR (95% CI)	−LR (95% CI)	+PV (95% CI)	−PV (95% CI)	Youden's Index
Stacking: no selection	0.852 (0.805, 0.898)	0.607 (0.468, 0.735)	0.867 (0.821, 0.905)	4.562 (3.162, 6.582)	0.453 (0.326, 0.630)	0.479 (0.359, 0.601)	0.916 (0.876, 0.900)	0.474
Stacking: LASSO	0.907 (0.891, 0.943)	0.768 (0.636, 0.870)	0.874 (0.829, 0.911)	6.099 (4.334, 8.582)	0.266 (0.165, 0.429)	0.551 (0.434, 0.664)	0.949 (0.915, 0.973)	0.642
Stacking: SCAD	0.909 (0.873, 0.944)	0.839 (0.717, 0.924)	0.849 (0.801, 0.889)	5.555 (4.110, 7.509)	0.189 (0.104, 0.345)	0.528 (0.419, 0.635)	0.963 (0.931, 0.983)	0.688
Stacking: MCP	0.907 (0.872, 0.943)	0.786 (0.656, 0.844)	0.863 (0.817, 0.901)	5.748 (4.151, 7.960)	0.258 (0.150, 0.411)	0.537 (0.423, 0.647)	0.952 (0.918, 0.975)	0.649
Voting: no selection	0.903 (0.887, 0.919)	0.613 (0.553, 0.670)	0.912 (0.900, 0.927)	6.991 (5.726, 8.536)	0.425 (0.366, 0.492)	0.608 (0.549, 0.665)	0.914 (0.897, 0.929)	0.525
Voting: LASSO	0.891 (0.871, 0.911)	0.542 (0.482, 0.601)	0.959 (0.947, 0.969)	8.885 (6.988, 11.296)	0.809 (0.552, 0.673)	0.664 (0.599, 0.724)	0.902 (0.885, 0.918)	0.481
Voting: SCAD	0.932 (0.918, 0.945)	0.845 (0.798, 0.885)	0.836 (0.814, 0.855)	5.143 (4.501, 5.876)	0.185 (0.141, 0.244)	0.681 (0.612, 0.741)	0.533 (0.486, 0.580)	0.681
Voting: MCP	0.924 (0.910, 0.938)	0.810 (0.759, 0.854)	0.854 (0.834, 0.873)	5.565 (4.817, 6.428)	0.223 (0.175, 0.283)	0.553 (0.504, 0.601)	0.953 (0.939, 0.964)	0.664

Areas under the receiver operating characteristic curve (AUC), confident interval (CI), positive likelihood ratio (+LR), negative likelihood ratios (−LR), positive predictive values (+PV), negative predictive values (−PV).

Table 3. Prediction performance of large for gestational age by the ensemble methods.

Method	AUC (95% CI)	Sensitivity (95% CI)	Specificity (95% CI)	+LR (95% CI)	−LR (95% CI)	+PV (95% CI)	−PV (95% CI)	Youden's Index
Stacking: no selection	0.785 (0.697, 0.874)	0.485 (0.308, 0.665)	0.947 (0.915, 0.969)	9.121 (5.044, 16.495)	0.544 (0.390, 0.758)	0.500 (0.319, 0.681)	0.944 (0.911, 0.967)	0.432
Stacking: LASSO	0.811 (0.728, 0.894)	0.455 (0.281, 0.636)	0.944 (0.911, 0.967)	8.048 (4.443, 14.578)	0.578 (0.423, 0.790)	0.469 (0.291, 0.653)	0.940 (0.907, 0.964)	0.398
Stacking: SCAD	0.785 (0.696, 0.873)	0.455 (0.281, 0.636)	0.944 (0.911, 0.967)	8.048 (4.443, 14.578)	0.578 (0.423, 0.790)	0.469 (0.291, 0.653)	0.940 (0.907, 0.964)	0.398
Stacking: MCP	0.775 (0.688, 0.863)	0.485 (0.308, 0.665)	0.937 (0.903, 0.962)	7.681 (4.389, 13.441)	0.550 (0.394, 0.767)	0.457 (0.288, 0.634)	0.943 (0.911, 0.967)	0.421
Voting: no selection	0.823 (0.740, 0.906)	0.485 (0.308, 0.665)	0.950 (0.919, 0.972)	9.729 (5.309, 17,831)	0.542 (0.389, 0.756)	0.516 (0.331, 0.698)	0.944 (0.912, 0.967)	0.435
Voting: LASSO	0.811 (0.728, 0.895)	0.515 (0.335, 0.692)	0.940 (0.907, 0.964)	8.614 (4.936, 15.035)	0.516 (0.362, 0.734)	0.486 (0.314, 0.660)	0.946 (0.915, 0.969)	0.455
Voting: SCAD	0.799 (0.713, 0.885)	0.515 (0.335, 0.692)	0.944 (0.911, 0.967)	9.121 (5.168, 16.099)	0.514 (0.361, 0.731)	0.500 (0.319, 0.681)	0.947 (0.915, 0.969)	0.459
Voting: MCP	0.774 (0.687, 0.861)	0.636 (0.451, 0.796)	0.900 (0.861, 0.932)	6.385 (4.168, 9.780)	0.404 (0.257, 0.635)	0.412 (0.276, 0.558)	0.958 (0.927, 0.978)	0.537

Areas under the receiver operating characteristic curve (AUC), confident interval (CI), positive likelihood ratio (+LR), negative likely ratios (−LR), positive predictive values (+PV), negative predictive values (−PV).

4. Discussion and Conclusions

We proposed using ensemble methods to combine the strengths from nonlinear and quadratic mixed-effects models and 26 empirical formulas of EFWs to predict macrosomia and LGA of newborns from sonographic ultrasound measurements. The prediction performance of the ensemble methods was studied with the data from the Scandinavia SGA study. We showed that the prediction performance varied among the empirical formulas and mixed-effects models. The three-parameter mixed-effects logistic model combined with empirical formula 11 in Table A1 gave the best prediction results in predicting macrosomia. In predicting LGA, the prediction performance also varied. The best prediction results were obtained from the quadratic mixed-effects model combined with empirical formula 6 in Table A1. These results showed that it was difficult to select any individual statistical learning model combined with only one empirical formula of EFWs, to predict macrosomia or LGA from sonographic ultrasound measurements.

We subsequently proposed applying ensemble methods to aggregate the prediction results from mixed-effects models and empirical formulas of EFWs, to achieve better prediction performance. Our investigation showed that, with the aid of either the SCAD or MCP for model selection, both stacking and voting methods improved the prediction accuracies in predicting macrosomia, as opposed to those from individual statistical models and empirical formulas. The voting method with the MCP for model selection predicted LGA more accurately than the individual statistical models and empirical formulas. In this study, the ensemble prediction algorithms were created from all the prenatal ultrasound measures and birth weights. However, the algorithms can be used to make prediction on macrosomia or LGA with the ultrasound measures only from the first or second trimester, although the ultrasound measures collected in the third trimester or before birth can substantially improve the prediction accuracy. Our current study is a feasibility study that demonstrates the ensemble methods can be integrated with ultrasound examinations to assist obstetricians in clinical diagnosis on whether a pregnant woman will give birth to a large infant, and to further guide clinical interventions for the condition. However, measurable clinical benefits are unclear until they are demonstrated in prospective clinical studies.

Our current study has several limitations. The proportion of macrosomia or LGA infants in the Scandinavia SGA dataset is small (15% for macrosomia and 11% LGA of n = 1115 infants). This may largely influence the prediction accuracy given by the individual models and empirical formulas. However, using machine learning methods specifically ensemble methods, can accommodate such imbalanced data, and improve prediction accuracy [23]. In addition, the initial objective of the SGA study was to characterize the intra-uterine growth restriction and assess the associated risk factors of SGA, but the study was not designed for studying macrosomia or LGA. As a consequence, the risk factors associated with macrosomia or LGA were not thoroughly collected. This may be the reason why, in our study, we did not receive benefits from adding covariates into the mixed-effects models. Lastly, The SGA study was conducted in 1980s, with out-of-date sonographic ultrasound examination technologies, so the prediction models developed in this study may not be directly applied to predict macrosomia or LGA with the ultrasound measures from most recent state-of-the-art ultrasound technologies. However, the ensemble methods can still be applied to aggregate any available ultrasound prediction models. Also, the subjects in this study were the Caucasians from Europe that were mostly not obese (11.6% overweight rate and 2.1% obese rate in the study). New studies and data on a diverse population should be able to substantially improve the prediction of macrosomia and LGA among both the whites and minorities, as well as the overweight and obese population.

Author Contributions: S.Y., H.Z., F.S., and B.Z. conceived of the presented methodology. S.Y., F.S., and B.Z. verified the analytical methods and conducted data analysis. S.Y., F.S., and B.Z. took the lead in writing the manuscript. H.Z., S.W., and J.G. provided critical feedback, helped shape the research and analysis, and helped in manuscript writing. All authors proved the manuscript contents. All authors have read and agreed to the published version of the manuscript.

Funding: Dr. Suzhen Wang's research was partially supported by the National Natural Science Foundation of China (No. 81872719), the National Bureau of Statistics Foundation Project (No. 2018LY79), the Natural Science Foundation of Shandong Province (No. ZR201807090257), and the Poverty Alleviation Fund Project of Weifang Medical University (No. FP1801001). Dr. Fuyan Shi's research was partially supported by the National Natural Science Foundation of China (No. 81803337), the Shandong Provincial Government Fund for Overseas Study (No. 27, 2019, Lu-Jiao), the Shandong Science and Technology Development Plan Project (No. 2015 WS0067), and the Weifang Medical University Doctoral Foundation Project (No. 2017BSQD51). Dr. Hui Zhang receives support from the Robert H. Lurie Comprehensive Cancer Center of Northwestern University in Chicago, IL, which is supported in part by a NCI Cancer Center Support Grant #P30CA060553, and Mesulam Center for Cognitive Neurology and Alzheimer's Disease of Northwestern University, which is supported in part by a NIA Center Support Grant #P30AG13854.

Appendix A

Table A1. Empirical formulas used for estimating fetal weight from sonographic ultrasound measurements (Melamed et al. [5]).

Formula	Reference	Equation
1	Campbell and Wilkin [25]	$\ln EFW = -4.564 + 0.383 \cdot AC - 0.00331 \cdot AC^2$
2	Hadlock et al. [5]	$\ln EFW = 2.695 + 0.253 \cdot AC - 0.00275 \cdot AC^2$
3	Jordaan [26]	$\log_{10} EFW = 0.6328 + 0.1881 \cdot AC - 0.0043 \cdot AC^2 + 0.000036239 \cdot AC^3$
4	Warsof et al. [27]	$\log_{10} EFW = 1.1633 + 0.092 \cdot AC - 0.000019 \cdot AC$
5	Higginbottom et al. [28]	$EFW = 0.0816 \cdot AC^3$
6	Hadlock et al. [5]	$\log_{10} EFW = 1.304 + 0.05281 \cdot AC + 0.1938 \cdot FL - 0.004 \cdot AC \cdot FL$
7	Woo et al. [29]	$\log_{10} EFW = 0.59 + 0.08 \cdot AC + 0.28 \cdot FL - 0.00716 \cdot AC \cdot FL$
8	Warsof et al. [30]	$\ln EFW = 2.792 + 0.108 \cdot FL + 0.0036 \cdot AC^2 - 0.0027 \cdot AC \cdot FL$
9	Vintzileos et al. [31]	$\log_{10} EFW = 1.879 + 0.084 \cdot BPD + 0.026 \cdot AC$
10	Warsof et al. [27]	$\log_{10} EFW = 1.401 + 0.144 \cdot BPD + 0.032 \cdot AC - 0.000111 \cdot AC \cdot BPD^2$
11	Shepard et al. [32]	$\log_{10} EFW = 1.2508 + 0.166 \cdot BPD + 0.046 \cdot AC - 0.002546 \cdot BPD \cdot AC$
12	Jordaan [26]	$\log_{10} EFW = 1.9317 + 0.0377 \cdot AC + 0.0950 \cdot BPD - 0.0015 \cdot BPD \cdot AC$
13	Hadlock et al. [5]	$\log_{10} EFW = 1.1134 + 0.05845 \cdot AC - 0.000604 \cdot AC^2 - 0.007365 \cdot BPD^2 + 0.000595 \cdot BPD \cdot AC + 0.1694 \cdot BPD$
14	Woo et al. [29]	$\log_{10} EFW = 1.63 + 0.16 \cdot BPD + 0.00111 \cdot AC^2 - 0.0000859 \cdot BPD \cdot AC^2$
15	Mirghani et al. [33]	$\log_{10} EFW = 2.1315 + 0.0056541 \cdot AC \cdot BPD - 0.00015515 \cdot BPD \cdot AC^2 + 0.000019782 \cdot AC^3 + 0.052594 \cdot BPD$
16	Hadlock et al. [5]	$\log_{10} EFW = 1.182 + 0.0273 \cdot HC + 0.07057 \cdot AC - 0.00063 \cdot AC^2 - 0.0002184 \cdot HC \cdot AC$
17	Jordaan [26]	$\log_{10} EFW = 0.9119 + 0.0488 \cdot HC + 0.0824 \cdot AC - 0.001599 \cdot HC \cdot AC$
18	Jordaan [26]	$\log_{10} EFW = 2.3231 + 0.02904 \cdot AC + 0.0079 \cdot HC - 0.0058 \cdot BPD$
19	Hadlock et al. [5]	$\log_{10} EFW = 1.335 - 0.0034 \cdot AC \cdot FL + 0.0316 \cdot BPD + 0.0457 \cdot AC + 0.1623 \cdot FL$
20	Woo et al. [29]	$\log_{10} EFW = 1.54 + 0.15 \cdot BPD + 0.00111 \cdot AC^2 - 0.0000764 \cdot BPD \cdot AC^2 + 0.05 \cdot FL - 0.000992 \cdot FL \cdot AC$
21	Shinozuka et al. [34]	$EFW = 0.23966 \cdot AC^2 \cdot FL + 1.6230 \cdot BPD^3$
22	Mirghani et al. [33]	$\log_{10} EFW = 2.7193 + 0.0094962 \cdot AC \cdot BPD - 0.1432 \cdot FL - 0.00076742 \cdot AC \cdot BPD^2 + 0.001745 \cdot FL \cdot BPD^2$
23	Hadlock et al. [5]	$\log_{10} EFW = 1.326 - 0.00326 \cdot AC \cdot FL + 0.0107 \cdot HC + 0.0438 \cdot AC + 0.158 \cdot FL$
24	Combs et al. [35]	$EFW = 0.23718 \cdot AC^2 \cdot FL + 0.03312 \cdot HC^3$
25	Ott et al. [36]	$\log_{10} EFW = 0.9339 + 0.04355 \cdot HC + 0.05392 \cdot AC - 0.0008582 \cdot HC \cdot AC + 1.2594 \cdot (FL/AC)$
26	Hadlock et al. [5]	$\log_{10} EFW = 1.3596 + 0.0064 \cdot HC + 0.0424 \cdot AC + 0.174 \cdot FL + 0.00061 \cdot BPD \cdot AC - 0.00386 \cdot AC \cdot FL$

Abdominal circumference (AC), femur length (FL), biparietal diameter (BPD), and head circumference (HC) are expressed in centimeters, and EFW is expressed in grams, unless stated otherwise. This is an identical table to the Table 1 in Melamed et al. [5].

Table A2. Prediction performance of the three-parameter mixed-effects logistic model without covariance when combined with the 26 estimated fetal weight empirical formulas * in predicting macrosomia.

Formulas	AUC (95% CI)	Sensitivity (95% CI)	Specificity (95% CI)	+LR (95% CI)	−LR (95% CI)	+PV (95% CI)	−PV (95% CI)	Youden's Index
1	0.884 (0.839, 0.930)	0.250 (0.144, 0.384)	0.982 (0.958, 0.994)	13.900 (5.217, 37.033)	0.764 (0.656, 0.889)	0.737 (0.488, 0.910)	0.867 (0.824, 0.902)	0.232
2	0.885 (0.840, 0.930)	0.464 (0.330, 0.603)	0.946 (0.913, 0.969)	8.605 (4.881, 15.169)	0.566 (0.443, 0.724)	0.634 (0.469, 0.779)	0.898 (0.857, 0.930)	0.410
3	All predicted birth weights were under 4000 g.							
4	0.886 (0.842, 0.931)	0.571 (0.432, 0.703)	0.914 (0.874, 0.944)	6.619 (4.243, 10.325)	0.469 (0.346, 0.636)	0.571 (0.432, 0.703)	0.914 (0.874, 0.944)	0.485
5	0.883 (0.838, 0.928)	0.536 (0.397, 0.670)	0.932 (0.895, 0.958)	7.838 (4.765, 12.895)	0.498 (0.375, 0.661)	0.612 (0.462, 0.748)	0.909 (0.869, 0.940)	0.467
6	0.882 (0.835, 0.928)	0.464 (0.330, 0.603)	0.924 (0.887, 0.953)	6.146 (3.734, 10.116)	0.579 (0.453, 0.741)	0.553 (0.401, 0.698)	0.895 (0.854, 0.928)	0.389
7	0.882 (0.837, 0.926)	0.857 (0.738, 0.936)	0.799 (0.747, 0.844)	4.255 (3.290, 5.504)	0.179 (0.094, 0.341)	0.462 (0.363, 0.562)	0.965 (0.933, 0.985)	0.656
8	0.872 (0.824, 0.920)	0.429 (0.297, 0.568)	0.932 (0.895, 0.958)	6.271 (3.695, 10.643)	0.613 (0.488, 0.771)	0.558 (0.399, 0.709)	0.890 (0.848, 0.924)	0.360
9	0.907 (0.871, 0.942)	0.821 (0.696, 0.911)	0.845 (0.797, 0.886)	5.311 (3.931, 7.174)	0.211 (0.120, 0.371)	0.517 (0.408, 0.624)	0.959 (0.926, 0.980)	0.667
10	0.906 (0.867, 0.945)	0.536 (0.397, 0.670)	0.953 (0.921, 0.975)	11.456 (6.388, 20.544)	0.487 (0.367, 0.646)	0.698 (0.539, 0.828)	0.911 (0.872, 0.941)	0.489
11	0.904 (0.867, 0.942)	0.821 (0.696, 0.911)	0.849 (0.801, 0.889)	5.437 (4.011, 7.370)	0.210 (0.120, 0.370)	0.523 (0.414, 0.630)	0.959 (0.927, 0.980)	0.670
12	0.910 (0.873, 0.946)	0.643 (0.504, 0.766)	0.921 (0.883, 0.950)	8.123 (5.201, 12.689)	0.388 (0.272, 0.552)	0.621 (0.484, 0.745)	0.928 (0.890, 0.955)	0.564
13	0.908 (0.869, 0.946)	0.696 (0.559, 0.812)	0.910 (0.870, 0.941)	7.744 (5.129, 11.693)	0.334 (0.224, 0.497)	0.609 (0.479, 0.729)	0.937 (0.901, 0.963)	0.607
14	0.908 (0.870, 0.946)	0.214 (0.116, 0.344)	0.989 (0.969, 0.998)	19.857 (5.792, 68.082)	0.792 (0.692, 0.911)	0.800 (0.519, 0.898)	0.862 (0.819, 0.898)	0.203
15	0.910 (0.874, 0.947)	0.732 (0.597, 0.842)	0.910 (0.870, 0.941)	9.141 (5.424, 12.220)	0.294 (0.191, 0.455)	0.621 (0.493, 0.738)	0.944 (0.909, 0.968)	0.642
16	0.905 (0.865, 0.969)	0.429 (0.297, 0.568)	0.968 (0.939, 0.985)	13.238 (6.507, 26.933)	0.591 (0.470, 0.742)	0.727 (0.545, 0.867)	0.894 (0.853, 0.926)	0.396
17	0.871 (0.824, 0.917)	0.339 (0.218, 0.478)	0.946 (0.913, 0.969)	6.288 (3.406, 11.608)	0.698 (0.578, 0.844)	0.559 (0.379, 0.728)	0.877 (0.834, 0.912)	0.285
18	0.888 (0.848, 0.928)	0.054 (0.011, 0.149)	0.996 (0.980, 1.000)	14.893 (1.578, 140.579)	0.950 (0.892, 1.011)	0.750 (0.194, 0.994)	0.839 (0.795, 0.877)	0.050
19	0.901 (0.860, 0.943)	0.679 (0.540, 0.797)	0.924 (0.887, 0.953)	8.983 (5.734, 12.074)	0.348 (0.237, 0.509)	0.644 (0.509, 0.764)	0.935 (0.899, 0.961)	0.603
20	0.910 (0.871, 0.948)	0.607 (0.468, 0.735)	0.935 (0.900, 0.961)	9.377 (5.722, 15.367)	0.420 (0.303, 0.583)	0.654 (0.509, 0.780)	0.922 (0.884, 0.950)	0.542
21	0.905 (0.865, 0.945)	0.429 (0.297, 0.568)	0.950 (0.917, 0.972)	8.510 (4.702, 15.403)	0.602 (0.479, 0.756)	0.632 (0.460, 0.782)	0.892 (0.851, 0.925)	0.378
22	0.901 (0.865, 0.937)	0.179 (0.089, 0.304)	0.982 (0.959, 0.994)	9.929 (3.529, 27.934)	0.836 (0.740, 0.946)	0.667 (0.384, 0.882)	0.856 (0.812, 0.892)	0.161
23	0.902 (0.861, 0.943)	0.464 (0.330, 0.603)	0.939 (0.904, 0.964)	7.592 (4.426, 13.025)	0.571 (0.446, 0.730)	0.605 (0.444, 0.750)	0.897 (0.856, 0.929)	0.403
24	0.906 (0.886, 0.945)	0.232 (0.130, 0.364)	0.993 (0.974, 0.999)	32.268 (7.488, 133.049)	0.773 (0.669, 0.894)	0.867 (0.595, 0.983)	0.865 (0.823, 0.901)	0.225
25	0.906 (0.866, 0.946)	0.393 (0.265, 0.532)	0.960 (0.930, 0.980)	9.929 (5.109, 19.294)	0.632 (0.511, 0.781)	0.667 (0.482, 0.820)	0.887 (0.846, 0.920)	0.353
26	0.903 (0.863, 0.944)	0.661 (0.522, 0.782)	0.932 (0.895, 0.958)	9.667 (6.025, 15.512)	0.364 (0.252, 0.526)	0.661 (0.522, 0.782)	0.932 (0.895, 0.958)	0.592

* See Table A1 for specifications of empirical formulas. Areas under the receiver operating characteristic curve (AUC), confident interval (CI), positive likelihood ratio (+LR), negative likelihood ratios (−LR), positive predictive values (+PV), negative predictive values (−PV).

Table A3. Prediction performance of the three-parameter mixed-effects logistic model with covariance when combined with the 26 estimated fetal weight empirical formulas* in predicting macrosomia.

Formulas	AUC (95% CI)	Sensitivity (95% CI)	Specificity (95% CI)	+LR (95% CI)	−LR (95% CI)	+PV (95% CI)	−PV (95% CI)	Youden's Index
1	0.885 (0.840, 0.931)	0.232 (0.130, 0.364)	0.982 (0.958, 0.994)	12.907 (4.793, 34.758)	0.782 (0.676, 0.904)	0.722 (0.465, 0.903)	0.864 (0.821, 0.900)	0.215
2	0.885 (0.830, 0.930)	0.500 (0.363, 0.637)	0.942 (0.908, 0.967)	8.688 (5.047, 14.953)	0.531 (0.408, 0.690)	0.636 (0.478, 0.776)	0.903 (0.863, 0.935)	0.442
3	All predicted birth weights were under 4000 g.							
4	0.885 (0.840, 0.930)	0.607 (0.468, 0.735)	0.917 (0.878, 0.947)	7.339 (4.705, 11.446)	0.428 (0.309, 0.594)	0.596 (0.458, 0.724)	0.921 (0.882, 0.950)	0.524
5	0.883 (0.837, 0.928)	0.518 (0.380, 0.653)	0.931 (0.895, 0.958)	7.577 (4.586, 12.520)	0.518 (0.394, 0.680)	0.604 (0.453, 0.742)	0.906 (0.866, 0.937)	0.450
6	0.880 (0.834, 0.927)	0.464 (0.330, 0.603)	0.928 (0.891, 0.956)	6.454 (3.886, 10.717)	0.577 (0.451, 0.738)	0.565 (0.411, 0.711)	0.896 (0.855, 0.929)	0.392
7	0.882 (0.838, 0.926)	0.839 (0.717, 0.924)	0.799 (0.747, 0.844)	4.166 (3.211, 5.407)	0.201 (0.110, 0.367)	0.456 (0.358, 0.557)	0.961 (0.927, 0.982)	0.638
8	0.880 (0.834, 0.927)	0.464 (0.330, 0.603)	0.928 (0.891, 0.956)	6.454 (3.886, 10.717)	0.577 (0.451, 0.738)	0.565 (0.411, 0.711)	0.896 (0.855, 0.929)	0.392
9	0.906 (0.870, 0.942)	0.804 (0.676, 0.898)	0.845 (0.797, 0.886)	5.195 (3.534, 7.039)	0.232 (0.136, 0.396)	0.511 (0.402, 0.619)	0.955 (0.921, 0.977)	0.649
10	0.907 (0.867, 0.946)	0.500 (0.363, 0.637)	0.950 (0.917, 0.972)	9.929 (5.594, 17.622)	0.527 (0.405, 0.685)	0.667 (0.505, 0.804)	0.904 (0.864, 0.935)	0.500
11	0.904 (0.867, 0.942)	0.821 (0.696, 0.911)	0.849 (0.801, 0.889)	5.437 (4.011, 7.370)	0.210 (0.120, 0.370)	0.523 (0.414, 0.630)	0.959 (0.926, 0.980)	0.670
12	0.910 (0.873, 0.946)	0.643 (0.504, 0.766)	0.921 (0.553, 0.950)	8.123 (5.201, 12.689)	0.388 (0.272, 0.552)	0.621 (0.484, 0.745)	0.928 (0.890, 0.955)	0.564
13	0.907 (0.868, 0.945)	0.679 (0.540, 0.797)	0.914 (0.874, 0.944)	7.860 (5.150, 11.996)	0.352 (0.240, 0.516)	0.613 (0.481, 0.734)	0.934 (0.897, 0.960)	0.592
14	0.909 (0.871, 0.947)	0.214 (0.116, 0.344)	0.986 (0.964, 0.996)	14.893 (4.984, 44.498)	0.797 (0.695, 0.915)	0.750 (0.476, 0.927)	0.862 (0.819, 0.898)	0.200
15	0.910 (0.874, 0.947)	0.714 (0.578, 0.827)	0.910 (0.870, 0.941)	7.943 (5.277, 11.956)	0.314 (0.207, 0.476)	0.615 (0.486, 0.733)	0.941 (0.905, 0.966)	0.624
16	0.905 (0.865, 0.944)	0.411 (0.281, 0.550)	0.968 (0.939, 0.985)	12.687 (6.205, 25.937)	0.609 (0.489, 0.759)	0.719 (0.533, 0.863)	0.891 (0.850, 0.924)	0.378
17	0.871 (0.825, 0.917)	0.339 (0.218, 0.478)	0.946 (0.913, 0.969)	6.288 (3.406, 11.608)	0.698 (0.578, 0.844)	0.559 (0.379, 0.728)	0.877 (0.834, 0.912)	0.285
18	0.885 (0.845, 0.924)	0.232 (0.130, 0.364)	0.975 (0.949, 0.990)	9.219 (3.851, 22.069)	0.788 (0.681, 0.911)	0.650 (0.408, 0.846)	0.863 (0.820, 0.899)	0.207
19	0.901 (0.860, 0.943)	0.679 (0.540, 0.797)	0.928 (0.891, 0.956)	9.432 (5.960, 14.927)	0.346 (0.236, 0.507)	0.655 (0.519, 0.775)	0.935 (0.899, 0.961)	0.607
20	0.909 (0.871, 0.948)	0.589 (0.450, 0.719)	0.932 (0.895, 0.958)	8.622 (5.303, 14.018)	0.441 (0.322, 0.604)	0.635 (0.490, 0.764)	0.918 (0.880, 0.948)	0.521
21	0.905 (0.865, 0.944)	0.429 (0.297, 0.568)	0.950 (0.917, 0.972)	8.510 (4.702, 15.403)	0.602 (0.479, 0.756)	0.632 (0.460, 0.782)	0.892 (0.851, 0.925)	0.378
22	0.903 (0.867, 0.939)	0.179 (0.089, 0.304)	0.982 (0.959, 0.994)	9.929 (3.529, 27.934)	0.836 (0.740, 0.946)	0.667 (0.384, 0.882)	0.856 (0.812, 0.892)	0.161
23	0.902 (0.861, 0.943)	0.482 (0.347, 0.620)	0.935 (0.900, 0.961)	7.446 (4.415, 12.560)	0.554 (0.429, 0.714)	0.600 (0.443, 0.743)	0.900 (0.859, 0.932)	0.417
24	0.906 (0.867, 0.946)	0.232 (0.130, 0.364)	0.993 (0.974, 0.999)	32.269 (7.488, 39.049)	0.773 (0.669, 0.894)	0.867 (0.595, 0.983)	0.865 (0.823, 0.901)	0.225
25	0.906 (0.866, 0.946)	0.393 (0.265, 0.532)	0.964 (0.935, 0.983)	10.921 (5.477, 21.778)	0.630 (0.510, 0.778)	0.688 (0.500, 0.839)	0.887 (0.846, 0.921)	0.357
26	0.903 (0.863, 0.944)	0.643 (0.504, 0.766)	0.932 (0.895, 0.958)	9.406 (5.844, 15.139)	0.383 (0.269, 0.546)	0.655 (0.514, 0.778)	0.928 (0.891, 0.956)	0.575

* See Table A1 for specifications of empirical formulas. Areas under the receiver operating characteristic curve (AUC), confident interval (CI), positive likelihood ratio (+LR), negative likelihood ratios (−LR), positive predictive values (+PV), negative predictive values (−PV).

Table A4. Prediction performance of the quadratic mixed-effects model without covariance when combined with the 26 estimated fetal weight empirical formulas* in predicting macrosomia.

Formulas	AUC (95% CI)	Sensitivity (95% CI)	Specificity (95% CI)	+LR (95% CI)	−LR (95% CI)	+PV (95% CI)	−PV (95% CI)	Youden's Index
1	0.861 (0.816, 0.906)	0.679 (0.540, 0.797)	0.845 (0.797, 0.886)	4.387 (3.158, 6.094)	0.380 (0.259, 0.558)	0.469 (0.357, 0.583)	0.929 (0.890, 0.957)	0.524
2	0.882 (0.841, 0.923)	0.839 (0.717, 0.924)	0.777 (0.723, 0.825)	3.763 (2.938, 4.820)	0.207 (0.113, 0.378)	0.431 (0.337, 0.530)	0.960 (0.925, 0.982)	0.616
3	0.877 (0.835, 0.919)	0.357 (0.234, 0.496)	0.953 (0.921, 0.975)	7.637 (4.041, 14.454)	0.674 (0.554, 0.821)	0.606 (0.421, 0.771)	0.880 (0.838, 0.915)	0.310
4	0.858 (0.813, 0.903)	0.786 (0.656, 0.884)	0.727 (0.670, 0.778)	2.874 (2.271, 3.637)	0.295 (0.178, 0.489)	0.367 (0.281, 0.459)	0.944 (0.904, 0.971)	0.512
5	0.889 (0.849, 0.930)	0.768 (0.636, 0.870)	0.827 (0.778, 0.870)	4.447 (3.311, 5.980)	0.281 (0.174, 0.453)	0.473 (0.367, 0.580)	0.947 (0.910, 0.971)	0.595
6	0.882 (0.840, 0.923)	0.839 (0.717, 0.924)	0.770 (0.716, 0.818)	3.646 (2.857, 4.651)	0.209 (0.114, 0.381)	0.423 (0.330, 0.521)	0.960 (0.925, 0.981)	0.609
7	0.874 (0.932, 0.917)	0.982 (0.904, 0.999)	0.482 (0.422, 0.542)	1.896 (1.684, 2.135)	0.037 (0.005, 0.259)	0.276 (0.215, 0.344)	0.993 (0.959, 0.999)	0.464
8	0.869 (0.825, 0.913)	0.911 (0.804, 0.970)	0.716 (0.659, 0.768)	3.205 (2.614, 3.929)	0.975 (0.944, 0.992)	0.392 (0.308, 0.482)	0.975 (0.944, 0.992)	0.627
9	0.903 (0.868, 0.938)	0.964 (0.877, 0.996)	0.662 (0.603, 0.717)	2.852 (2.401, 3.387)	0.054 (0.014, 0.211)	0.365 (0.287, 0.448)	0.989 (0.962, 0.999)	0.626
10	0.902 (0.867, 0.937)	0.839 (0.717, 0.924)	0.805 (0.754, 0.851)	4.321 (3.313, 5.634)	0.199 (0.109, 0.364)	0.465 (0.365, 0.567)	0.961 (0.928, 0.982)	0.645
11	0.895 (0.858, 0.932)	0.982 (0.904, 0.999)	0.579 (0.519, 0.638)	2.334 (2.024, 2.691)	0.031 (0.004, 0.216)	0.320 (0.251, 0.395)	0.994 (0.966, 0.999)	0.561
12	0.905 (0.870, 0.939)	0.875 (0.759, 0.948)	0.788 (0.735, 0.834)	4.123 (3.220, 5.279)	0.159 (0.079, 0.318)	0.454 (0.358, 0.552)	0.969 (0.937, 0.987)	0.663
13	0.899 (0.863, 0.935)	0.893 (0.781, 0.960)	0.745 (0.689, 0.795)	3.496 (2.805, 4.357)	0.144 (0.067, 0.307)	0.413 (0.324, 0.506)	0.972 (0.940, 0.990)	0.637
14	0.898 (0.863, 0.934)	0.643 (0.504, 0.766)	0.892 (0.850, 0.926)	5.957 (4.032, 8.801)	0.400 (0.281, 0.570)	0.545 (0.418, 0.669)	0.925 (0.887, 0.954)	0.535
15	0.904 (0.869, 0.939)	0.875 (0.759, 0.948)	0.763 (0.708, 0.811)	3.686 (2.920, 4.652)	0.164 (0.082, 0.329)	0.426 (0.334, 0.522)	0.968 (0.935, 0.987)	0.637
16	0.898 (0.863, 0.934)	0.857 (0.738, 0.936)	0.799 (0.747, 0.844)	4.255 (3.290, 5.504)	0.179 (0.094, 0.341)	0.462 (0.363, 0.562)	0.965 (0.933, 0.985)	0.656
17	0.879 (0.836, 0.921)	0.804 (0.676, 0.898)	0.788 (0.735, 0.834)	3.786 (2.917, 4.915)	0.249 (0.146, 0.425)	0.433 (0.336, 0.533)	0.952 (0.916, 0.976)	0.591
18	0.901 (0.865, 0.938)	0.804 (0.676, 0.898)	0.838 (0.789, 0.879)	4.964 (3.688, 6.682)	0.234 (0.138, 0.399)	0.500 (0.393, 0.607)	0.955 (0.921, 0.977)	0.642
19	0.895 (0.856, 0.933)	0.875 (0.759, 0.948)	0.748 (0.693, 0.798)	3.475 (2.773, 4.354)	0.167 (0.083, 0.335)	0.412 (0.322, 0.506)	0.967 (0.934, 0.987)	0.623
20	0.900 (0.864, 0.936)	0.875 (0.759, 0.948)	0.755 (0.700, 0.805)	3.577 (2.845, 4.498)	0.165 (0.082, 0.332)	0.419 (0.328, 0.514)	0.968 (0.935, 0.987)	0.630
21	0.898 (0.861, 0.935)	0.857 (0.738, 0.936)	0.752 (0.697, 0.801)	3.453 (2.741, 4.350)	0.190 (0.100, 0.362)	0.410 (0.320, 0.505)	0.963 (0.929, 0.984)	0.609
22	0.903 (0.868, 0.938)	0.875 (0.759, 0.948)	0.758 (0.704, 0.808)	3.631 (2.882, 4.574)	0.165 (0.082, 0.330)	0.422 (0.331, 0.518)	0.968 (0.935, 0.987)	0.634
23	0.896 (0.858, 0.934)	0.839 (0.717, 0.924)	0.791 (0.739, 0.838)	4.023 (3.114, 5.197)	0.203 (0.111, 0.371)	0.448 (0.350, 0.548)	0.961 (0.927, 0.982)	0.631
24	0.898 (0.861, 0.935)	0.786 (0.656, 0.884)	0.831 (0.782, 0.873)	4.647 (3.463, 6.238)	0.258 (0.156, 0.427)	0.484 (0.377, 0.591)	0.951 (0.915, 0.974)	0.617
25	0.900 (0.864, 0.936)	0.821 (0.696, 0.911)	0.795 (0.743, 0.841)	4.006 (3.084, 5.205)	0.225 (0.128, 0.395)	0.447 (0.349, 0.548)	0.957 (0.922, 0.979)	0.616
26	0.897 (0.859, 0.934)	0.857 (0.738, 0.936)	0.758 (0.707, 0.808)	3.557 (2.813, 4.496)	0.188 (0.099, 0.359)	0.417 (0.326, 0.513)	0.963 (0.929, 0.984)	0.616

* See Table A1 for specifications of empirical formulas. Areas under the receiver operating characteristic curve (AUC), confident interval (CI), positive likelihood ratio (+LR), negative likelihood ratios (−LR), positive predictive values (+PV), negative predictive values (−PV).

Table A5. Prediction performance of the quadratic mixed-effects model with covariance when combined with the 26 estimated fetal weight empirical formulas* in predicting macrosomia.

Formulas	AUC (95% CI)	Sensitivity (95% CI)	Specificity (95% CI)	+LR (95% CI)	−LR (95% CI)	+PV (95% CI)	−PV (95% CI)	Youden's Index
1	0.860 (0.815, 0.905)	0.661 (0.522, 0.782)	0.845 (0.797, 0.886)	4.272 (3.062, 5.958)	0.401 (0.278, 0.580)	0.463 (0.350, 0.578)	0.925 (0.886, 0.954)	0.506
2	0.882 (0.841, 0.923)	0.839 (0.717, 0.924)	0.781 (0.727, 0.828)	3.825 (2.980, 4.909)	0.206 (0.113, 0.376)	0.435 (0.340, 0.534)	0.960 (0.926, 0.982)	0.620
3	0.877 (0.835, 0.919)	0.357 (0.234, 0.496)	0.953 (0.921, 0.975)	7.637 (4.041, 14.434)	0.674 (0.554, 0.821)	0.606 (0.421, 0.771)	0.880 (0.838, 0.915)	0.310
4	0.857 (0.812, 0.903)	0.786 (0.656, 0.884)	0.730 (0.674, 0.781)	2.912 (2.298, 3.691)	0.293 (0.177, 0.487)	0.370 (0.283, 0.463)	0.944 (0.905, 0.971)	0.516
5	0.889 (0.849, 0.930)	0.768 (0.636, 0.870)	0.827 (0.778, 0.870)	4.447 (3.311, 5.972)	0.281 (0.174, 0.453)	0.473 (0.367, 0.580)	0.947 (0.910, 0.971)	0.595
6	0.881 (0.839, 0.923)	0.839 (0.717, 0.924)	0.770 (0.716, 0.820)	3.646 (2.857, 4.651)	0.209 (0.114, 0.381)	0.423 (0.330, 0.521)	0.960 (0.925, 0.981)	0.609
7	0.873 (0.830, 0.916)	0.982 (0.904, 0.999)	0.478 (0.418, 0.539)	1.883 (1.673, 2.119)	0.037 (0.005, 0.261)	0.275 (0.214, 0.342)	0.993 (0.959, 1.000)	0.461
8	0.868 (0.824, 0.912)	0.911 (0.804, 0.970)	0.712 (0.655, 0.765)	3.165 (2.585, 3.874)	0.125 (0.054, 0.290)	0.389 (0.305, 0.478)	0.975 (0.943, 0.992)	0.623
9	0.902 (0.867, 0.937)	0.964 (0.877, 0.996)	0.669 (0.610, 0.724)	2.914 (2.447, 3.470)	0.053 (0.014, 0.209)	0.370 (0.292, 0.454)	0.989 (0.962, 0.999)	0.633
10	0.902 (0.867, 0.937)	0.839 (0.717, 0.924)	0.806 (0.754, 0.851)	4.321 (3.313, 5.634)	0.199 (0.109, 0.364)	0.465 (0.365, 0.567)	0.961 (0.928, 0.982)	0.645
11	0.893 (0.856, 0.931)	0.982 (0.904, 0.999)	0.579 (0.519, 0.638)	2.334 (2.024, 2.691)	0.031 (0.004, 0.216)	0.320 (0.251, 0.395)	0.994 (0.966, 1.000)	0.561
12	0.905 (0.870, 0.939)	0.875 (0.759, 0.948)	0.784 (0.731, 0.831)	4.054 (3.173, 5.179)	0.159 (0.079, 0.320)	0.500 (0.354, 0.548)	0.969 (0.937, 0.987)	0.659
13	0.898 (0.862, 0.934)	0.893 (0.781, 0.960)	0.748 (0.693, 0.798)	3.546 (2.840, 4.427)	0.143 (0.067, 0.306)	0.417 (0.327, 0.510)	0.972 (0.940, 0.990)	0.641
14	0.898 (0.875, 0.948)	0.643 (0.504, 0.766)	0.892 (0.850, 0.926)	5.957 (4.032, 8.801)	0.400 (0.281, 0.570)	0.545 (0.418, 0.669)	0.925 (0.887, 0.954)	0.535
15	0.903 (0.869, 0.938)	0.875 (0.759, 0.948)	0.759 (0.704, 0.808)	3.631 (2.882, 4.574)	0.165 (0.082, 0.330)	0.422 (0.331, 0.518)	0.968 (0.935, 0.987)	0.634
16	0.898 (0.862, 0.934)	0.857 (0.738, 0.936)	0.799 (0.747, 0.844)	4.255 (3.290, 5.504)	0.179 (0.094, 0.341)	0.462 (0.363, 0.562)	0.965 (0.933, 0.985)	0.656
17	0.878 (0.836, 0.921)	0.786 (0.656, 0.884)	0.788 (0.735, 0.834)	3.702 (2.842, 4.823)	0.272 (0.164, 0.451)	0.427 (0.330, 0.528)	0.948 (0.911, 0.973)	0.573
18	0.901 (0.864, 0.938)	0.804 (0.676, 0.898)	0.842 (0.793, 0.883)	5.077 (3.760, 6.856)	0.233 (0.137, 0.397)	0.506 (0.398, 0.613)	0.955 (0.921, 0.977)	0.645
19	0.894 (0.856, 0.932)	0.875 (0.759, 0.948)	0.745 (0.689, 0.795)	3.426 (2.739, 4.285)	0.168 (0.084, 0.337)	0.408 (0.320, 0.502)	0.967 (0.934, 0.987)	0.620
20	0.900 (0.865, 0.936)	0.875 (0.759, 0.948)	0.755 (0.700, 0.805)	3.577 (2.845, 4.498)	0.165 (0.082, 0.332)	0.419 (0.328, 0.514)	0.968 (0.935, 0.987)	0.630
21	0.897 (0.860, 0.934)	0.857 (0.738, 0.936)	0.755 (0.700, 0.805)	3.504 (2.777, 4.422)	0.189 (0.099, 0.360)	0.414 (0.323, 0.509)	0.963 (0.929, 0.984)	0.613
22	0.903 (0.868, 0.938)	0.875 (0.759, 0.948)	0.755 (0.700, 0.805)	3.577 (2.845, 4.498)	0.165 (0.082, 0.332)	0.419 (0.328, 0.514)	0.968 (0.935, 0.987)	0.630
23	0.895 (0.857, 0.933)	0.821 (0.696, 0.911)	0.791 (0.739, 0.838)	3.937 (3.037, 5.104)	0.226 (0.128, 0.397)	0.442 (0.345, 0.543)	0.957 (0.921, 0.979)	0.613
24	0.898 (0.861, 0.935)	0.786 (0.656, 0.884)	0.831 (0.782, 0.873)	4.647 (3.463, 6.238)	0.258 (0.156, 0.427)	0.484 (0.377, 0.591)	0.951 (0.915, 0.974)	0.617
25	0.899 (0.863, 0.936)	0.821 (0.696, 0.911)	0.799 (0.747, 0.844)	4.078 (3.132, 5.310)	0.957 (0.922, 0.979)	0.451 (0.352, 0.553)	0.957 (0.922, 0.979)	0.620
26	0.897 (0.859, 0.934)	0.857 (0.738, 0.936)	0.755 (0.700, 0.805)	3.504 (2.777, 4.422)	0.189 (0.099, 0.360)	0.414 (0.323, 0.509)	0.963 (0.929, 0.984)	0.613

* See Table A1 for specifications of empirical formulas. Areas under the receiver operating characteristic curve (AUC), confident interval (CI), positive likelihood ratio (+LR), negative likelihood ratios (−LR), positive predictive values (+PV), negative predictive values (−PV).

Table A6. Prediction performance of the three-parameter mixed-effects logistic model without covariance when combined with the 26 estimated fetal weight empirical formulas* in predicting large for gestational age.

Formulas	AUC (95% CI)	Sensitivity (95% CI)	Specificity (95% CI)	+LR (95% CI)	−LR (95% CI)	+PV (95% CI)	−PV (95% CI)	Youden's Index
1	0.865 (0.810, 0.919)	0.424 (0.255, 0.608)	0.930 (0.895, 0.956)	6.081 (3.429, 10.783)	0.612 (0.461, 0.831)	0.400 (0.239, 0.579)	0.936 (0.903, 0.961)	0.354
2	0.867 (0.812, 0.922)	0.455 (0.281, 0.636)	0.940 (0.907, 0.964)	7.601 (4.241, 13.622)	0.580 (0.424, 0.793)	0.454 (0.281, 0.636)	0.940 (0.907, 0.964)	0.395
3	0.867 (0.811, 0.923)	0.485 (0.308, 0.665)	0.940 (0.907, 0.964)	8.108 (4.587, 14.330)	0.548 (0.393, 0.764)	0.471 (0.298, 0.649)	0.943 (0.911, 0.967)	0.425
4	0.868 (0.814, 0.922)	0.455 (0.281, 0.636)	0.940 (0.907, 0.964)	7.601 (4.241, 13.622)	0.580 (0.424, 0.793)	0.454 (0.281, 0.636)	0.940 (0.907, 0.964)	0.395
5	0.868 (0.812, 0.923)	0.455 (0.281, 0.636)	0.944 (0.911, 0.967)	8.048 (4.443, 14.578)	0.578 (0.423, 0.790)	0.469 (0.291, 0.653)	0.940 (0.907, 0.964)	0.398
6	0.873 (0.818, 0.927)	0.515 (0.335, 0.692)	0.937 (0.903, 0.962)	8.161 (4.724, 14.100)	0.518 (0.364, 0.737)	0.472 (0.304, 0.645)	0.946 (0.914, 0.969)	0.452
7	0.891 (0.839, 0.944)	0.455 (0.281, 0.636)	0.937 (0.903, 0.962)	7.201 (4.057, 12.780)	0.582 (0.426, 0.796)	0.441 (0.272, 0.621)	0.940 (0.907, 0.964)	0.391
8	0.876 (0.820, 0.932)	0.485 (0.308, 0.665)	0.944 (0.911, 0.967)	8.585 (4.805, 15.339)	0.546 (0.392, 0.761)	0.485 (0.308, 0.665)	0.944 (0.911, 0.967)	0.428
9	0.894 (0.854, 0.934)	0.455 (0.281, 0.636)	0.934 (0.899, 0.959)	6.841 (3.889, 12.034)	0.584 (0.427, 0.780)	0.429 (0.263, 0.606)	0.940 (0.907, 0.964)	0.388
10	0.886 (0.846, 0.927)	0.485 (0.308, 0.665)	0.930 (0.895, 0.956)	6.949 (4.041, 11.950)	0.554 (0.397, 0.772)	0.432 (0.271, 0.605)	0.943 (0.910, 0.966)	0.415
11	0.895 (0.856, 0.935)	0.485 (0.308, 0.665)	0.940 (0.907, 0.964)	8.108 (4.587, 14.330)	0.548 (0.393, 0.764)	0.471 (0.298, 0.649)	0.943 (0.911, 0.967)	0.425
12	0.891 (0.849, 0.933)	0.515 (0.335, 0.692)	0.950 (0.919, 0.972)	10.337 (5.707, 18.724)	0.510 (0.359, 0.726)	0.531 (0.347, 0.709)	0.947 (0.915, 0.969)	0.465
13	0.890 (0.849, 0.932)	0.485 (0.308, 0.665)	0.944 (0.911, 0.967)	8.585 (4.805, 15.339)	0.546 (0.392, 0.761)	0.485 (0.308, 0.665)	0.944 (0.911, 0.967)	0.428
14	0.886 (0.845, 0.926)	0.545 (0.364, 0.719)	0.944 (0.911, 0.967)	9.658 (5.533, 16.856)	0.482 (0.331, 0.701)	0.514 (0.340, 0.686)	0.950 (0.919, 0.972)	0.489
15	0.892 (0.852, 0.931)	0.485 (0.308, 0.665)	0.940 (0.907, 0.964)	8.108 (4.587, 14.330)	0.548 (0.393, 0.764)	0.471 (0.298, 0.649)	0.943 (0.911, 0.967)	0.425
16	0.883 (0.842, 0.924)	0.485 (0.308, 0.665)	0.937 (0.903, 0.962)	7.681 (4.389, 13.441)	0.550 (0.394, 0.767)	0.457 (0.288, 0.634)	0.943 (0.911, 0.967)	0.422
17	0.861 (0.803, 0.919)	0.455 (0.281, 0.636)	0.934 (0.899, 0.959)	6.841 (3.889, 12.034)	0.584 (0.427, 0.780)	0.429 (0.263, 0.606)	0.940 (0.907, 0.964)	0.388
18	0.871 (0.818, 0.924)	0.515 (0.335, 0.692)	0.937 (0.903, 0.962)	8.161 (4.724, 14.100)	0.518 (0.364, 0.737)	0.472 (0.304, 0.645)	0.946 (0.914, 0.969)	0.452
19	0.887 (0.841, 0.933)	0.515 (0.335, 0.692)	0.937 (0.903, 0.962)	8.161 (4.724, 14.100)	0.518 (0.364, 0.737)	0.472 (0.304, 0.645)	0.946 (0.914, 0.969)	0.452
20	0.892 (0.853, 0.932)	0.545 (0.364, 0.719)	0.944 (0.911, 0.967)	9.658 (5.533, 16.856)	0.482 (0.331, 0.701)	0.514 (0.340, 0.686)	0.950 (0.919, 0.972)	0.489
21	0.890 (0.850, 0.931)	0.424 (0.255, 0.608)	0.937 (0.903, 0.962)	6.721 (3.728, 12.117)	0.615 (0.458, 0.825)	0.424 (0.255, 0.608)	0.937 (0.903, 0.962)	0.361
22	0.884 (0.840, 0.929)	0.485 (0.308, 0.665)	0.940 (0.907, 0.964)	8.108 (4.587, 14.330)	0.548 (0.393, 0.764)	0.471 (0.298, 0.649)	0.943 (0.911, 0.967)	0.425
23	0.882 (0.836, 0.929)	0.485 (0.308, 0.665)	0.940 (0.907, 0.964)	8.108 (4.587, 14.330)	0.548 (0.393, 0.764)	0.471 (0.298, 0.649)	0.943 (0.911, 0.967)	0.425
24	0.887 (0.846, 0.929)	0.455 (0.281, 0.636)	0.937 (0.903, 0.962)	7.201 (4.057, 12.780)	0.582 (0.426, 0.796)	0.441 (0.272, 0.621)	0.940 (0.907, 0.964)	0.391
25	0.889 (0.847, 0.931)	0.455 (0.281, 0.636)	0.937 (0.903, 0.962)	7.201 (4.057, 12.780)	0.582 (0.426, 0.796)	0.441 (0.272, 0.621)	0.940 (0.907, 0.964)	0.391
26	0.885 (0.840, 0.930)	0.515 (0.335, 0.692)	0.940 (0.907, 0.964)	8.614 (4.936, 15.035)	0.516 (0.362, 0.734)	0.456 (0.243, 0.656)	0.946 (0.915, 0.969)	0.455

* See Table A1 for specifications of empirical formulas. Areas under the receiver operating characteristic curve (AUC), confident interval (CI), positive likelihood ratio (+LR), negative likelihood ratios (−LR), positive predictive values (+PV), negative predictive values (−PV).

Table A7. Prediction performance of the three-parameter mixed-effects logistic model with covariance when combined with the 26 estimated fetal weight empirical formulas* in predicting large for gestational age.

Formulas	AUC (95% CI)	Sensitivity (95% CI)	Specificity (95% CI)	+LR (95% CI)	−LR (95% CI)	+PV (95% CI)	−PV (95% CI)	Youden's index
1	0.868 (0.814, 0.922)	0.455 (0.281, 0.636)	0.934 (0.899, 0.959)	6.841 (3.889, 12.034)	0.584 (0.427, 0.799)	0.429 (0.263, 0.606)	0.940 (0.907, 0.964)	0.388
2	0.867 (0.812, 0.922)	0.455 (0.281, 0.636)	0.940 (0.907, 0.964)	7.601 (4.241, 13.622)	0.580 (0.424, 0.793)	0.454 (0.281, 0.636)	0.940 (0.907, 0.964)	0.395
3	0.867 (0.811, 0.923)	0.515 (0.335, 0.692)	0.940 (0.907, 0.964)	8.614 (4.936, 15.035)	0.516 (0.362, 0.734)	0.456 (0.243, 0.656)	0.946 (0.915, 0.969)	0.455
4	0.868 (0.814, 0.922)	0.455 (0.281, 0.636)	0.937 (0.903, 0.962)	7.201 (4.057, 12.780)	0.582 (0.426, 0.796)	0.441 (0.272, 0.621)	0.940 (0.907, 0.964)	0.391
5	0.868 (0.812, 0.923)	0.455 (0.281, 0.636)	0.940 (0.907, 0.964)	7.601 (4.241, 13.622)	0.580 (0.424, 0.793)	0.454 (0.281, 0.636)	0.940 (0.907, 0.964)	0.395
6	0.873 (0.818, 0.927)	0.545 (0.364, 0.719)	0.944 (0.911, 0.967)	9.658 (5.533, 16.856)	0.482 (0.331, 0.701)	0.514 (0.340, 0.686)	0.950 (0.919, 0.972)	0.489
7	0.891 (0.839, 0.944)	0.455 (0.281, 0.636)	0.940 (0.907, 0.964)	7.601 (4.241, 13.622)	0.580 (0.424, 0.793)	0.454 (0.281, 0.636)	0.940 (0.907, 0.964)	0.395
8	0.876 (0.820, 0.932)	0.485 (0.308, 0.665)	0.947 (0.915, 0.969)	9.121 (5.044, 16.495)	0.544 (0.390, 0.758)	0.500 (0.319, 0.681)	0.944 (0.911, 0.967)	0.432
9	0.894 (0.854, 0.934)	0.455 (0.281, 0.636)	0.937 (0.903, 0.962)	7.201 (4.057, 12.780)	0.582 (0.426, 0.796)	0.441 (0.272, 0.621)	0.940 (0.907, 0.964)	0.391
10	0.886 (0.846, 0.927)	0.455 (0.281, 0.636)	0.934 (0.899, 0.959)	6.841 (3.889, 12.034)	0.584 (0.427, 0.799)	0.429 (0.263, 0.606)	0.940 (0.907, 0.964)	0.388
11	0.895 (0.856, 0.935)	0.485 (0.308, 0.665)	0.940 (0.907, 0.964)	8.108 (4.587, 14.330)	0.548 (0.393, 0.764)	0.471 (0.298, 0.649)	0.943 (0.911, 0.967)	0.425
12	0.891 (0.849, 0.933)	0.515 (0.335, 0.692)	0.950 (0.919, 0.972)	10.337 (5.707, 18.724)	0.510 (0.359, 0.726)	0.465 (0.255, 0.664)	0.947 (0.915, 0.969)	0.465
13	0.890 (0.849, 0.932)	0.455 (0.281, 0.636)	0.940 (0.907, 0.964)	7.601 (4.241, 13.622)	0.580 (0.424, 0.793)	0.454 (0.281, 0.636)	0.940 (0.907, 0.964)	0.395
14	0.886 (0.845, 0.926)	0.485 (0.308, 0.665)	0.940 (0.907, 0.964)	8.108 (4.587, 14.330)	0.548 (0.393, 0.764)	0.471 (0.298, 0.649)	0.943 (0.911, 0.967)	0.425
15	0.892 (0.852, 0.931)	0.455 (0.281, 0.636)	0.944 (0.911, 0.967)	8.048 (4.443, 14.578)	0.578 (0.423, 0.790)	0.469 (0.291, 0.653)	0.940 (0.907, 0.964)	0.398
16	0.883 (0.842, 0.924)	0.485 (0.308, 0.665)	0.937 (0.903, 0.962)	7.681 (4.389, 13.441)	0.550 (0.394, 0.767)	0.457 (0.288, 0.634)	0.943 (0.911, 0.967)	0.422
17	0.861 (0.803, 0.919)	0.424 (0.255, 0.608)	0.937 (0.903, 0.962)	6.721 (4.728, 12.117)	0.615 (0.458, 0.825)	0.424 (0.255, 0.608)	0.937 (0.903, 0.962)	0.361
18	0.871 (0.818, 0.924)	0.455 (0.281, 0.636)	0.934 (0.899, 0.959)	6.841 (3.889, 12.034)	0.584 (0.427, 0.780)	0.429 (0.263, 0.606)	0.940 (0.907, 0.964)	0.388
19	0.887 (0.841, 0.933)	0.485 (0.308, 0.665)	0.940 (0.907, 0.964)	8.108 (4.587, 14.330)	0.548 (0.393, 0.764)	0.471 (0.298, 0.649)	0.943 (0.911, 0.967)	0.425
20	0.892 (0.853, 0.932)	0.515 (0.335, 0.692)	0.944 (0.911, 0.967)	9.121 (5.168, 16.099)	0.514 (0.361, 0.731)	0.500 (0.247, 0.659)	0.947 (0.915, 0.969)	0.459
21	0.890 (0.850, 0.931)	0.455 (0.281, 0.636)	0.937 (0.903, 0.962)	7.201 (4.057, 12.780)	0.582 (0.426, 0.796)	0.441 (0.272, 0.621)	0.940 (0.907, 0.964)	0.391
22	0.884 (0.840, 0.929)	0.545 (0.364, 0.719)	0.944 (0.911, 0.967)	9.658 (5.533, 16.846)	0.482 (0.331, 0.701)	0.514 (0.340, 0.686)	0.950 (0.919, 0.972)	0.489
23	0.882 (0.836, 0.929)	0.485 (0.308, 0.665)	0.940 (0.907, 0.964)	8.108 (4.587, 14.330)	0.548 (0.393, 0.764)	0.471 (0.298, 0.649)	0.943 (0.911, 0.967)	0.425
24	0.887 (0.846, 0.929)	0.424 (0.255, 0.608)	0.934 (0.899, 0.959)	6.385 (3.572, 11.412)	0.617 (0.459, 0.828)	0.412 (0.246, 0.593)	0.937 (0.903, 0.961)	0.358
25	0.889 (0.847, 0.931)	0.485 (0.308, 0.665)	0.937 (0.903, 0.962)	7.681 (4.389, 13.441)	0.550 (0.394, 0.767)	0.457 (0.288, 0.634)	0.943 (0.911, 0.967)	0.422
26	0.885 (0.840, 0.930)	0.485 (0.308, 0.665)	0.940 (0.907, 0.964)	8.108 (4.587, 14.330)	0.548 (0.393, 0.764)	0.471 (0.298, 0.649)	0.943 (0.911, 0.967)	0.425

* See Table A1 for specifications of empirical formulas. Areas under the receiver operating characteristic curve (AUC), confident interval (CI), positive likelihood ratio (+LR), negative likelihood ratios (−LR), positive predictive values (+PV), negative predictive values (−PV).

Table A8. Prediction performance of the quadratic mixed-effects model without covariance when combined with the 26 estimated fetal weight empirical formulas* in predicting large for gestational age.

Formulas	AUC (95% CI)	Sensitivity (95% CI)	Specificity (95% CI)	+LR (95% CI)	−LR (95% CI)	+PV (95% CI)	−PV (95% CI)	Youden's Index
1	0.864 (0.810, 0.919)	0.455 (0.281, 0.636)	0.937 (0.903, 0.962)	7.201 (4.057, 12.780)	0.582 (0.426, 0.796)	0.441 (0.272, 0.621)	0.940 (0.907, 0.964)	0.391
2	0.867 (0.812, 0.922)	0.455 (0.281, 0.636)	0.937 (0.903, 0.962)	7.201 (4.057, 12.780)	0.582 (0.426, 0.796)	0.441 (0.272, 0.621)	0.940 (0.907, 0.964)	0.391
3	0.867 (0.811, 0.923)	0.455 (0.281, 0.636)	0.937 (0.903, 0.962)	7.201 (4.057, 12.780)	0.582 (0.426, 0.796)	0.441 (0.272, 0.621)	0.940 (0.907, 0.964)	0.391
4	0.868 (0.814, 0.922)	0.485 (0.308, 0.665)	0.940 (0.907, 0.964)	8.108 (4.587, 14.330)	0.548 (0.393, 0.764)	0.471 (0.298, 0.649)	0.943 (0.911, 0.967)	0.425
5	0.868 (0.812, 0.923)	0.455 (0.281, 0.636)	0.937 (0.903, 0.962)	7.201 (4.057, 12.780)	0.582 (0.426, 0.796)	0.441 (0.272, 0.621)	0.940 (0.907, 0.964)	0.391
6	0.873 (0.818, 0.927)	0.576 (0.392, 0.745)	0.950 (0.919, 0.972)	11.554 (6.510, 20.505)	0.446 (0.300, 0.665)	0.559 (0.379, 0.728)	0.953 (0.923, 0.974)	0.526
7	0.891 (0.839, 0.944)	0.455 (0.281, 0.636)	0.937 (0.903, 0.962)	7.201 (4.057, 12.780)	0.582 (0.426, 0.796)	0.441 (0.272, 0.621)	0.940 (0.907, 0.964)	0.391
8	0.876 (0.820, 0.932)	0.545 (0.364, 0.719)	0.947 (0.915, 0.969)	10.261 (5.806, 18.136)	0.480 (0.330, 0.698)	0.529 (0.351, 0.702)	0.950 (0.919, 0.972)	0.492
9	0.894 (0.854, 0.934)	0.455 (0.281, 0.636)	0.937 (0.903, 0.962)	7.201 (4.057, 12.780)	0.582 (0.426, 0.796)	0.441 (0.272, 0.621)	0.940 (0.907, 0.964)	0.391
10	0.886 (0.846, 0.927)	0.455 (0.281, 0.636)	0.937 (0.903, 0.962)	7.201 (4.057, 12.780)	0.582 (0.426, 0.796)	0.441 (0.272, 0.621)	0.940 (0.907, 0.964)	0.391
11	0.895 (0.856, 0.935)	0.455 (0.281, 0.636)	0.937 (0.903, 0.962)	7.201 (4.057, 12.780)	0.582 (0.426, 0.796)	0.441 (0.272, 0.621)	0.940 (0.907, 0.964)	0.391
12	0.891 (0.849, 0.933)	0.515 (0.335, 0.692)	0.944 (0.911, 0.967)	9.121 (5.168, 16.099)	0.514 (0.361, 0.731)	0.500 (0.247, 0.659)	0.947 (0.915, 0.969)	0.459
13	0.890 (0.849, 0.932)	0.485 (0.308, 0.665)	0.940 (0.907, 0.964)	8.108 (4.587, 14.330)	0.548 (0.393, 0.764)	0.471 (0.298, 0.649)	0.943 (0.911, 0.967)	0.425
14	0.886 (0.845, 0.926)	0.424 (0.255, 0.608)	0.930 (0.895, 0.956)	6.081 (3.429, 10.783)	0.619 (0.461, 0.831)	0.400 (0.239, 0.579)	0.936 (0.903, 0.961)	0.354
15	0.892 (0.852, 0.931)	0.485 (0.308, 0.665)	0.940 (0.907, 0.964)	8.108 (4.587, 14.330)	0.548 (0.393, 0.764)	0.471 (0.298, 0.649)	0.943 (0.911, 0.967)	0.425
16	0.883 (0.842, 0.924)	0.455 (0.281, 0.636)	0.937 (0.903, 0.962)	7.201 (4.057, 12.780)	0.582 (0.426, 0.796)	0.441 (0.272, 0.621)	0.940 (0.907, 0.964)	0.391
17	0.861 (0.803, 0.919)	0.485 (0.308, 0.665)	0.940 (0.907, 0.964)	8.108 (4.587, 14.330)	0.548 (0.393, 0.764)	0.471 (0.298, 0.649)	0.943 (0.911, 0.967)	0.425
18	0.871 (0.818, 0.924)	0.485 (0.308, 0.665)	0.943 (0.911, 0.967)	8.585 (4.805, 15.339)	0.546 (0.392, 0.761)	0.485 (0.308, 0.665)	0.943 (0.911, 0.967)	0.428
19	0.887 (0.841, 0.933)	0.515 (0.335, 0.692)	0.944 (0.911, 0.967)	9.121 (5.168, 16.099)	0.514 (0.361, 0.731)	0.500 (0.247, 0.659)	0.947 (0.915, 0.969)	0.459
20	0.892 (0.853, 0.932)	0.455 (0.281, 0.636)	0.937 (0.903, 0.962)	7.201 (4.057, 12.780)	0.582 (0.426, 0.796)	0.441 (0.272, 0.621)	0.940 (0.907, 0.964)	0.391
21	0.890 (0.850, 0.931)	0.485 (0.308, 0.665)	0.937 (0.903, 0.962)	7.681 (4.389, 13.441)	0.550 (0.394, 0.767)	0.457 (0.288, 0.634)	0.943 (0.911, 0.967)	0.422
22	0.884 (0.840, 0.929)	0.485 (0.308, 0.665)	0.940 (0.907, 0.964)	8.108 (4.587, 14.330)	0.548 (0.393, 0.764)	0.471 (0.298, 0.649)	0.943 (0.911, 0.967)	0.425
23	0.882 (0.836, 0.929)	0.485 (0.308, 0.665)	0.940 (0.907, 0.964)	8.108 (4.587, 14.330)	0.548 (0.393, 0.764)	0.471 (0.298, 0.649)	0.943 (0.911, 0.967)	0.425
24	0.887 (0.846, 0.929)	0.485 (0.308, 0.665)	0.940 (0.907, 0.964)	8.108 (4.587, 14.330)	0.548 (0.393, 0.764)	0.471 (0.298, 0.649)	0.943 (0.911, 0.967)	0.425
25	0.889 (0.847, 0.931)	0.515 (0.335, 0.692)	0.940 (0.907, 0.964)	8.614 (4.936, 15.035)	0.516 (0.362, 0.734)	0.456 (0.243, 0.656)	0.946 (0.915, 0.969)	0.455
26	0.885 (0.840, 0.930)	0.485 (0.308, 0.665)	0.940 (0.907, 0.964)	8.108 (4.587, 14.330)	0.548 (0.393, 0.764)	0.471 (0.298, 0.649)	0.943 (0.911, 0.967)	0.425

* See Table A1 for specifications of empirical formulas. Areas under the receiver operating characteristic curve (AUC), confident interval (CI), positive likelihood ratio (+LR), negative likelihood ratios (−LR), positive predictive values (+PV), negative predictive values (−PV).

Table A9. Prediction performance of the quadratic mixed-effects model with covariance when combined with the 26 estimated fetal weight empirical formulas* in predicting large for gestational age.

Formulas	AUC (95% CI)	Sensitivity (95% CI)	Specificity (95% CI)	+LR (95% CI)	−LR (95% CI)	+PV (95% CI)	−PV (95% CI)	Youden's index
1	0.865 (0.810, 0.919)	0.455 (0.281, 0.636)	0.937 (0.903, 0.962)	7.201 (4.057, 12.780)	0.582 (0.426, 0.796)	0.441 (0.272, 0.621)	0.940 (0.907, 0.964)	0.391
2	0.867 (0.812, 0.922)	0.455 (0.281, 0.636)	0.937 (0.903, 0.962)	7.201 (4.057, 12.780)	0.582 (0.426, 0.796)	0.441 (0.272, 0.621)	0.940 (0.907, 0.964)	0.391
3	0.867 (0.811, 0.923)	0.455 (0.281, 0.636)	0.934 (0.899, 0.959)	6.841 (3.889, 12.034)	0.584 (0.427, 0.799)	0.429 (0.263, 0.606)	0.940 (0.907, 0.964)	0.388
4	0.868 (0.814, 0.922)	0.485 (0.308, 0.665)	0.937 (0.903, 0.962)	7.681 (4.389, 13.441)	0.550 (0.394, 0.767)	0.457 (0.288, 0.634)	0.943 (0.911, 0.967)	0.422
5	0.868 (0.812, 0.923)	0.455 (0.281, 0.636)	0.937 (0.903, 0.962)	7.201 (4.057, 12.780)	0.582 (0.426, 0.796)	0.441 (0.272, 0.621)	0.940 (0.907, 0.964)	0.391
6	0.873 (0.818, 0.927)	0.576 (0.392, 0.745)	0.950 (0.919, 0.972)	11.554 (6.510, 20.505)	0.446 (0.300, 0.665)	0.559 (0.379, 0.728)	0.953 (0.923, 0.974)	0.526
7	0.891 (0.839, 0.944)	0.455 (0.281, 0.636)	0.937 (0.903, 0.962)	7.201 (4.057, 12.780)	0.582 (0.426, 0.796)	0.441 (0.272, 0.621)	0.940 (0.907, 0.964)	0.391
8	0.876 (0.820, 0.932)	0.515 (0.335, 0.692)	0.947 (0.915, 0.969)	9.691 (5.424, 17.316)	0.512 (0.360, 0.727)	0.515 (0.335, 0.692)	0.947 (0.915, 0.969)	0.462
9	0.894 (0.854, 0.934)	0.455 (0.281, 0.636)	0.937 (0.903, 0.962)	7.201 (4.057, 12.780)	0.582 (0.426, 0.796)	0.441 (0.272, 0.621)	0.940 (0.907, 0.964)	0.391
10	0.886 (0.846, 0.927)	0.455 (0.281, 0.636)	0.937 (0.903, 0.962)	7.201 (4.057, 12.780)	0.582 (0.426, 0.796)	0.441 (0.272, 0.621)	0.940 (0.907, 0.964)	0.391
11	0.895 (0.856, 0.935)	0.455 (0.281, 0.636)	0.937 (0.903, 0.962)	7.201 (4.057, 12.780)	0.582 (0.426, 0.796)	0.441 (0.272, 0.621)	0.940 (0.907, 0.964)	0.391
12	0.891 (0.849, 0.933)	0.515 (0.335, 0.692)	0.944 (0.911, 0.967)	9.121 (5.168, 16.099)	0.514 (0.361, 0.731)	0.500 (0.247, 0.659)	0.947 (0.915, 0.969)	0.459
13	0.890 (0.849, 0.932)	0.485 (0.308, 0.665)	0.940 (0.907, 0.964)	8.108 (4.587, 14.330)	0.548 (0.393, 0.764)	0.471 (0.298, 0.649)	0.943 (0.911, 0.967)	0.425
14	0.886 (0.845, 0.926)	0.424 (0.255, 0.608)	0.930 (0.895, 0.956)	6.081 (3.429, 10.783)	0.619 (0.461, 0.831)	0.400 (0.239, 0.579)	0.936 (0.903, 0.961)	0.354
15	0.892 (0.852, 0.931)	0.455 (0.281, 0.636)	0.940 (0.907, 0.964)	7.601 (4.241, 13.622)	0.580 (0.424, 0.793)	0.454 (0.281, 0.636)	0.940 (0.907, 0.964)	0.395
16	0.883 (0.842, 0.924)	0.455 (0.281, 0.636)	0.937 (0.903, 0.962)	7.201 (4.057, 12.780)	0.582 (0.426, 0.796)	0.441 (0.272, 0.621)	0.940 (0.907, 0.964)	0.391
17	0.861 (0.803, 0.919)	0.455 (0.281, 0.636)	0.937 (0.903, 0.962)	7.201 (4.057, 12.780)	0.582 (0.426, 0.796)	0.441 (0.272, 0.621)	0.940 (0.907, 0.964)	0.391
18	0.871 (0.818, 0.924)	0.485 (0.308, 0.665)	0.944 (0.911, 0.967)	8.585 (4.805, 15.339)	0.546 (0.392, 0.761)	0.485 (0.308, 0.665)	0.944 (0.911, 0.967)	0.428
19	0.887 (0.841, 0.933)	0.515 (0.335, 0.692)	0.944 (0.911, 0.967)	9.121 (5.168, 16.099)	0.514 (0.361, 0.731)	0.500 (0.247, 0.659)	0.947 (0.915, 0.969)	0.459
20	0.892 (0.853, 0.932)	0.455 (0.281, 0.636)	0.940 (0.907, 0.964)	7.601 (4.241, 13.622)	0.580 (0.424, 0.793)	0.454 (0.281, 0.636)	0.940 (0.907, 0.964)	0.395
21	0.890 (0.850, 0.931)	0.485 (0.308, 0.665)	0.937 (0.903, 0.962)	7.681 (4.389, 13.441)	0.550 (0.394, 0.767)	0.457 (0.288, 0.634)	0.943 (0.911, 0.967)	0.422
22	0.884 (0.840, 0.929)	0.485 (0.308, 0.665)	0.940 (0.907, 0.964)	8.108 (4.587, 14.330)	0.548 (0.393, 0.764)	0.471 (0.298, 0.649)	0.943 (0.911, 0.967)	0.425
23	0.882 (0.836, 0.929)	0.485 (0.308, 0.665)	0.940 (0.907, 0.964)	8.108 (4.587, 14.330)	0.548 (0.393, 0.764)	0.471 (0.298, 0.649)	0.943 (0.911, 0.967)	0.425
24	0.887 (0.846, 0.929)	0.485 (0.308, 0.665)	0.940 (0.907, 0.964)	8.108 (4.587, 14.330)	0.548 (0.393, 0.764)	0.471 (0.298, 0.649)	0.943 (0.911, 0.967)	0.425
25	0.889 (0.847, 0.931)	0.515 (0.335, 0.692)	0.944 (0.911, 0.967)	9.121 (5.168, 16.099)	0.514 (0.361, 0.731)	0.500 (0.247, 0.659)	0.947 (0.915, 0.969)	0.459
26	0.885 (0.840, 0.930)	0.485 (0.308, 0.665)	0.940 (0.907, 0.964)	8.108 (4.587, 14.330)	0.548 (0.393, 0.764)	0.471 (0.298, 0.649)	0.943 (0.911, 0.967)	0.425

* See Table A1 for specifications of empirical formulas. Areas under the receiver operating characteristic curve (AUC), confident interval (CI), positive likelihood ratio (+LR), negative likelihood ratios (−LR), positive.

References

1 Esakoff, T.F.; Cheng, Y.W.; Sparks, T.N.; Caughey, A.B. The association between birthweight 4000 g or greater and perinatal outcomes in patients with and without gestational diabetes mellitus. *Am. J. Obstet. Gynecol.* **2009**, *200*, e1–e4. [CrossRef] [PubMed]

2 Boulet, S.L.; Alexander, G.R.; Salihu, H.M.; Pass, M. Macrosomic births in the United States: Determinants, outcomes, and proposed grades of risk. *Am. J. Obstet. Gynecol.* **2003**, *188*, 1372–1378. [CrossRef] [PubMed]

3 Meshari, A.A.; De Silva, S.; Rahman, I. Fetal macrosomia—maternal risks and fetal outcome. *Int. J. Gynaecol. Obstet.* **1990**, *32*, 215–222. [CrossRef]

4. Zhang, J.; Kim, S.; Grewal, J.; Albert, P.S. Predicting large fetuses at birth: Do multiple ultrasound examinations and longitudinal statistical modelling improve prediction? *Paediatr. Perinat. Epidemiol.* **2012**, *26*, 199–207. [CrossRef]

5. Hadlock, F.P.; Harrist, R.B.; Carpenter, R.J.; Deter, R.L.; Park, S.K. Sonographic estimation of fetal weight. The value of femur length in addition to head and abdomen measurements. *Radiology* **1984**, *150*, 535–540. [CrossRef]

6. Liang, K.Y.; Zeger, S.L. Longitudinal data analysis using generalized linear models. *Biometrika* **1986**, *73*, 13–22. [CrossRef]

7. Melamed, N.; Yogev, Y.; Meizner, I.; Mashiach, R.; Bardin, R.; Ben-Haroush, A. Sonographic fetal weight estimation: Which model should be used? *J. Ultrasound Med.* **2009**, *28*, 617–629. [CrossRef]

8. Siemer, J.; Egger, N.; Hart, N.; Meurer, B.; Müller, A.; Dathe, O.; Goecke, T.; Schild, R.L. Fetal weight estimation by ultrasound: Comparison of 11 different formulae and examiners with differing skill levels. *Ultraschall Med.* **2008**, *29*, 159–164. [CrossRef]

9. Aviram, A.; Yogev, Y.; Ashwal, E.; Hiersch, L.; Hadar, E.; Gabbay-Benziv, R. Prediction of large for gestational age by various sonographic fetal weight estimation formulas - Which should we use? *J. Perinatol.* **2017**, *37*, 513–517. [CrossRef]

10. Pinheiro, J.C.; Bates, D.M. *Mixed Effects Models in S and S-Plus*, 1st ed.; Springer: New York, NY, USA, 2000; pp. 217–304.

11. Bakketeig, L.S.; Jacobsen, G.; Hoffman, H.J.; Lindmark, G.; Bergsjø, P.; Molne, K.; Rødsten, J. Pre-pregnancy risk factors for small-for-gestational age births among parous women in Scandinavia. *Acta. Obstet. Gynecol. Scand.* **1993**, *72*, 273–279. [CrossRef]

12. Loughna, P.; Chitty, L.; Evans, T.; Chudleigh, T. Fetal Size and Dating: Charts Recommended for Clinical Obstetric Practice. *Ultrasound* **2009**, *17*, 161–167. [CrossRef]

13. Davidian, M.; Giltinan, D.M. Nonlinear models for repeated measurement data: An overview and update. *J. Agric. Biol. Environ. Stat.* **2003**, *8*, 387. [CrossRef]

14. Zhou, Z.H. *Ensemble Methods: Foundations and Algorithms*, 1st ed.; Chapman & Hall: Boca Raton, FL, USA, 2012; pp. 67–98.

15. Ruta, D.; Gabrys, B. Classifier selection for majority voting. *Inf. Fusion* **2005**, *6*, 63–81. [CrossRef]

16. Ruta, D.; Gabrys, B. Analysis of the Correlation Between Majority Voting Error and the Diversity Measures in Multiple Classifier Systems. In Proceedings of the Soft Computing and Intelligent Systems for Industry, Proceedings of Fourth International ICSC Symposium, Paisley, Scotland, 26–29 June 2001; p. 2001.

17 Windeatt, T. Diversity measures for multiple classifier system analysis and design. *Inf. Fusion* **2005**, *6*, 21–36. [CrossRef]

18 Tibshirani, R. Regression Selection and Shrinkage via the Lasso. *J. R. Stat. Soc. B* **1996**, *58*, 267–288. [CrossRef]

19 Fan, J.; Li, R. Variable selection via nonconcave penalized likelihood and its oracle properties. *J. Am. Stat. Assoc.* **2001**, *96*, 1348–1360. [CrossRef]

20. Zhang, C.H. Nearly unbiased variable selection under minimax concave penalty. *Ann. Stat.* **2010**, *38*, 894–942. [CrossRef]

21. Wolpert, D.H. Stacked generalization. *Neural Netw.* **1992**, *5*, 241–259. [CrossRef]

22. Breiman, L. Stacked regressions. *Mach. Learn.* **1996**, *24*, 49–64. [CrossRef]

23. van der Laan, M.J.; Polley, E.C.; Hubbard, A.E. Super Learner. *Stat. Appl. Genet. Mol. Biol.* **2007**, *6*, e25. [CrossRef]

24. Debray, T.P.A.; Koffijberg, H.; Nieboer, D.; Vergouwe, Y.; Steyerberg, E.W.; Moons, K.G.M. Meta-analysis and aggregation of multiple published prediction models. *Stat. Med.* **2014**, *33*, 2341–2362. [CrossRef] [PubMed]

25. Campbel, S.; Wilkin, D. Ultrasonic measurement of fetal abdomen circumference in the estimation of fetal weight. *Br. J. Obstet. Gynaecol.* **1975**, *82*, 689–697. [CrossRef] [PubMed]
26. Jordaan, H. Estimation of fetal weight by ultrasound. *J. Clin. Ultrasound.* **1983**, *11*, 59–66. [CrossRef] [PubMed]
27. Warsof, S.L.; Gohari, P.; Berkowitz, R.L.; Hobbins, J.C. The estimation of fetal weight by computer-assisted analysis. *Am. J. Obstet. Gynecol.* **1977**, *128*, 881–892. [CrossRef]
28. Higginbottom, J.; Slater, J.; Porter, G.; Whitfield, C.R. Estimation of fetal weight from ultrasound measurement trunk circumference. *Br. J. Obstet. Gynaecol.* **1975**, *82*, 698–701. [CrossRef] [PubMed]
29. Woo, J.S.; Wan, C.W.; Cho, K.M. Computer-assisted evaluation of ultrasonic fetal weight prediction using multiple regression equations with and without the fetal femur length. *J. Ultrasound Med.* **1985**, *4*, 65–67. [CrossRef]
30. Warsof, S.L.; Wolf, P.; Coulehan, J.; Queenan, J.T. Comparison of fetal weight estimation formulas with and without head measurements. *Obstet. Gynecol.* **1986**, *67*, 569–573.
31. Vintzileos, A.M.; Campbell, W.A.; Rodis, J.F.; Bors-Koefoed, R.; Nochimson, D.J. Fetal weight estimation formulas with head, abdominal, femur, and thigh circumference measurements. *Am. J. Obstet. Gynecol.* **1987**, *157*, 410–414. [CrossRef]
32. Shepard, M.J.; Richards, V.A.; Berkowitz, R.L.; Warsof, S.L.; Hobbins, J.C. An evaluation of two equations for predicting fetal weight by ultrasound. *Am. J. Obstet. Gynecol.* **1982**, *142*, 47–54. [CrossRef]
33. Mirghani, H.M.; Weerasinghe, S.; Ezimokhai, M.; Smith, J.R. Ultrasonic estimation of fetal weight at term: An evaluation of eight formulae. *J. Obstet. Gynaecol. Res.* **2005**, *31*, 409–413. [CrossRef]
34. Shinozuka, N.; Okai, T.; Kohzuma, S.; Mukubo, M.; Shih, C.T.; Maeda, T.; Kuwabara, Y.; Mizuno, M. Formulas for fetal weight estimation by ultrasound measurements based on neonatal specific gravities and volumes. *Am. J. Obstet. Gynecol.* **1987**, *157*, 1140–1145. [CrossRef]
35. Combs, C.A.; Jaekle, R.K.; Rosenn, B.; Pope, M.; Miodovnik, M.; Siddiqi, T.A. Sonographic estimation of fetal weight based on a model of fetal volume. *Obstet. Gynecol.* **1993**, *82*, 365–370. [PubMed]
36. Ott, W.J.; Doyle, S.; Flamm, S.; Wittman, J. Accurate Ultrasonic Estimation of Fetal Weight: Prospective Analysis of New Ultrasonic Formulas. *Am. J. Perinatol.* **1986**, *3*, 307–310. [CrossRef] [PubMed]

8

Preoperative Health-Related Quality of Life Predicts Minimal Clinically Important Difference and Survival after Surgical Resection of Hepatocellular Carcinoma

Chong-Chi Chiu [1,2,3], King-Teh Lee [4,5], Jhi-Joung Wang [6], Ding-Ping Sun [2], Hao-Hsien Lee [1], Chien-Cheng Huang [7,8] and Hon-Yi Shi [5,9,10,*]

1 Department of General Surgery, Chi Mei Medical Center, Liouying 73657, Taiwan; chiuchongchi@yahoo.com.tw (C.-C.C.); hao_hsien@hotmail.com (H.-H.L.)
2 Department of General Surgery, Chi Mei Medical Center, Tainan 71004, Taiwan; sdp0127@gmail.com
3 Department of Electrical Engineering, Southern Taiwan University of Science and Technology, Tainan 71005, Taiwan
4 Division of Hepatobiliary Surgery, Department of Surgery, Kaohsiung Medical University Hospital, Kaohsiung 80708, Taiwan; ktlee@kmu.edu.tw
5 Department of Healthcare Administration and Medical Informatics, Kaohsiung Medical University, Kaohsiung 80708, Taiwan
6 Department of Medical Research, Chi Mei Medical Center, Tainan 71004, Taiwan; 400002@mail.chimei.org.tw
7 Department of Emergency Medicine, Chi Mei Medical Center, Tainan 71004, Taiwan; honyi6165@yahoo.com
8 Department of Senior Services, Southern Taiwan University of Science and Technology, Tainan 71005, Taiwan
9 Department of Business Management, National Sun Yat-sen University, Kaohsiung 80424, Taiwan
10 Department of Medical Research, Kaohsiung Medical University Hospital, Kaohsiung 80708, Taiwan
* Correspondence: hshi@kmu.edu.tw

Abstract: Despite the growing use of minimal clinically important difference (MCID) as a cancer outcome measure, no study has reported clinically significant outcomes in cancer patients. We defined MCID and evaluated the use of preoperative HRQoL for predicting MCID and survival after surgical resection of hepatocellular carcinoma (HCC). In total, 369 patients completed the Functional Assessment of Cancer Therapy-Hepatobiliary (FACT-Hep) and the SF-36 at baseline and at two years post-operative at three tertiary academic hospitals. The corresponding MCID values were 3.6 (SF-36 physical component summary), 4.2 (SF-36 mental component summary), 5.4 (FACT-General total score), and 6.7 (FACT-Hep total score). The predictors of achieving postoperative MCID were significantly higher in patients who had low preoperative HRQoL score, advanced age, high education level, and high BMI ($p < 0.05$). However, patients with a high preoperative HRQoL score, high education level, high BMI, and low Charlson comorbidity index score were significantly associated with survival ($p < 0.05$). Preoperative HRQoL scores were predictive of MCID and overall survival after surgical resection of HCC. The findings of this study may be useful for managing the preoperative expectations of candidates for HCC resection and for developing shared decision-making procedures for patients undergoing surgical resection of HCC.

Keywords: hepatocellular carcinoma; health-related quality of life; minimal clinically important difference; survival

---

1. Introduction

Hepatic resection is the mainstay curative treatment for patients with hepatocellular carcinoma (HCC), even in some patients with early-stage HCC [1–3]. Health-related quality of life (HRQoL) is a recognized indicator of healthcare outcomes and, since the 1990s, evaluations of cancer treatment outcomes have increasingly emphasized assessment of HRQoL [4,5]. Disease-specific and generic HRQoL measures are often reported together and provide complementary assessments of patient well-being before and after an intervention. It is important not to mix up the concept of quality of life with a recently growing area of HRQoL. Quality of life is an essential concept in the field of international development since it allows analysis of development on a measure broader than the standard of living [6,7]. Within development theory, however, there are varying ideas concerning what constitutes desirable change for a particular society, and the different ways that institutions define the quality of life, therefore, shapes how these organizations work for its improvement as a whole. The Functional Assessment of Cancer Therapy-Hepatobiliary (FACT-Hep) measure is one of the most widely used patient-reported questionnaires for measuring HRQoL in cancer research [8]. Unfortunately, research has shown that most of the studies that have used the FACT-Hep lack any reporting of clinical significance, even though guidelines for assessing clinical significance do exist.

A clinically important difference is a change that a patient or clinician would consider meaningful or worthwhile, such that an intervention or treatment would be considered worthy of repeating or such that patients would consider the change as an improvement in HRQoL. As such, measures of clinical significance such as the minimal clinically important difference (MCID) are increasingly used as a standard clinical outcome measure [6,7]. The MCID is defined as the smallest outcome change that the patient perceives as clinically important [9]. Despite the growing use of MCID as a cancer outcome measure, no study has reported clinically significant outcomes after surgical resection of HCC.

For cancer patients and their families, clinical data for HRQoL outcomes provide a useful indicator of the expected course of recovery and the expected effects of treatment. Thus, HRQoL data can help them make informed treatment decisions [10,11]. Baseline assessments of HRQoL have proven useful for predicting survival in various cancers, including colorectal, esophageal, breast, oropharyngeal, and lung cancers [10–13]. For varying severity of cancer, HRQoL has shown higher sensitivity compared to conventional prognostic indicators and compared to physician assessments [11,14]. Gotay et al. assessed the use of patient-reported HRQoL as a prognostic indicator of cancer outcomes [15]. Out of 39 clinical trials reviewed by the authors, 36 reported at least one HRQoL domain that was a significant predictor of survival. However, comparisons of results published in the literature are difficult because studies differ in the HRQoL measures applied and studied populations differ in patient attributes such as the type, site, and stage of disease [14–17]. Given the variability in reported overall survival rates and overall study heterogeneity, the evidence base for overall survival and determinants of overall survival after surgical resection of HCC are still evolving, and continued investigation is warranted.

A growing body of evidence indicates that preoperative functional status or HRQoL are important determinants of cancer surgery outcomes [14–17]. To the best of our knowledge, no prior study has systematically evaluated the role of preoperative HRQoL in achieving MCID and in overall survival after surgical resection of HCC. Therefore, the purpose of this study was to investigate the use of preoperative HRQoL scores for predicting achievement of MCID and for predicting overall survival after surgical resection of HCC.

2. Materials and Methods

2.1. Subjects and Data Collection

This study recruited all patients who had received surgical resection of HCC performed at one of three southern Taiwan medical centers between February 2013 and February 2017. For accurate assessment of postoperative outcome measures, the analysis was limited to patients who had received surgical resection performed by a director of surgery in a medical institution or by a senior attending doctor specializing in HCC surgery or treatment. Inclusion criteria were the following: (1) a histologic or combined radiographic and laboratory diagnosis of HCC, (2) ability to communicate in Chinese or Taiwanese, and (3) agreement to participate in a questionnaire survey performed in the hospital ward or by telephone. Major exclusion criteria included concurrent malignancy or participation in another quality-of-life study that might have interfered with this study. Figure 1 shows that, during the sample selection period, 496 subjects were eligible for participation. Of these, 62 were excluded due to benign tumor or cognitive impairment. Therefore, 369 subjects were assessed preoperatively (baseline) and at 2 years postoperatively. Baseline demographic and clinical data were collected through questionnaire surveys and medical records reviews. This study was approved by the Institutional Review Board of Chi Mei Medical Center (10002-L01).

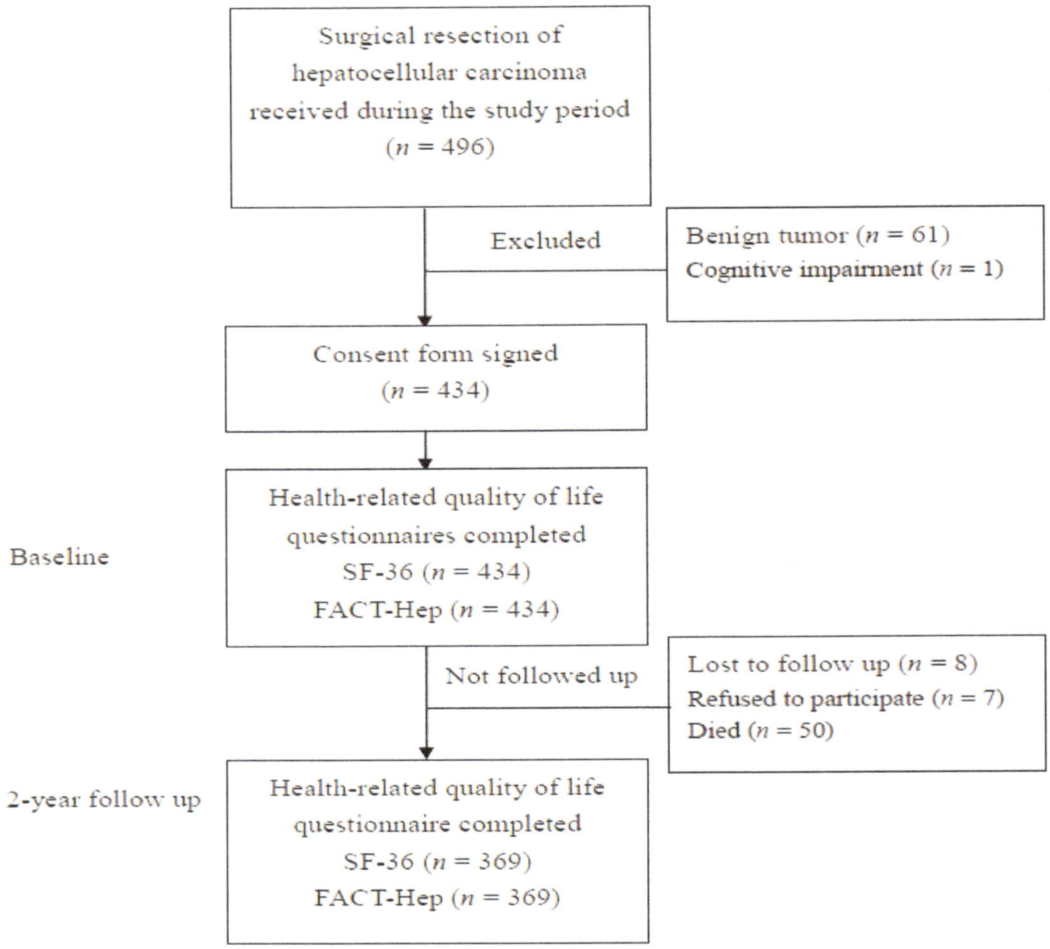

Figure 1. Flow chart showing population changes during the study, including subjects who met initial exclusion criteria, those who later declined to participate and those who lost to follow-up. SF-36: 36-Item Short Form Survey; FACT-Hep: Functional Assessment of Cancer Therapy-Hepatobiliary.

2.2. *Study Protocol*

Patients were asked to complete the questionnaires during follow-up visits at our outpatient clinic. To maximize compliance and minimize volunteer bias, a research assistant was available to help patients complete the questionnaires during each outpatient session. All HRQoL data were collected by the same research assistant. Patients were informed that their questionnaire responses would not be revealed to their attending surgeons and, hence, would not affect their treatment.

2.3. *Measures of HRQoL*

The Short Form-36 (SF-36) Health Survey measures eight dimensions: physical function, role limitation due to physical health, bodily pain, general health, vitality, social function, role limitation due to emotional health, and mental health. To compare the overall physical and mental functioning of the study population with those in the general Taiwan population, physical component summary scores (PCS) and mental component summary scores (MCS) were calculated by norm-based scoring methods and used as dependent variables [18]. Based on a previous study [19], the PCS and MCS were computed in comparison with the general population of Taiwan. Values below 50 indicated that the examined PCS or MCS were below the average values for the general Taiwan population, and vice versa.

The FACT-Hep measure contains five dimensions: physical well-being, social/family well-being, functional well-being, emotional well-being, and additional concerns. The subscales for the physical well-being, social/family well-being, and functional well-being dimensions each contained seven items with a subscale score range of 0–28 points; the subscale for emotional well-being contained six items with a subscale score range of 0–24 points; the subscale for additional concerns about HCC contained 18 items with a subscale score range of 0–72 points [8]. The Functional Assessment of Cancer Therapy-General (Fact-G) and additional concerns for HCC scores were summed to obtain the FACT-Hep total score, which ranged from 0 to 180. Higher scores on all FACT-Hep dimensions were interpreted as better HRQoL and fewer symptoms.

2.4. Statistical Analysis

Studies show that a distribution-based method can reliably derive MCID calculated as one-half the standard deviation (SD) in outcome score change from baseline to the two-year follow up for a given instrument in a patient cohort [9,20]. Therefore, this methodology was used to determine MCID values for the SF-36 PCS, SF-36 MCS, FACT-G total score, and FACT-Hep total score.

Multivariable logistic regression models were used to identify predictors of the achievement of MCID after surgical resection of HCC. A Cox multivariable proportional hazard regression model was also used to evaluate how other prognostic factors affect survival. Survival distribution was estimated by Kaplan–Meier method. Significant differences in survival probability were stratified by a log-rank test. Hazard ratios (HRs) and 95% confidence intervals (CIs) were estimated from regression coefficients.

Variables included in the multivariable analyses were gender, age, marital status, education, body mass index (BMI), Charlson co-morbidity index (CCI) score, co-residence with family, smoking, drinking, tumor stage, chemotherapy, radiotherapy, and average length of stay (ALOS). Multivariable analyses also included preoperative HRQoL score. Variables that fell out of the model were excluded from the tables of multivariable results. Statistical analyses were performed using SPSS software (IBM SPSS Statistics for Windows, Version 20.0, Armonk, NY, USA). All statistical tests were two tailed with a significance level of 0.05.

3. Results

3.1. Patient Demographics

The SF-36 and FACT-Hep measures were completed by 369 HCC surgery patients preoperatively and at two years postoperatively. We compared the patients who remained in the study throughout the two-year period with those who were lost or dead to follow up between the baseline and the second year after discharge. There was no difference in terms of gender, age, marital status, education, BMI, CCI score, co-residence with family, smoking, drinking, tumor stage, chemotherapy, radiotherapy, ALOS, or in any preoperative HRQoL parameters mentioned above (data not shown). Table 1 presents their demographic and clinical characteristics.

Table 1. Demographic and clinical characteristics of 369 patients with hepatic resection for hepatocellular carcinoma.

Variable		N (%) or Mean ± SD
Gender	Male	271 (73.4)
	Female	98 (26.6)
Age, years		60.2 ± 10.8
Marital status	Married	335 (90.8)
	Divorced or widowed	34 (9.2)
Education		8.7 ± 3.6
	No formal education	26 (7.1)
	Primary school	122 (33.1)
	Junior high school	75 (20.3)
	Senior high school	92 (24.9)
	College or above	54 (14.6)
Body mass index, kg/m^2		25.0 ± 3.5
	Normal (18.5~24.9 kg/m^2)	218 (59.1)
	Overweight (25.0~29.9 kg/m^2)	124 (33.6)
	Obese (≥30.0 kg/m^2)	27 (7.3)
Charlson co-morbidity index, score		1.6 ± 1.3
Co-residence with family	Yes	358 (97.0)
	No	11 (3.0)
Smoking	Yes	71 (19.2)
	No	298 (80.8)
Drinking	Yes	78 (21.1)
	No	291 (78.8)
Tumor stage	I	216 (58.6)
	II	102 (27.6)
	III	51 (13.8)
Chemotherapy	Yes	11 (3.0)
	No	358 (97.0)
Radiotherapy	Yes	5 (1.4)
	No	364 (98.6)
Average length of stay, days		13.0 ± 6.6

SD: standard deviation.

3.2. HRQoL Outcomes

The patients had a mean age of 60.2 ± 10.8 years, and 73.4% (271) patients were male. Table 2 shows that mean patient-reported HRQoL scores at two years after surgery were significantly higher than those before surgery ($p < 0.001$). The MCID values were 3.6 for the SF-36 PCS; 4.2 for the SF-36 MCS; 5.4 for the FACT-G total score; and 6.7 for the FACT-Hep total score.

Table 2. Mean ± standard deviation for SF-36 and Functional Assessment of Cancer Therapy-Hepatobiliary (FACT-Hep) before and after resection for hepatocellular carcinoma (n = 369) *.

Variable	Preoperative	2 Years Postoperative	2 Years Postoperative-Preoperative	p Value
SF-36 PCS	56.0 ± 8.7	61.7 ± 9.5	5.8 ± 7.2	$p < 0.001$
SF-36 MCS	48.5 ± 8.1	57.1 ± 9.8	8.5 ± 8.4	$p < 0.001$
FACT-G total	91.2 ± 10.4	98.7 ± 10.8	7.5 ± 10.9	$p < 0.001$
FACT-Hep total	156.9 ± 14.2	165.6 ± 15.8	9.7 ± 13.3	$p < 0.001$

* Both PCS and MCS scores were converted to obtain a mean of 50 and a standard deviation of 10 compared to the normal (nationwide) group. SF-36, 36-Item Short Form Survey; PCS, physical component summary; MCS, mental component summary; FACT-G, Functional Assessment of Cancer Therapy-General; FACT-Hep, Functional Assessment of Cancer Therapy-Hepatobiliary.

3.3. Multivariable Analyses

Multivariable analyses of HRQoL and survival were performed to identify predictors of the achievement of MCID after surgical resection for HCC. For each HRQoL measure, a high preoperative score negatively predicted achievement of MCID ($p < 0.001$) (Table 3). According to the SF-36 PCS data, the odds of achieving MCID were lower in males than in females (odds ratio (OR), 0.31; 95% CI, 0.12–0.83) but were higher in patients with advanced age (OR, 1.05; 95% CI, 1.01, 1.10), high education level (OR, 1.14; 95% CI, 1.01, 1.30), and high BMI (OR, 1.11; 95% CI, 1.09, 1.12) compared to their counterparts with young age, low education level, and low BMI, respectively. According to the SF-12 MCS data, the odds of achieving MCID were lower in patients with high BMI compared to those with low BMI (OR, 0.91; 95% CI, 0.84, 0.99); however, the odds of achieving MCID were higher in those with advanced age (OR, 1.01; 95% CI, 1.01, 1.02) and high CCI score (OR, 1.53; 95% CI, 1.13, 1.94) compared to their counterparts with young age and low CCI score, respectively. According to the FACT-G total data, the odds of achieving MCID were higher in patients with advanced age (OR, 1.04; 95% CI, 1.01, 1.07), high education level (OR, 1.12; 95% CI, 1.04, 1.21), and high BMI (OR, 1.19; 95% CI, 1.09, 1.29) compared to their counterparts with young age, low education level, and low BMI, respectively. According to the FACT-Hep total data, the odds of achieving MCID were higher in patients with advanced age (OR, 1.05; 95% CI, 1.02, 1.07), high education level (OR, 1.11; 95% CI, 1.03, 1.19), and high BMI (OR, 1.09; 95% CI, 1.01, 1.18) compared to their counterparts with young age, low education level, and low BMI.

Table 3. Odds of achieving minimal clinical important difference (MCID) in health-related quality of life according to multivariate logistic regression model *.

Variables	Odds Ratio (95% CI)	*p* Value
SF-36 PCS		
Preoperative SF-36 PCS score	0.90 (0.84, 0.96)	<0.001
Age	1.05 (1.01, 1.10)	0.041
Gender (male vs. female)	0.31 (0.12, 0.83)	0.019
Education	1.14 (1.01, 1.30)	0.040
Body mass index	1.11 (1.09, 1.12)	0.045
SF-36 MCS		
Preoperative SF-36 MCS score	0.80 (0.73, 0.88)	<0.001
Age	1.01 (1.01, 1.02)	<0.001
Body mass index	0.91 (0.84, 0.99)	0.034
Charlson co-morbidity index	1.53 (1.13, 1.94)	<0.001
FACT-G total		
Preoperative FACT-G total score	0.92 (0.90, 0.95)	<0.001
Age	1.04 (1.01, 1.07)	0.007
Education	1.12 (1.04, 1.21)	0.002
Body mass index	1.19 (1.09, 1.29)	<0.001
FACT-Hep total		
Preoperative FACT-Hep total score	0.97 (0.95, 0.98)	<0.001
Age	1.05 (1.02, 1.07)	0.001
Education	1.11 (1.03, 1.19)	0.007
Body mass index	1.09 (1.01, 1.18)	0.020

* The full model was adjusted for preoperative functional status, gender, age, marital status, education, body mass index, Charlson co-morbidity index, co-residence with family, smoking, drinking, tumor stage, chemotherapy, radiotherapy, and average length of stay. SF-36, 36-Item Short Form Survey; PCS, physical component summary; MCS, mental component summary; FACT-G, Functional Assessment of Cancer Therapy-General; FACT-Hep, Functional Assessment of Cancer Therapy-Hepatobiliary.

Multivariate analyses of each pre-operative HRQoL score showed that a high score was a positive predictor of overall survival (Table 4). Lower pre-operative HRQoL scores were significantly associated with post-operative morbidity ($p < 0.05$). Education level, BMI, and CCI also showed significant associations with overall survival ($p < 0.001$).

Table 4. Overall survival analysis by Cox multivariable proportional hazard regression model *.

Variable	HR (95% CI)	*p* Value
Preoperative SF-36 PCS score	1.05 (1.03, 1.08)	<0.001
Preoperative SF-36 MCS score	1.03 (1.01, 1.05)	<0.001
Preoperative SF-36 physical function	1.06 (1.01, 1.10)	<0.001
Preoperative SF-36 role physical	1.03 (1.00, 1.05)	<0.001
Preoperative SF-36 bodily pain	1.02 (1.01, 1.03)	0.008
Preoperative SF-36 general health	1.07 (1.01, 1.14)	<0.001
Preoperative SF-36 vitality	1.02 (1.01, 1.04)	0.001
Preoperative SF-36 social function	1.02 (1.01, 1.03)	0.003
Preoperative SF-36 role emotional	1.04 (1.01, 1.06)	<0.001
Preoperative SF-36 mental health	1.03 (1.00, 1.05)	<0.001
Preoperative FACT physical well-being	1.04 (1.00, 1.07)	<0.001
Preoperative FACT social/family well-being	1.01 (1.01, 1.02)	0.010
Preoperative FACT functional well-being	1.03 (1.01, 1.06)	<0.001
Preoperative FACT emotional well-being	1.03 (1.01, 1.05)	<0.001
Preoperative FACT additional concerns	1.02 (1.00, 1.04)	<0.001
Preoperative FACT-G total score	1.07 (1.01, 1.14)	<0.001
Preoperative FACT-Hep total score	1.10 (1.02, 1.19)	<0.001
Education	1.10 (1.02, 1.18)	0.012
Body mass index	1.02 (1.01, 1.04)	0.002
Charlson co-morbidity index	0.83 (0.70, 0.99)	0.040

* The full model was adjusted for preoperative functional status, gender, age, marital status, education, body mass index, Charlson co-morbidity index, co-residence with family, smoking, drinking, tumor stage, chemotherapy, radiotherapy, and average length of stay. SF-36, 36-Item Short Form Survey; PCS, physical component summary; MCS, mental component summary; FACT-G, Functional Assessment of Cancer Therapy-General; FACT-Hep, Functional Assessment of Cancer Therapy-Hepatobiliary; HR, hazard ratio; CI, confidence interval.

4. Discussion

This study investigated how patient-reported preoperative HRQoL affects two outcomes of surgical resection of HCC: MCID and overall survival. Multivariate analyses showed that each preoperative HRQoL score was predictive of both MCID and overall survival. Low preoperative HRQoL score, advanced age, high education level, and high BMI were significantly associated with achievement of postoperative MCID ($p < 0.05$). Additionally, high preoperative HRQoL score, high education level, high BMI, and low CCI had significant positive associations overall survival ($p < 0.05$). It demonstrates that, at baseline, preoperative HRQoL scores relates to postoperative mortality. Lower scores in physical and functional domains are associated with an increased risk of postoperative mortality. The importance of preoperative HRQoL scores for predicting outcomes of surgical resection in HCC patients is now well recognized [9,21]. The current study found that, for a given HRQoL outcome measure, a high preoperative score was significantly for not achieving a postoperative MCID in the outcome measure. The likely explanation for this finding is that patients who already have high HRQoL scores before surgery and less potential for achieving a HRQoL score improvement that meets the criteria for an MCID.

This study aimed to calculate and report the MCID value of commonly used HRQoL scales. Changes in HRQoL by time and/or treatment may not correlate with the direction (positive vs. negative) as well as the magnitude of clinical improvements in outcomes as they are perceived by the patients. Furthermore, cancer treatment has a more significant impact on HRQoL among HCC surgical patients. The MCID for (SF-36 PCS, SF-36 MCS, and FACT-G total score) value changes differed across domains, and they differed for perceived improvement and deterioration. We knew that domain scores related to physical function diminished from pre-treatment to on- or immediately after treatment, and emotional function improved. Additionally, the initial anxiety of the diagnosis and treatment initiation period may have been ameliorated by subsequent familiarity and supportive psychosocial care provided by the clinical service teams after patients finished the initial questionnaire. Thus, this might explain why those patients with a low preoperative score did achieve a postoperative MCID in the outcome measure and regarded as "efficacy" when compared with that achieved by those patients who had full pre-operative familiarity and mental support and thus noted with a high preoperative score.

The significant associations revealed by the HRQoL instruments investigated in this study underscore the relationship between HRQoL measures and medical outcomes. The study showed that preoperative HRQoL scores accurately predict postoperative MCID and overall survival, which is consistent with the literature [11,15,17]. Therefore, counseling is essential for apprising HCC resection candidates of expected postoperative improvements and impairments. If medical outcomes are considered benchmarks, then the preoperative HRQoL score, which is an important predictor of postoperative MCID and overall survival, is crucial.

Until now, no studies have described the implications of significant changes in disease-specific and generic HRQoL outcome measures in patients who have undergone HCC surgery. Steel et al. evaluated the clinical meaningfulness of FACT-Hep scores in HCC patients [22]. The authors combined distribution-based analyses with cross-sectional anchor-based analyses to obtain minimally important differences (MIDs) in FACT-G subscale scores (2–3 points), FACT-G total scores (6–7 points), Hepatobiliary Cancer Subscale scores (MID 5–6 points), and FACT-Hep scores (MID 8–9 points). However, data for clinically significant improvements in HCC surgery outcomes, particularly patient-reported outcomes, are very limited [4–6]. For patients who undergo surgical resection of HCC, the current study obtained MCID values of 3.6 for SF-36 PCS; 4.2 for SF-36 MCS; 5.4 for FACT-G total score; and 6.7 for FACT-Hep total score. These data are a novel addition to the literature and provide a useful reference for further studies of HRQoL outcomes after surgical resection of HCC. Notably, this study used patient-reported data for the period from before surgery until two years after surgery. A distribution-based method was used to calculate MCID. Since MCID values may change depending on the time point studied and the psychometric method used for analysis, further studies are needed to investigate MCID after surgical resection of HCC using different time points and mixed anchor/distribution-based methods of deriving MCID values.

The evidence base for overall survival after surgical resection of HCC is growing but is still relatively limited. The overall survival rates reported in the literature are somewhat variable, and the studied populations have been heterogeneous. Quinten et al. investigated the prognostic relationship between HRQoL and survival in a dataset for 30 randomized controlled trials performed by the European Organization for Research and Treatment of Cancer [11]. Their study showed that, in each cancer site, at least one HRQoL domain had an additive prognostic value that exceeded the prognostic values of clinical and sociodemographic variables. A systematic literature review by Quinten et al. confirmed that baseline HRQoL and at least one HRQoL domain were significantly associated with overall survival [11]. The current study found that preoperative HRQoL scores, education level, and BMI had significant positive associations with overall survival ($p < 0.05$) whereas CCI score had a significant negative association with overall survival ($p < 0.05$).

The HRQoL factors identified in this study varied from those in previous studies [9,20,22]. One possible explanation is differences in study populations. Our study focused on patients in both early and advanced stages of HCC whereas previous studies have only focused on patients in advanced stages of the disease. Secondly, patients with different cultural backgrounds may have different perceptions of HRQoL. Thirdly, patients in recent studies have more treatment options compared to patients in earlier studies, which can result in different perceptions of the implications of HCC and thus different perceptions of HRQoL. Fourthly, even studies that use the same HRQoL measure may have very different data analysis methodologies.

The findings of this study have important implications for preoperative counseling of patients, management of patient expectations, and stratification of outcomes. Healthcare providers increasingly emphasize shared decision making and are now using predictive modeling to inform surgery patients about potential clinical outcomes and the likelihood of success [11,22]. The results of the present study suggest that healthcare providers should consider routinely administering HRQoL instruments preoperatively as screening tools and for informing shared decision-making strategies. Patients with low HRQoL scores can be referred for counseling to modify their outcome expectations or referred for targeted interventions to optimize their HCC resection outcomes.

Certain limitations of this study are noted. Firstly, the patient data were derived from a multi-institutional HCC registry containing data contributed by multiple surgeons. As such, other than institutional best practices, surgical techniques and rehabilitation protocols were not standardized. However, since patient-reported HRQoL outcomes were obtained at the time of each clinical encounter, the reports of functional status are assumedly accurate. Another limitation is that sensitivity of the MCID values was not analyzed. The MCID can be calculated according to a consensus of or by using an anchor-based method or a distribution-based method [9,23]. Each methodology for deriving MCID has its associated pitfalls, and none has consistently proven to be superior. The applied methodology should be selected according to the characteristics of the data and the disease under study [23]. Additionally, the role of the FACT-Hep for assessing outcomes after surgical resection of HCC has not been robustly studied or validated. As such, the responsiveness of the HRQoL outcomes for this population subset is not clear; for example, the reliability (and change over time) of emotional, psychological, and social responses after surgical resection of HCC needs further study.

5. Conclusions

In conclusion, this study revealed that HRQoL scores are independent predictors of MCID and overall survival after surgical resection of HCC. The MCID values were 3.6 for the SF-36 PCS; 4.2 for the SF-36 MCS; 5.4 for the FACT-G total score; and 6.7 for the FACT-Hep total score. The findings of this study may be useful for preoperative management of patient expectations and for developing shared decision-making measures for patients undergoing surgical resection of HCC.

Author Contributions: Study concept and design: C.-C.C., and H.-Y.S.; acquisition of data: K.-T.L., J.-J.W., D.-P.S., H.-H.L., and C.-C.H.; analysis and interpretation of data: C.-C.C., and H.-Y.S.; drafting of the manuscript: C.-C.C., and H.-Y.S.; revised the manuscript: K.-T.L., J.-J.W., D.-P.S., H.-H.L., and C.-C.H.; approved the manuscript: all authors.

Acknowledgments: We thank all the individuals who participated in this study, without which this study would not have been possible.

References

1. Dhir, M.; Melin, A.A.; Douaiher, J.; Lin, C.; Zhen, W.K.; Hussain, S.M.; Geschwind, J.F.; Doyle, M.B.; Abou-Alfa, G.K.; Are, C. A Review and update of treatment options and controversies in the management of hepatocellular carcinoma. *Ann. Surg.* **2016**, *263*, 1112–1125. [CrossRef]
2. Robertson, F.P.; Fuller, B.J.; Davidson, B.R. An evaluation of ischaemic preconditioning as a method of reducing ischaemia reperfusion injury in liver surgery and transplantation. *J. Clin. Med.* **2017**, *6*, 69. [CrossRef] [PubMed]
3. Glantzounis, G.K.; Paliouras, A.; Stylianidi, M.C.; Milionis, H.; Tzimas, P.; Roukos, D.; Pentheroudakis, G.; Felekouras, E. The role of liver resection in the management of intermediate and advanced stage hepatocellular carcinoma. A systematic review. *Eur. J. Surg. Oncol.* **2018**, *44*, 195–208. [CrossRef]
4. Nishikawa, H.; Enomoto, H.; Yoh, K.; Iwata, Y.; Sakai, Y.; Kishino, K.; Ikeda, N.; Takashima, T.; Aizawa, N.; Takata, R.; et al. Health-related quality of life after treatment for bladder cancer in England. *J. Clin. Med.* **2018**, *7*, 553. [CrossRef] [PubMed]

5. Chiu, C.C.; Lee, K.T.; Wang, J.J.; Sun, D.P.; Lee, H.H.; Shi, H.Y. Health-related quality of life before and after surgical resection of hepatocellular carcinoma: A prospective study. *Asian Pac. J. Cancer Prev.* **2018**, *19*, 65–72.
6. Shapiro, C.L. Highlights of recent findings on quality-of-life management for patients with cancer and their survivors. *JAMA Oncol.* **2016**, *2*, 1401–1402. [CrossRef]
7. Costa, D.S. Reflective, causal, and composite indicators of quality of life: A conceptual or an empirical distinction? *Qual. Life Res.* **2015**, *24*, 2057–2065. [CrossRef]
8. Heffernan, N.; Cella, D.; Webster, K.; Odom, L.; Martone, M.; Passik, S.; Bookbinder, M.; Fong, Y.; Jarnagin, W.; Blumgart, L. Measuring health-related quality of life in patients with hepatobiliary cancers: The functional assessment of cancer therapy-hepatobiliary questionnaire. *J. Clin. Oncol.* **2002**, *20*, 2229–2239. [CrossRef] [PubMed]
9. Jayadevappa, R.; Cook, R.; Chhatre, S. Minimal important difference to infer changes in health-related quality of life-a systematic review. *Clin. Epidemiol.* **2017**, *89*, 188–198. [CrossRef]
10. Quinten, C.; Martinelli, F.; Coens, C.; Sprangers, M.A.; Ringash, J.; Gotay, C.; Bjordal, K.; Greimel, E.; Reeve, B.B.; Maringwa, J.; et al. A global analysis of multitrial data investigating quality of life and symptoms as prognostic factors for survival in different tumor sites. *Cancer* **2014**, *120*, 302–311. [CrossRef]
11. Quinten, C.; Coens, C.; Mauer, M.; Comte, S.; Sprangers, M.A.; Cleeland, C.; Osoba, D.; Bjordal, K.; Bottomley, A.; EORTC Clinical Groups. Baseline quality of life as a prognostic indicator of survival: A meta-analysis of individual patient data from EORTC clinical trials. *Lancet Oncol.* **2009**, *10*, 865–871. [CrossRef]
12. Grande, G.E.; Farquhar, M.C.; Barclay, S.I.; Todd, C.J. Quality of life measures (EORTC QLQ-C30 and SF-36) as predictors of survival in palliative colorectal and lung cancer patients. *Palliat. Support. Care* **2009**, *7*, 289–297. [CrossRef] [PubMed]
13. Dunne, D.F.; Jack, S.; Jones, R.P.; Jones, L.; Lythgoe, D.T.; Malik, H.Z.; Poston, G.J.; Palmer, D.H.; Fenwick, S.W. Randomized clinical trial of prehabilitation before planned liver resection. *Br. J. Surg.* **2016**, *103*, 504–512. [CrossRef] [PubMed]
14. Quinten, C.; Maringwa, J.; Gotay, C.C.; Martinelli, F.; Coens, C.; Reeve, B.B.; Flechtner, H.; Greimel, E.; King, M.; Osoba, D.; et al. Patient self-reports of symptoms and clinician ratings as predictors of overall cancer survival. *J. Natl. Cancer Inst.* **2011**, *103*, 1851–1858. [CrossRef] [PubMed]
15. Robinson, D.W.J.; Eisenberg, D.F.; Cella, D.; Zhao, N.; de Boer, C.; DeWitte, M. The prognostic significance of patient-reported outcomes in cancer clinical trials. *J. Clin. Oncol.* **2008**, *26*, 1355–1363.
16. Lin, S.; Hoffmann, K.; Schemmer, P. Treatment of hepatocellular carcinoma: A systematic review. *Liver Cancer* **2012**, *1*, 144–158. [CrossRef] [PubMed]
17. Pompili, C.; Salati, M.; Refai, M.; Berardi, R.; Onofri, A.; Mazzanti, P.; Brunelli, A. Preoperative quality of life predicts survival following pulmonary resection in stage I non-small-cell lung cancer. *Eur. J. Cardiothorac. Surg.* **2013**, *43*, 905–910. [CrossRef]
18. Ware, J.E.J.; Sherbourne, C.D. The MOS 36-item short-form health survey (SF-36). I. Conceptual framework and item selection. *Med. Care* **1992**, *30*, 473–483. [CrossRef]
19. Huang, I.C.; Wu, A.W.; Frangakis, C. Do the SF-36 and WHOQOL-BREF measure the same constructs? Evidence from the Taiwan population. *Qual. Life Res.* **2006**, *5*, 15–24. [CrossRef]
20. Blondel, B.; Schwab, F.; Ungar, B.; Smith, J.; Bridwell, K.; Glassman, S.; Shaffrey, C.; Farcy, J.P.; Lafage, V. Impact of magnitude and percentage of global sagittal plane correction on health-related quality of life at 2-years follow-up. *Neurosurgery* **2012**, *71*, 341–348. [CrossRef] [PubMed]
21. Doll, K.M.; Snavely, A.C.; Kalinowski, A.; Irwin, D.E.; Bensen, J.T.; Bae-Jump, V.; Boggess, J.F.; Soper, J.T.; Brewster, W.R.; Gehrig, P.A. Preoperative quality of life and surgical outcomes in gynecologic oncology patients: A new predictor of operative risk? *Gynecol. Oncol.* **2014**, *133*, 546–551. [CrossRef] [PubMed]
22. Steel, J.L.; Eton, D.T.; Cella, D.; Olek, M.C.; Carr, B.I. Clinically meaningful changes in health-related quality of life in patients diagnosed with hepatobiliary carcinoma. *Ann. Oncol.* **2006**, *17*, 304–312. [CrossRef] [PubMed]
23. McGlothlin, A.E.; Lewis, R.J. Minimal clinically important difference: Defining what really matters to patients. *JAMA* **2014**, *312*, 1342–1343. [CrossRef] [PubMed]

9

Postprandial Hypotension as a Risk Factor for the Development of New Cardiovascular Disease: A Prospective Cohort Study with 36 Month Follow-Up in Community-Dwelling Elderly People

Aelee Jang

Department of Nursing, University of Ulsan, 93, Daehak-ro, Nam-gu, Ulsan 44610, Korea; aeleejang@ulsan.ac.kr;

Abstract: Postprandial hypotension (PPH) is common among the elderly. However, it is unknown whether the presence of PPH can predict the development of new cardiovascular disease (CVD) in the elderly during the long-term period. This study aimed to prospectively evaluate the presence of PPH and the development of new CVD within a 36 month period in 94 community-dwelling elderly people without a history of CVD. PPH was diagnosed in 47 (50.0%) participants at baseline and in 7 (7.4%) during the follow-up period. Thirty participants (31.9%) developed new CVD within 36 months. We performed a time-dependent Cox regression analysis with PPH, hypertension, diabetes, and body mass index (BMI) as time-varying covariates. In the univariate analyses, the presence of PPH, higher BMI, hypertension, diabetes mellitus, and higher systolic and diastolic blood pressure were associated with the development of new CVD. The multivariate analysis indicated that the relationship between PPH and the development of new CVD remained (adjusted hazard ratio 11.18, 95% confidence interval 2.43–51.38, $p = 0.002$) even after controlling for other variables as covariates. In conclusion, the presence of PPH can predict the development of new CVD. Elderly people with PPH may require close surveillance to prevent CVD.

Keywords: cardiovascular disease; postprandial; hypotension; blood pressure; elderly

---

1. Introduction

Postprandial hypotension (PPH) is a common but often unrecognized disorder in the elderly [1]. PPH is defined as a ≥20 mmHg decrease in systolic blood pressure (SBP) within 2 h after a meal [2]. The prevalence of PPH is 20–91% in hospitalized geriatric patients [3–6]. The pathogenesis of PPH is unclear, but an inadequate cardiovascular response to postprandial splanchnic blood pooling is regarded as a primary mechanism [2]. In the elderly, sympathetic activation to decrease the effective circulating volume is often suppressed; hence, a continuous pooling of blood in the splanchnic bed may result in a significant decrease in blood pressure (BP) after a meal [7,8]. Changes in cardiovascular function and the neurohormonal response with aging can also contribute to diverse comorbidities associated with the dysregulation of BP homeostasis [9].

Cardiovascular diseases (CVDs), such as stroke, transient ischemic attack, angina, and myocardial infarction, are the main cause of mortality and work disability in the elderly [10,11]. Early recognition of subclinical risk factors is essential for the proper surveillance and prevention of new CVD. PPH is also recognized as an important clinical issue, particularly as a significant risk factor for subsequent CVD, but this has not yet been accurately confirmed [2,12]. Some studies have suggested an association between PPH and CVD and mortality [9,13]. However, it is difficult to determine the casual relationship between PPH and CVD development owing to differences in patient selection, study design, and diagnosis criteria among previous studies [9,14–16]. Furthermore, the diagnosis of PPH was heterogeneous in previous studies, such as with regard to the time interval between meal consumption and BP measurement [5]. Therefore, to investigate whether the presence of PPH can predict the development of new CVD in the elderly, this study aimed to prospectively evaluate the existence of PPH and the development of new CVD among community-dwelling elderly people in a period of 36 months.

2. Materials and Methods

2.1. Study Design and Participants

This prospective cohort study enrolled 94 participants from three senior community centers in South Korea between 2011 and 2015. The inclusion criteria were (1) age ≥65 years, (2) ability to eat independently and maintain a sitting position for 2 h after a meal, and (3) ability to perform activities of daily living independently. The exclusion criteria included (1) impaired cognitive function, (2) psychiatric illness, (3) recent hospitalization owing to acute illness within 1 month prior to the study, (4) medical history of CVD (congestive heart failure, myocardial infarction, angina, or cerebrovascular accidents, including transient ischemic attack), or (5) use of medications affecting gastrointestinal motility. After evaluating the presence of PPH at baseline, the new onset of PPH was evaluated during the follow-up period of 36 months. Body mass index (BMI) and the presence of hypertension and diabetes were also assessed regularly. This study was conducted following the guidelines of the Declaration of Helsinki of 1975, revised in 2013, and was approved by the institutional review board of Pusan National University Hospital (E-2014007), located in B city, South Korea. All participants provided written informed consent.

2.2. Evaluation of PPH and Acquisition of Demographic Data

BP was measured using an automated sphygmomanometer (A&D UA-851; A&D Company, Japan) following the European Society of Hypertension guidelines [17]. BP was measured by a well-trained nurse with the participant in a sitting position. Baseline BP was measured before a meal. Participants were asked to refrain from eating food, drinking coffee or alcohol, and smoking 4 h before measurement. All participants took any prescription medications after the evaluation of PPH, including antihypertensive drugs and hypoglycemic agents. BP was measured twice with a 5 min interval before a meal, and the average of the two measurements was used as the baseline BP. To measure postprandial BP, participants were provided the same standardized meal comprising 210 g rice, 100 g soup, and 70 g side dishes, which was approximately 500 kcal. After the participant consumed the meal, postprandial BP was measured every 15 min for 2 h. PPH was defined as a decrease in SBP of ≥20 mmHg from the baseline within 2 h after a meal [2]. We analyzed the reliability of measurements and found that the intraclass correlation coefficients (ICCs) for intra-rater reliability for SBP and diastolic blood pressure (DBP) were 0.995 (95% confidence interval (CI) 0.975–0.998, $p < 0.001$) and 0.989 (95% CI 0.942–0.996, $p < 0.001$), respectively.

Demographic and clinical information was also obtained by interviewing the participants using a questionnaire. Information on age, living conditions, alcohol intake, and smoking habits was collected, and information on medical history was obtained from hospital records after consent was obtained from the participants and their families. Bodyweight and height were measured using an automated measuring machine (G-Tech International Co., Ltd., Uijeongbu, Korea) to determine the BMI.

2.3. Surveillance of CVD Development

The primary endpoint was the occurrence of new CVD within 36 months. CVD in this study included coronary heart disease (such as congestive heart failure, angina, and myocardial infarction) and cerebrovascular disease (such as stroke and transient ischemic attack) according to the World Health Organization definition of CVD [18]. Participants were regularly followed every 3 months, and CVD-related information was obtained from them or their families during their visits to the centers or via telephone calls. If the participant was diagnosed with a new disease, additional information was also obtained from the medical record or prescription from the hospital at which the participant was diagnosed with new conditions, including the new onset of hypertension, diabetes, and CVDs.

2.4. Statistical Analysis

The reliability of BP measurements was calculated by determining the ICC (two-way random effects model). Variables are expressed as frequencies and percentages for categorical data, and means ± standard deviation for numerical data. Group differences were assessed using the chi-squared test or Fisher's exact test for categorical data and the independent t test or Mann–Whitney U test for numerical data as appropriate. To determine whether the distribution was normal, we used the Shapiro–Wilk test. Time to CVD was estimated using Kaplan–Meier curves. Survival curves were compared between groups using the log-rank test. Cox regression models with time-varying covariates were used to identify prognostic factors that were independently related to CVD. The main predictors were baseline PPH and PPH as a time-varying covariate (incorporating new onset PPH during the follow-up and duration of PPH as a time-varying covariate). In addition, hypertension, diabetes mellitus, and BMI were monitored during the follow-up period. These predicting variables were considered as time-varying covariates in time-dependent Cox regression models. All statistical analyses were performed using SPSS version 24.0 (IBM Corp., Armonk, NY, USA) and R version 3.5.1, and p-values <0.05 were considered statistically significant.

3. Results

3.1. Baseline Characteristics

The participants comprised 79 (84.0%) females and 15 (16.0%) males. The mean age was 73.1 ± 4.8 years, and the mean BMI was 23.7 ± 2.5 kg/m^2. Among the participants, 67 (71.3%) had lower than middle school education, and 62 (66.0%) were currently living with their family or spouse. The most common comorbidity was hypertension (50.0%), followed by diabetes mellitus (19.1%). At baseline, 47 (50%) participants were diagnosed with PPH, but there were no significant differences in baseline characteristics, with the exception of BP, between participants with and without PPH (Table 1).

Table 1. Baseline characteristics of participants with and without PPH.

Characteristics	Total (n = 94)	PPH (n = 47)	Non-PPH (n = 47)	p-Value
Age (years)	73.1 ± 4.8	73.6 ± 4.4	72.7 ± 5.1	0.355 [1]
Sex				0.778 [3]
Male	15 (16.0)	8 (17.0)	7 (14.9)	
Female	79 (84.0)	39 (83.0)	40 (85.1)	
Body Mass Index (kg/m^2)	23.7 ± 2.5	23.8 ± 2.7	23.5 ± 2.4	0.642 [2]
Education Level				0.509 [3]
Elementary School	67 (71.3)	36 (76.6)	31 (66.0)	
Middle School	13 (13.8)	5 (10.6)	8 (17.0)	
High School	14 (14.9)	6 (12.8)	8 (17.0)	
Living Status				1.000 [3]
Living Alone	32 (34.0)	16 (34.0)	16 (34.0)	
With Family or Spouse	62 (66.0)	31 (66.0)	31 (66.0)	
Alcohol Drinking				0.370 [3]
Yes	13 (13.8)	5 (10.6)	8 (17.0)	
No	81 (86.2)	42 (89.4)	39 (83.0)	
Smoking				1.000 [4]
Yes	4 (4.3)	2 (4.3)	2 (4.3)	
No	90 (95.7)	45 (95.7)	45 (95.7)	
Hypertension	47 (50.0)	26 (55.3)	21 (44.7)	0.302 [3]
Diabetes Mellitus	18 (19.1)	11 (23.4)	7 (14.9)	0.294 [3]
Baseline SBP (mmHg)	128.6 ± 20.2	140.1 ± 17.2	117.1 ± 16.1	<0.001 [2]
<120	34 (36.2)	6 (12.8)	28 (59.6)	<0.001 [3]
≥120 to <140	31 (33.0)	15 (31.9)	16 (34.0)	
≥140	29 (30.9)	26 (55.3)	3 (6.4)	
Baseline DBP (mmHg)	75.2 ± 9.9	78.7 ± 7.5	71.7 ± 10.9	<0.001 [2]
<80	64 (68.1)	23 (48.9)	41 (87.2)	<0.001 [3]
≥80	30 (31.9)	24 (51.1)	6 (12.8)	
Postprandial SBP Change (mmHg)				<0.001 [3]
<10	26 (27.7)	0 (0.0)	26 (55.3)	
≥10 to <20	21 (22.3)	0 (0.0)	21 (44.7)	
≥20	47 (50.0)	47 (100.0)	0 (0.0)	
Postprandial DBP Change (mmHg)				<0.001 [3]
<10	41 (43.6)	9 (19.1)	32 (68.1)	
≥10	53 (56.4)	38 (80.9)	15 (31.9)	

Values are either frequency with percentage in parentheses or mean ± standard deviation. PPH, postprandial hypotension; SBP, systolic blood pressure; DBP, diastolic blood pressure. [1] P values were derived from independent t tests. [2] P values were derived from Mann–Whitney's U test. [3] P values were derived using chi-square tests. [4] P values were derived using Fisher's exact test. Shapiro–Wilk's test was employed for test of normality assumption.

3.2. Incidence of CVD

During the follow-up, 30 (31.9%) patients developed new CVD, of whom 4 passed away owing to acute myocardial infarction (n = 2) and ischemic stroke (n = 2). The CVD incidence was significantly higher in the group with PPH than the group without PPH at baseline (55.3% vs. 8.5%, $p < 0.001$, Figure 1).

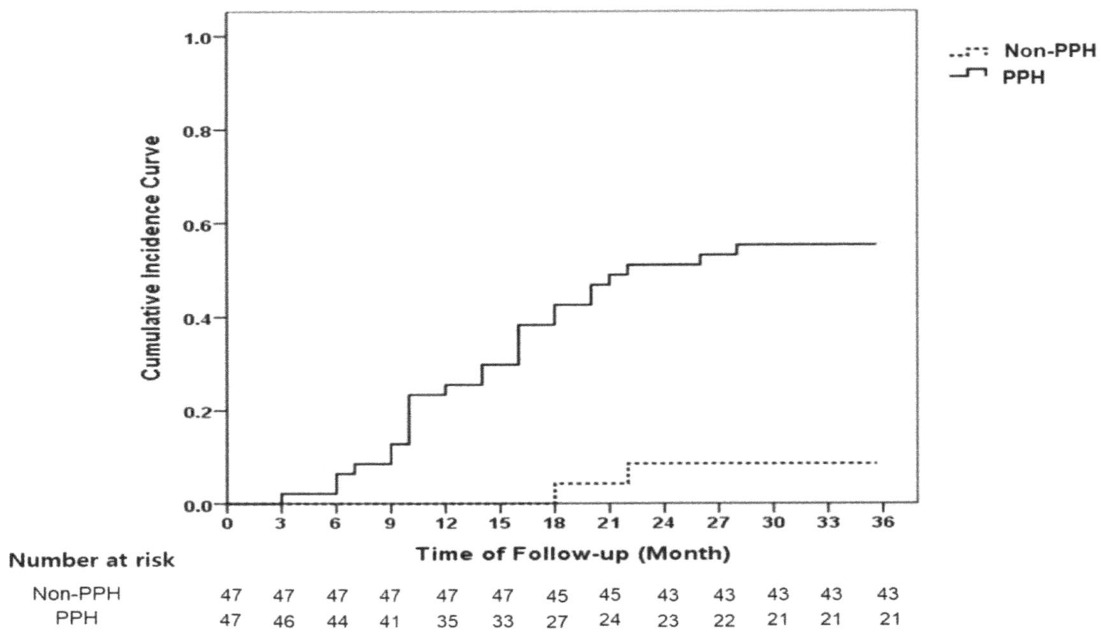

Figure 1. Kaplan–Meier curve of the incidence of new CVD between participants with and without PPH at baseline. The 3 year incidence of CVD was significantly higher in the group with PPH than in the group without PPH at baseline (55.3% vs. 8.5%, log-rank test, $p < 0.001$). PPH, postprandial hypotension; CVD, cardiovascular disease.

Table 2 indicates the differences between groups with respect to CVD development. The presence of PPH at baseline (86.7% in the CVD group vs. 32.8% in the non-CVD group, $p < 0.001$), higher BMI (24.5 ± 2.1 in the CVD group vs. 23.3 ± 2.7 in the non-CVD group), hypertension (66.7% in the CVD group vs. 42.2% in the non-CVD group), higher baseline SBP (139.3 ± 20.9 mmHg in the CVD group vs. 123.6 ± 17.9 mmHg in the non-CVD group), and higher baseline DBP (79.0 ± 8.6 mmHg in the CVD group vs. 73.4 ± 10.1 mmHg in the non-CVD group) were significantly related to the development of new CVD. The percentage of participants with an SBP change of ≥20 mmHg (86.7% vs. 32.8%, respectively, $p < 0.001$) and a DBP change of ≥10 mmHg (73.3% vs. 48.4%, respectively, $p = 0.023$) were significantly higher among participants who developed new CVD than among those who did not.

Table 2. Differences of characteristics between participants who developed and did not develop new CVD.

	Total (n = 94)	CVD (n = 30)	Non-CVD (n = 64)	p-Value
PPH				<0.001 [3]
Yes	47 (50.0)	26 (86.7)	21 (32.8)	
No	47 (50.0)	4 (13.3)	43 (67.2)	
Age (years)	73.1 ± 4.8	73.0 ± 4.1	73.2 ± 5.1	0.849 [1]
Sex				1.000 [4]
Male	15 (16.0)	5 (16.7)	10 (15.6)	
Female	79 (84.0)	25 (83.3)	54 (84.4)	
Body mass index (kg/m^2)	23.7 ± 2.5	24.5 ± 2.1	23.3 ± 2.7	0.013 [2]
Education level				0.534 [4]
Elementary school	67 (71.3)	24 (80.0)	43 (67.2)	
Middle school	13 (13.8)	3 (10.0)	10 (15.6)	
High school	14 (14.9)	3 (10.0)	11 (17.2)	
Living status				0.571 [3]
Living alone	32 (34.0)	9 (30.0)	23 (35.9)	
With family or spouse	62 (66.0)	21 (70.0)	41 (64.1)	

Table 2. *Cont.*

	Total (n = 94)	CVD (n = 30)	Non-CVD (n = 64)	p-Value
Alcohol drinking				0.336 [4]
Yes	13 (13.8)	6 (20.0)	7 (10.9)	
No	81 (86.2)	24 (80.0)	57 (89.1)	
Smoking				0.590 [4]
Yes	4 (4.3)	2 (6.7)	2 (3.1)	
No	90 (95.7)	28 (93.3)	62 (96.9)	
Hypertension	47 (50.0)	20 (66.7)	27 (42.2)	0.027 [3]
Diabetes mellitus	18 (19.1)	9(30.0)	9 (14.1)	0.067 [3]
Baseline SBP (mmHg)	128.6 ± 20.2	139.3 ± 20.9	123.6 ± 17.9	<0.001 [2]
<120	34 (36.2)	5 (16.7)	29 (45.3)	<0.001 [3]
≥120 to <140	31 (33.0)	7 (23.3)	24 (37.5)	
≥140	29 (30.9)	18 (60.0)	11 (17.2)	
Baseline DBP (mmHg)	75.2 ± 9.9	79.0 ± 8.6	73.4 ± 10.1	0.005 [2]
<80	64 (68.1)	15 (50.0)	49 (76.6)	0.010 [3]
≥80	30 (31.9)	15 (50.0)	15 (23.4)	
Postprandial SBP change (mmHg)				<0.001 [3]
<10	26 (27.7)	3 (10.0)	23 (35.9)	
≥10 to <20	21 (22.3)	1 (3.3)	20 (31.3)	
≥20	47 (50.0)	26 (86.7)	21 (32.8)	
Postprandial DBP change (mmHg)				0.023 [3]
<10	41 (43.6)	8 (26.7)	33 (51.6)	
≥10	53 (56.4)	22 (73.3)	31 (48.4)	

Values are either frequency with percentage in parentheses or mean ± standard deviation. PPH, postprandial hypotension; CVD, cardiovascular disease; SBP, systolic blood pressure; DBP, diastolic blood pressure. [1] P values were derived from independent t tests. [2] P values were derived from Mann–Whitney's U test. [3] P values were derived using chi-square tests. [4] P values were derived using Fisher's exact test. Shapiro–Wilk's test was employed for test of normality assumption.

3.3. *Predictive Factors for the Development of New CVD*

Ninety-four patients were available for the Cox regression models to assess the relationship between PPH and CVD using PPH as the time-varying covariate. There were 30 cases of CVD. We considered time-varying covariates, including PPH, hypertension, diabetes, and BMI, in the time-dependent Cox regression models. Among the 47 patients without PPH at baseline, 7 were diagnosed with PPH during the follow-up period. The main predictive factors were baseline PPH, with PPH as a time-varying covariate incorporating new onset PPH during follow-up, and the duration of PPH as a time-varying covariate. New onset hypertension and diabetes mellitus during the follow-up period were observed in 12 and 11 patients, respectively. In addition, BMI was measured at baseline, 1 year, and 2 years. All predictive variables were considered as time-varying covariates in time-dependent Cox regression models. In the univariate analyses, the presence of PPH, higher BMI, hypertension, diabetes mellitus, and higher SBP and DBP were found to be associated with the development of new CVD, while age, sex, education level, living status, alcohol consumption, and smoking were not. Patients with PPH were more likely to develop new CVD (crude hazard ratio (HR) 15.97, 95% CI 3.80–67.08, $p < 0.001$). The multivariate analysis that included significant factors in the univariate analyses as covariates revealed that the relationship between PPH and the development of new CVD remained (adjusted HR 11.18, 95% CI 2.43–51.38, $p = 0.002$) even after controlling for other variables as covariates in the multivariate analysis. Hypertension was also found to be a significant factor affecting CVD (adjusted HR 3.26, 95% CI 1.22–8.76, $p = 0.019$) (Table 3).

Table 3. Summary of time-dependent Cox regression analyses using time-varying covariates (a total of 94 subjects, 30 CVDs).

Characteristic	Univariate			Multivariate		
	HR	95% CI	*p*-Value	HR	95% CI	*p*-Value
PPH	15.97	3.80–67.08	<0.001	11.18	2.43–51.38	0.002
Age (years)	1.00	0.93–1.07	0.940			
Sex (female)	0.90	0.34–2.35	0.830			
BMI (kg/m^2)	1.14	1.01–1.29	0.030	1.10	0.96–1.26	0.173
Education level (vs. Elementary school)						
Middle school	0.61	0.19–2.04	0.430			
High school	0.57	0.17–1.88	0.350			
Living status (Living alone)	0.80	0.37–1.75	0.580			
Alcohol drinking	1.61	0.66–3.95	0.300			
Smoking	1.77	0.42–7.46	0.430			
Hypertension	4.61	1.77–12.05	0.002	3.26	1.22–8.73	0.019
Diabetes mellitus	3.20	1.56–6.56	0.002	1.80	0.84–3.89	0.132
Baseline SBP (mmHg)	1.03	1.02–1.05	<0.001	1.02	0.99–1.05	0.148
Baseline DBP (mmHg)	1.03	1.01–1.06	0.013	0.97	0.91–1.02	0.245

HR, hazard ratio; CVD, cardiovascular disease; BMI, body mass index; SBP, systolic blood pressure; DBP, diastolic blood pressure; PPH, postprandial hypotension.

4. Discussion

This study investigated the time-varying effect of PPH associated with new CVD in community-dwelling elderly people. The study indicated that approximately half (55.3%) of the participants with PPH developed new CVD within the 36 month follow-up period, whereas only 8.5% of participants without PPH developed CVD. After adjustment for other covariates, the time-varying effect of PPH on the development of new CVD was found to be significant (HR 11.18, 95% CI 2.43–51.38). These results suggest that elderly people with PPH were more likely to develop new CVD and, thus, required close surveillance.

The reported prevalence of PPH varies widely in previous studies depending on the patient population and diagnostic methods [5]. Studies of institutionalized elderly patients reported a PPH prevalence of 24–38% [3,4]. Meanwhile, the incidence of PPH among hospitalized geriatric patients was considerably high (up to 91%) [5,6]. However, studies investigating the incidence of PPH among healthy elderly people are relatively rare [19]. Unlike previous studies, the present study investigated PPH in relatively healthy elderly people who were not institutionalized or hospitalized. Although the study population comprised elderly patients, the PPH incidence was 50%, which seems to be slightly higher than that reported in previous studies. The development of PPH is highly dependent on meal composition. Carbohydrate-rich meals predispose patients to a more immediate decrease in BP than do meals containing primarily protein or fat [20]. Therefore, it is expected that PPH might be more prevalent in people from Asian regions owing to their carbohydrate-dominant diets. However, few studies have investigated PPH in Asian patients [21]. To date, this is the first prospective cohort study to investigate PPH and its association with CVD in relatively healthy Asian elderly people. In this study, a stringent diagnostic approach was used for PPH, such as provision of a standardized meal and more frequent BP measurements. Furthermore, in this study, variance in BP changes related to food composition was reduced by administering the same standardized meal to all participants. Therefore, this study may provide relevant insights into the epidemiology of PPH in Asian regions. Large cohort studies are recommended to further determine the prevalence of PPH in different patient populations using a standardized diagnostic method.

In this study, 30 (31.9%) participants developed new CVD during the 36 month follow-up. In one study on PPH as a predictor of new CVD [14], 40.8% of older nursing home residents developed CVD during a 29 month follow-up. The patients with new CVD exhibited a significantly greater decline in postprandial SBP than did those without ($p < 0.001$). The other previous study found a 59.2% occurrence of new CVD during a 4.7 year follow-up period in older low-level-care residents in long-term health facilities [9]. The occurrence of new CVD cases was lower in this study (31.9%) than in previous studies (40.1–59.2%) because this study was conducted in a relatively healthy cohort from a community setting. Furthermore, the previous studies did not fully exclude populations with a history of CVD. In contrast, this prospective study excluded people with a history of CVD to clearly demonstrate the relationship between PPH and CVD.

In this study, the presence of PPH, higher BMI, hypertension, diabetes mellitus, and higher SBP and DBP were predictive factors for the development of CVD in the univariate analysis using the time-dependent Cox proportional hazard model. After adjustment for these factors, the time-varying effect of PPH and hypertension on the occurrence of new CVD still remained in the elderly people. According to Aronow et al. [14], the mean maximal decrease in postprandial SBP was a significant risk factor for developing CVD. Similarly, in previous cross-sectional studies, PPH was considered an independent predictor of asymptomatic cerebrovascular damage in healthy participants and hospitalized patients with essential hypertension [15,16]. Despite the small sample size, this study is meaningful as a prospective cohort study for the risk factors of new CVD in the presence or absence of PPH among community-dwelling elderly people without a history of CVD.

The total mortality (7/94, 7.4%) and CVD-related mortality (4/94, 4.3%) rates in this study were relatively lower than those reported in previous studies (16.9–54.2%) [9,13,14]. Again, this is likely because this study included relatively healthy older adults (i.e., from a community setting) in contrast to previous studies, which generally included hospitalized geriatric patients or patients in nursing homes. The mean age of the participants in this study (73.1 years) was also relatively lower than that in previous studies (77.8–83.2 years) [9,13,14]. In a previous study of hypertensive elderly patients who were followed up at the cardiology clinic for 4 years, the total mortality rate was 16.9%, and a greater decrease in postprandial SBP was associated with a greater increase in CVD mortality. In that prospective study, CVD mortality constituted 50% of the total mortality rate, while PPH accounted for 52.9% of deaths owing to CVD [13], which was similar to the findings of the present study. In a study by Fisher et al. [9], PPH was the only risk factor for all-cause mortality, and 50% of deaths were attributed to CVD. Participants with a postprandial SBP difference of ≥20 mmHg had the lowest survival during the 4.7 year follow-up period. They also reported that PPH accounted for 47% of deaths in long-term healthcare facilities, which was lower than the 57.1% (4 of 7 deaths) found in the present study. Populations in long-term healthcare facilities typically require nursing care for monitoring and preventing serious diseases, including CVD. These perspectives may explain the difference in attributing the total mortality rate to CVD mortality between the present study and the previous study mentioned above [9]. Therefore, prevention and close monitoring are needed to reduce deaths due to new CVD by classifying patients diagnosed with PPH as high risk for CVD.

This study had some limitations. First, the sample size was relatively small. However, compared to previous studies, this study was conducted over a long-term follow-up with the time-varying effect of PPH. The post hoc power for investigating the primary objective of this study was approximately 99%. Second, despite efforts to recruit a similar ratio of males and females, the participants were predominantly female because of the higher proportion of elderly women in the Korean elderly population. Future studies should confirm CVD risk factors in sex-balanced populations with postprandial SBP reduction during long-term follow-up. Third, the level of physical activity was not considered in this study, which could affect the development of CVDs. Nevertheless, the participants had similar lifestyle patterns because they resided in the same town and enjoyed the same activity programs provided by the community welfare center. Therefore, their physical activity levels may be similar. Fourth, the pathophysiological relationship between PPH and CVD remains vague despite PPH being identified as an independent time-varying variable for the development of new CVD. Autonomic dysfunction may play a major role in the development of PPH-related new CVD because PPH has been reported to be pathologically associated with autonomic dysfunction. This needs further evaluation using animal models. Fifth, the positive association between PPH and CVD may only reflect the high baseline SBP on the risk of CVD because the baseline SBP level in the PPH group was much higher than that in the non-PPH group. Although hypertension was adjusted in the multivariate model, based on the small sample size, the effect of high baseline SBP may persist. As it is impossible to stratify the analysis by hypertension status at baseline, owing to the limited sample size, further research in the form of a well-designed, large-sample study in a normotensive elderly population is necessary to definitively establish the effect of PPH on the risk of CVD.

This study investigated the relationship between PPH and the development of new CVD in elderly people during a long-term follow-up period. The results also suggest that the underlying reason of CVD development could be the greater decline in postprandial SBP (such as that occurring in PPH). This study demonstrated that increases in SBP variations after a meal may be a manifestation of CVD development and may reflect the presence of subclinical cardiovascular damage.

5. Conclusions

This study revealed that PPH was an independent predictor of new CVD among community-dwelling elderly people during a 36 month follow-up. Thus, CVD development may be prevented or monitored based on the presence of PPH. However, longitudinal studies in larger samples are needed to clarify the prognostic significance of PPH in the development of new CVD.

References

1. Luciano, G.L.; Brennan, M.J.; Rothberg, M.B. Postprandial hypotension. *Am. J. Med.* **2010**, *123*, e1–e6. [CrossRef] [PubMed]
2. Jansen, R.W.; Lipsitz, L.A. Postprandial hypotension: Epidemiology, pathophysiology, and clinical management. *Ann. Intern. Med.* **1995**, *122*, 286–295. [CrossRef] [PubMed]
3. Aronow, W.S.; Ahn, C. Postprandial hypotension in 499 elderly persons in a long-term health care facility. *J. Am. Geriatr. Soc.* **1994**, *42*, 930–932. [CrossRef] [PubMed]
4. Le Couteur, D.G.; Fisher, A.A.; Davis, M.W.; McLean, A.J. Postprandial systolic blood pressure responses of older people in residential care: Association with risk of falling. *Gerontology* **2003**, *49*, 260–264. [CrossRef] [PubMed]
5. Van Orshoven, N.P.; Jansen, P.A.; Oudejans, I.; Schoon, Y.; Oey, P.L. Postprandial hypotension in clinical geriatric patients and healthy elderly: Prevalence related to patient selection and diagnostic criteria. *J. Aging Res.* **2010**, *2010*, 243752. [CrossRef] [PubMed]
6. Puisieux, F.; Bulckaen, H.; Fauchais, A.L.; Drumez, S.; Salomez-Granier, F.; Dewailly, P. Ambulatory blood pressure monitoring and postprandial hypotension in elderly persons with falls or syncopes. *J. Gerontol. A Biol. Sci. Med. Sci.* **2000**, *55*, M535–M540. [CrossRef]
7. Lipsitz, L.A.; Ryan, S.M.; Parker, J.A.; Freeman, R.; Wei, J.Y.; Goldberger, A.L. Hemodynamic and autonomic nervous system responses to mixed meal ingestion in healthy young and old subjects and dysautonomic patients with postprandial hypotension. *Circulation* **1993**, *87*, 391–400. [CrossRef]
8. Jang, A.L.; Hwang, S.K.; Kim, D.U. Effects of guar gum ingestion on postprandial blood pressure in older adults. *J. Nutr. Health. Aging.* **2015**, *19*, 299–304. [CrossRef]
9. Fisher, A.A.; Davis, M.W.; Srikusalanukul, W.; Budge, M.M. Postprandial hypotension predicts all-cause mortality in older, low-level care residents. *J. Am. Geriatr. Soc.* **2005**, *53*, 1313–1320. [CrossRef] [PubMed]
10. World Health Organization (WHO). The Top 10 Causes of Death. Available online: https://www.who.int/news-room/fact-sheets/detail/the-top-10-causes-of-death (accessed on 10 September 2019).
11. Virtanen, M.; Lallukka, T.; Ervasti, J.; Rahkonen, O.; Lahelma, E.; Pentti, J.; Pietiläinen, O.; Vahtera, J.; Kivimäki, M. The joint contribution of cardiovascular disease and socioeconomic status to disability retirement: A register linkage study. *Int. J. Cardiol.* **2017**, *230*, 222–227. [CrossRef] [PubMed]

12. Trahair, L.G.; Horowitz, M.; Jones, K.L. Postprandial hypotension: A systematic review. *J. Am. Med. Dir. Assoc.* **2014**, *15*, 394–409. [CrossRef] [PubMed]
13. Zanasi, A.; Tincani, E.; Evandri, V.; Giovanardi, P.; Bertolotti, M.; Rioli, G. Meal-induced blood pressure variation and cardiovascular mortality in ambulatory hypertensive elderly patients: Preliminary results. *J. Hypertens.* **2012**, *30*, 2125–2132. [CrossRef] [PubMed]
14. Aronow, W.S.; Ahn, C. Association of postprandial hypotension with incidence of falls, syncope, coronary events, stroke, and total mortality at 29-month follow-up in 499 older nursing home residents. *J. Am. Geriatr. Soc.* **1997**, *45*, 1051–1053. [CrossRef] [PubMed]
15. Tabara, Y.; Okada, Y.; Uetani, E.; Nagai, T.; Igase, M.; Kido, T.; Ochi, N.; Ohara, M.; Takita, R.; Kohara, K.; et al. Postprandial hypotension as a risk marker for asymptomatic lacunar infarction. *J. Hypertens.* **2014**, *32*, 1084–1090. [CrossRef] [PubMed]
16. Kohara, K.; Jiang, Y.; Igase, M.; Takata, Y.; Fukuoka, T.; Okura, T.; Kitami, Y.; Hiwada, K. Postprandial hypotension is associated with asymptomatic cerebrovascular damage in essential hypotensive patients. *Hypertension* **1999**, *33*, 565–568. [CrossRef] [PubMed]
17. Mancia, G.; Grassi, G. The new European society of hypertension/European society of cardiology (ESH/ESC) guidelines. *Ther. Adv. Cardiovasc. Dis.* **2008**, *2*, 5–12. [CrossRef] [PubMed]
18. World Health Organization (WHO). Cardiovascular Diseases (CVDs). Available online: https://www.who.int/news-room/fact-sheets/detail/cardiovascular-diseases-(cvds) (accessed on 15 September 2019).
19. Peitzman, S.J.; Berger, S.R. Postprandial blood pressure decrease in well elderly persons. *Arch. Intern. Med.* **1989**, *149*, 286–288. [CrossRef] [PubMed]
20. Gentilcore, D.; Hausken, T.; Meyer, J.H.; Chapman, I.M.; Horowitz, M.; Jones, K.L. Effects of intraduodenal glucose, fat, and protein on blood pressure, heart rate, and splanchnic blood flow in healthy older subjects. *Am. J. Clin. Nutr.* **2008**, *87*, 156–161. [CrossRef] [PubMed]
21. Son, J.T.; Lee, E. Prevalence and risk factors of postprandial hypotension in Korean elderly people. *J. Korean Acad. Nurs.* **2009**, *39*, 198–206. [CrossRef]

10

Predicting Long-Term Health-Related Quality of Life after Bariatric Surgery Using a Conventional Neural Network: A Study Based on the Scandinavian Obesity Surgery Registry

Yang Cao [1,*], Mustafa Raoof [2], Scott Montgomery [1,3,4], Johan Ottosson [2] and Ingmar Näslund [2]

1 Clinical Epidemiology and Biostatistics, School of Medical Sciences, Örebro University, 70182 Örebro, Sweden; scott.montgomery@oru.se
2 Department of Surgery, Faculty of Medicine and Health, Örebro University, 70182 Örebro, Sweden; mustafa.raoof@regionorebrolan.se (M.R.); johan.ottosson@regionorebrolan.se (J.O.); ingmar.naslund@regionorebrolan.se (I.N.)
3 Clinical Epidemiology Division, Department of Medicine, Karolinska Institutet, 17177 Stockholm, Sweden
4 Department of Epidemiology and Public Health, University College London, London WC1E 6BT, UK
* Correspondence: yang.cao@oru.se

Abstract: Severe obesity has been associated with numerous comorbidities and reduced health-related quality of life (HRQoL). Although many studies have reported changes in HRQoL after bariatric surgery, few were long-term prospective studies. We examined the performance of the convolution neural network (CNN) for predicting 5-year HRQoL after bariatric surgery based on the available preoperative information from the Scandinavian Obesity Surgery Registry (SOReg). CNN was used to predict the 5-year HRQoL after bariatric surgery in a training dataset and evaluated in a test dataset. In general, performance of the CNN model (measured as mean squared error, MSE) increased with more convolution layer filters, computation units, and epochs, and decreased with a larger batch size. The CNN model showed an overwhelming advantage in predicting all the HRQoL measures. The MSEs of the CNN model for training data were 8% to 80% smaller than those of the linear regression model. When the models were evaluated using the test data, the CNN model performed better than the linear regression model. However, the issue of overfitting was apparent in the CNN model. We concluded that the performance of the CNN is better than the traditional multivariate linear regression model in predicting long-term HRQoL after bariatric surgery; however, the overfitting issue needs to be mitigated using more features or more patients to train the model.

Keywords: prediction; deep learning; conventional neural network; health-related quality of life; bariatric surgery

---

1. Introduction

Severe obesity, defined as having a body mass index (BMI) greater than 40 kg/m^2 or greater than 35 kg/m^2 plus at least one obesity-related comorbidity [1,2], has been associated with numerous health outcomes and reduced health-related quality of life (HRQoL) [3–8]. HRQoL measures population health multi-dimensionally from physical, mental, emotional, and social functioning domains, which have already been identified as an important indication for bariatric surgery and recognized by the United States National Institutes of Health Conference as early as 1991 [9,10]. Although many studies have reported changes in HROoL after bariatric surgery, few are long-term prospective studies. A systematic review of seven prospective cohort studies with a follow-up time of ≥5 years revealed that bariatric surgery patients reported considerably improved HRQoL and the improvement was maintained over the long term [11]. However, many patients still experience reduced HRQoL after surgery. In our study, 39% of patients had significant improvements in physical functioning (PF) (increased by >25 in the original score or >0.25 in the scaled score), and the rest had no significant improvement and some patients (2%) even had significant deterioration (reduced by >25 in the original score or >0.25 in the scaled score). No relationship between the PF scores before and 5 years after surgery was identified (Figure S1).

Although some preoperative psychological factors, including personality change, severe psychiatric disorder, or depressive symptoms, are associated with postoperative HRQoL after bariatric surgery [12,13], whether long-term HRQoL after bariatric surgery can be predicted based on patients' baseline features has not been investigated. The present study examined the performance of the convolution neural network (CNN) for predicting 5-year HRQoL after bariatric surgery based on the available preoperative information from a national quality registry, and compared CNN with a conventional linear regression estimator.

2. Material and Methods

2.1. Patients and Features

Data for the patients registered in the Scandinavian Obesity Surgery Registry (SOReg) were used for the current study. The SOReg was launched in 2007 and covers 98% of bariatric surgery in Sweden since 2009. SOReg is validated regularly and has been shown to have high data quality [14]. In total, 27 - of 42 operating centers in Sweden participate in the HRQoL registration in SOReg. HRQoL was measured using the RAND-SF-36 and the obesity-related problems (OP) scale preoperatively and 1, 2, and 5 years after surgery. In the present study, preoperative and 5-year HRQoL data, including PF, role physical (RP), bodily pain (BP), general health (GH), vitality (VT), social functioning (SF), role emotional (RE), mental health (MH) scale, summary physical scale (PCS), summary mental scale (MCS), and OP, were used. All scale scores ranged from 0 to 100, with higher scores indicating better health status except for OP, where low values represent good health. Eight baseline features, including sex, age, BMI, sleep apnea syndrome (SAS), hypertension, diabetes, dyslipidemia, and depression, were also used as predictors.

In total, 6687 patients with complete information on 19 baseline features and 11 5-year HRQoL measures were used in the machine learning study.

The data that support the study are not publicly available because they contain information that could compromise research participant privacy and confidentiality. The authors will make the data available upon reasonable request and with permission of the Committee of Scandinavian Obesity Surgery Registry in Örebro, Sweden.

2.2. Feature Scaling

Before machine learning, the features in the dataset were scaled. The binary features were converted into dummy variables, and the continuous features were scaled to between 0 and 1 using a min-max scaler. In the sensitivity analysis, the normalizer and standardizer scalers were also used to evaluate the influence of scalers on the model's performance.

2.3. Conventional Neural Network

A CNN is a regularized version of a multi-layer perceptron neural network, which was inspired by a biological process where the connectivity pattern between neurons resembles the organization of the visual cortex [15]. Although not specifically developed for non-image data, CNN may achieve state-of-the-art results on regression prediction problems, especially for data with time series or spatial patterns. The CNN input is traditionally two-dimensional (2D) but can also be changed to be one-dimensional (1D), allowing it to develop an internal representation of a 1D sequence. In our study, we used a CNN with seven hidden layers, including two 1D convolution layers (with 10 filters for each), two 1D max pooling layers, one flattened layer, and two dense layers (with 1000 computation units). The rectified linear unit (relu) activation function was used for the convolution layers and dense layers, and the normal distribution was used to initialize weights in the layers. The mean squared error was used as the loss function and the an Adadelta algorithm was used as optimizer when compiling the model [16]. The structure of the CNN model is shown in Figure S2.

2.4. Model Validation and Evaluation

In total, 20% of the patients were randomly selected as a test dataset for the final evaluation of the data, and the rest of the patients were used as the training dataset. To find optimal high-level parameters (like the number, size, and type of layers in the networks) and lower-level parameters (like the number of epochs, choice of loss function and activation function, and optimization procedure) in the CNN model, the K-fold cross validation method was used during the training phase [17]. We split the training data into 5 partitions, instantiated 5 identical models, and trained each one on 4 partitions while validating on the remaining partition. The performance of each model was evaluated using the mean squared error (MSE) because of the existence of zero values in the outcome variables. We then computed the average performance over the 5 folds. In the end, the choice of the parameters was a compromise between the model's performance and computing time, i.e., the model with both the smallest validation error and a shorter computing time was deemed an optimal model. The training, validation, and final evaluation process is shown in Figure S3.

To avoid overuse of the deep learning method for prediction, we also applied a simple multivariate linear regression model as an estimator to predict the 5-year HRQoL scores, and compared the performance between the linear regression model and the CNN model.

2.5. Software and Hardware

The descriptive and inferential statistical analyses were performed using Stata 15.1 (StataCorp LLC, College Station, TX, USA). The CNN and multiple linear regression models were achieved using packages scikit-learn 0.21.2 and Keras 2.2.4 in Python 3.6 (Python Software Foundation, https://www.python.org/).

All of the computation was conducted in a computer with a 64-bit Windows 7 Enterprise operation system (Service Pack 1), Intel ®Core TM i5-4210U CPU @ 2.40 GHz, and 16.0 GB random access memory.

3. Results

3.1. Descriptive Analysis of the Data

In total, 6687 patients registered in SOReg between 2008 and 2012 with complete demographic and preoperative comorbidity information, and preoperative and 5-year HROoL scores were included in the study. The characteristics of the patients are shown in Table 1. Briefly, the average age and BMI of the patients were 42.7 years and 42.3 kg/m2, respectively. More than three quarters (77%) were female and 45% had at least one of the five comorbidities (SAS, hypertension, diabetes, depression, and dyslipidemia) before bariatric surgery.

Table 1. Characteristics of the patients (n = 6687) included in the study, mean (SD) or n (%).

	Preoperative		Five Years after Bariatric Surgery	
	Original	Scaled	Original	Scaled
Age (year)	42.7 (11.0)	0.494 (0.197)	47.7 (11.0)	0.494 (0.197)
BMI (kg/m^2)	42.3 (5.2)	0.241 (0.103)	30.3 (5.2)	0.358 (0.127)
Female	5259 (77%)	NA	5259 (77%)	NA
SAS	680 (10%)	NA	NA	NA
Hypertension	1851 (27%)	NA	NA	NA
Diabetes	990 (15%)	NA	NA	NA
Depression	884 (13%)	NA	NA	NA
Dyslipidemia	747 (11%)	NA	NA	NA
PF	61.6 (21.9)	0.616 (0.219)	84.2 (20.7)	0.842 (0.207)
RP	60.2 (38.9)	0.602 (0.389)	77.8 (36.6)	0.778 (0.366)
BP	56.0 (26.8)	0.560 (0.268)	65.1 (30.8)	0.651 (0.308)
GH	58.2 (21.4)	0.582 (0.214)	68.0 (24.7)	0.680 (0.247)
VT	47.3 (23.0)	0.473 (0.230)	54.5 (26.9)	0.545 (0.269)
SF	74.8 (26.1)	0.748 (0.261)	79.5(26.5)	0.795 (0.265)
RE	75.9 (36.2)	0.759 (0.362)	76.7 (37.9)	0.767 (0.379)
MH	71.5 (19.4)	0.715 (0.194)	72.0 (23.0)	0.720 (0.230)
PCS	38.3 (10.7)	0.567 (0.177)	47.6 (11.1)	0.653 (0.163)
MCS	46.8 (11.7)	0.621 (0.172)	44.6 (13.8)	0.621 (0.192)
OP	61.0 (26.3)	0.610 (0.263)	25.6 (27.4)	0.256 (0.274)

SD, standard deviation; NA, not applicable; BMI, body mass index; SAS, sleep apnea syndrome; PF, physical functioning; RP, role-physical; BP, bodily pain; GH, general health; VT, vitality; SF, social functioning; RE, role-emotional; MH, mental health; PCS, summary physical scale; MCS, summary mental scale; OP, obesity-related problems.

3.2. Performance of the CNN Model in the K-Fold Cross-Validation

We analyzed 11 HRQoL scores in the study. To make our description concise, we used the PF score as an example of our data analysis as follows.

In general, the performance of the CNN model (measured as the MSE) increased with more convolution layer filters, computation units, and epochs, and decreased with a larger batch size. Although the performance increased with the model's complexity, the computing time increased exponentially. When we set the number of computation units and filters to be large enough (1000 and 10, respectively) and the batch size was small enough (10), the performance of the CNN model in K-fold cross-validation is shown in Figure 1. The performance was not stable when the number of epochs was small and changed dramatically depending on the random seed used in training (Figure 1). When the number of epochs was >40, the model presented smaller MSE than the linear regression model (0.032 vs. 0.035, Figures 1 and 2). Although more epochs reduced the MSE in the CNN model, the computing time increased exponentially, indicating a higher cost in machine learning (Figure 1). The MSE of the linear regression model appeared constant when the number of epochs >40 (Figure 2), which means the prediction cannot be improved with more epochs. The cross-validation indicates that the CNN model may provide better prediction but at the expense of the computing time.

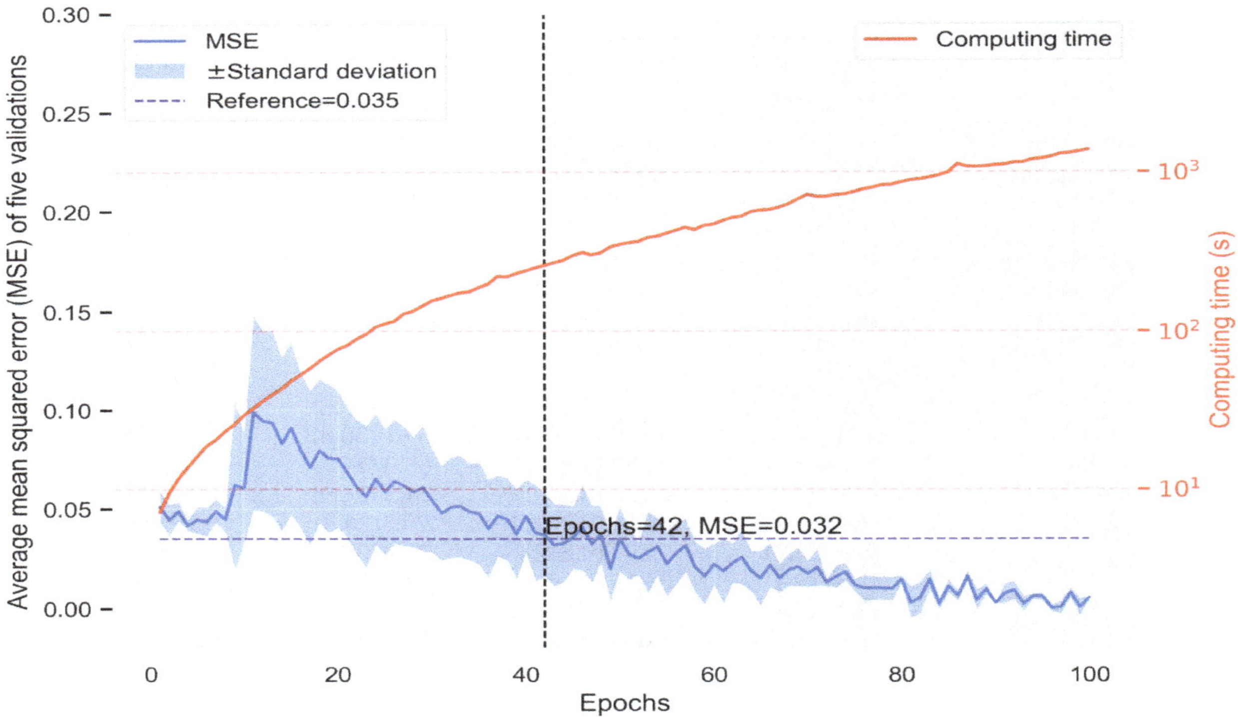

Figure 1. Performance of the convolution neural network (CNN) model in K-fold cross-validation.

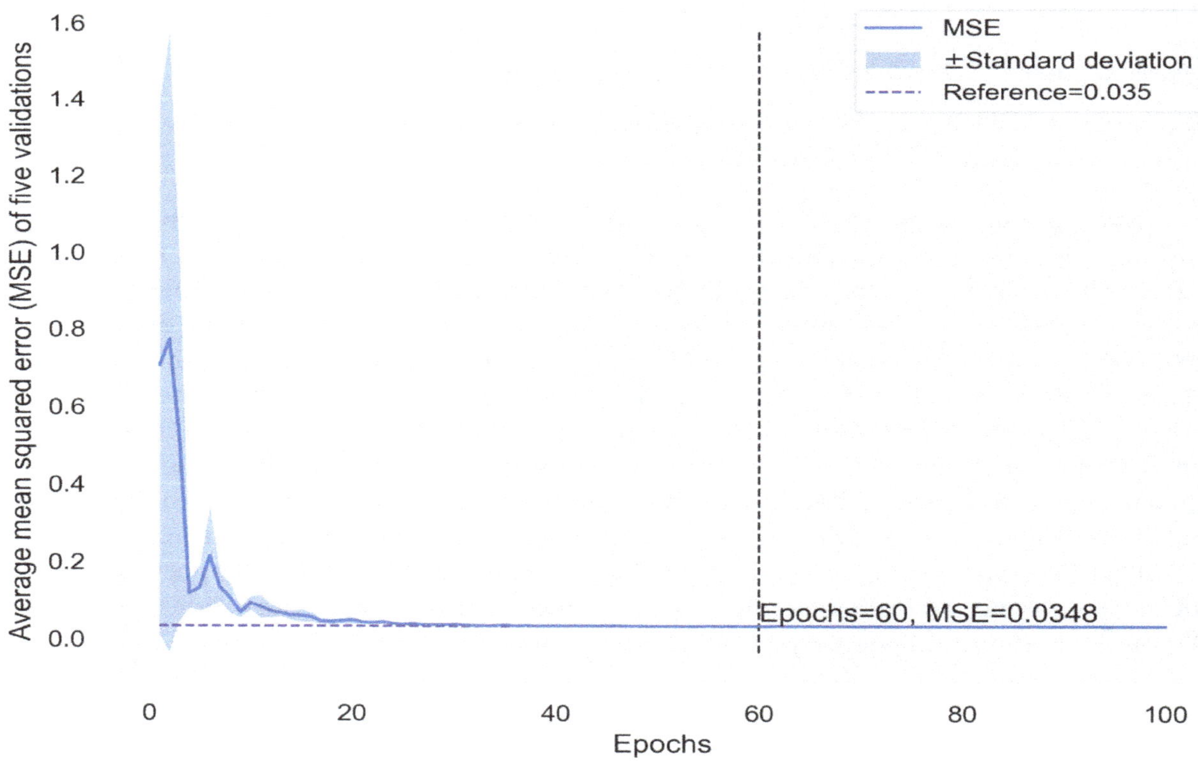

Figure 2. Performance of the simple multivariate linear regression model in K-fold cross-validation.

3.3. Performance of the CNN Model in the Final Evaluation

When the models were evaluated using the test data that were not seen previously by the models, in general, the CNN model presented a better performance (solid line in Figure 3b) than the linear regression model (solid line in Figure 3a) with epochs >40. Although overfitting was presented sporadically in the CNN model (comparing the solid line with the dotted line in Figure 3b), the performance improved gradually with an increased number of epochs while remaining constant in the linear regression model.

Finally, we used 40 epochs for the CNN model, and predicted PF scores for both the training data and the test data. Clear correlations can be seen between the predicted values and observed values in the training data, with an MSE of 0.032 for the CNN model (Figure 3d and Table 2) compared to the MSE of 0.033 seen in the linear regression model (Figure 3c and Table 2). For the test data, the CNN model had an MSE of 0.035 (Figure 3f and Table 2) compared with 0.034 (Figure 3e and Table 2) from the linear regression model. Although the CNN model provided better prediction than the linear regression model for the test data, the overfitting became apparent in some situations when the model learned patterns more specific to the training data.

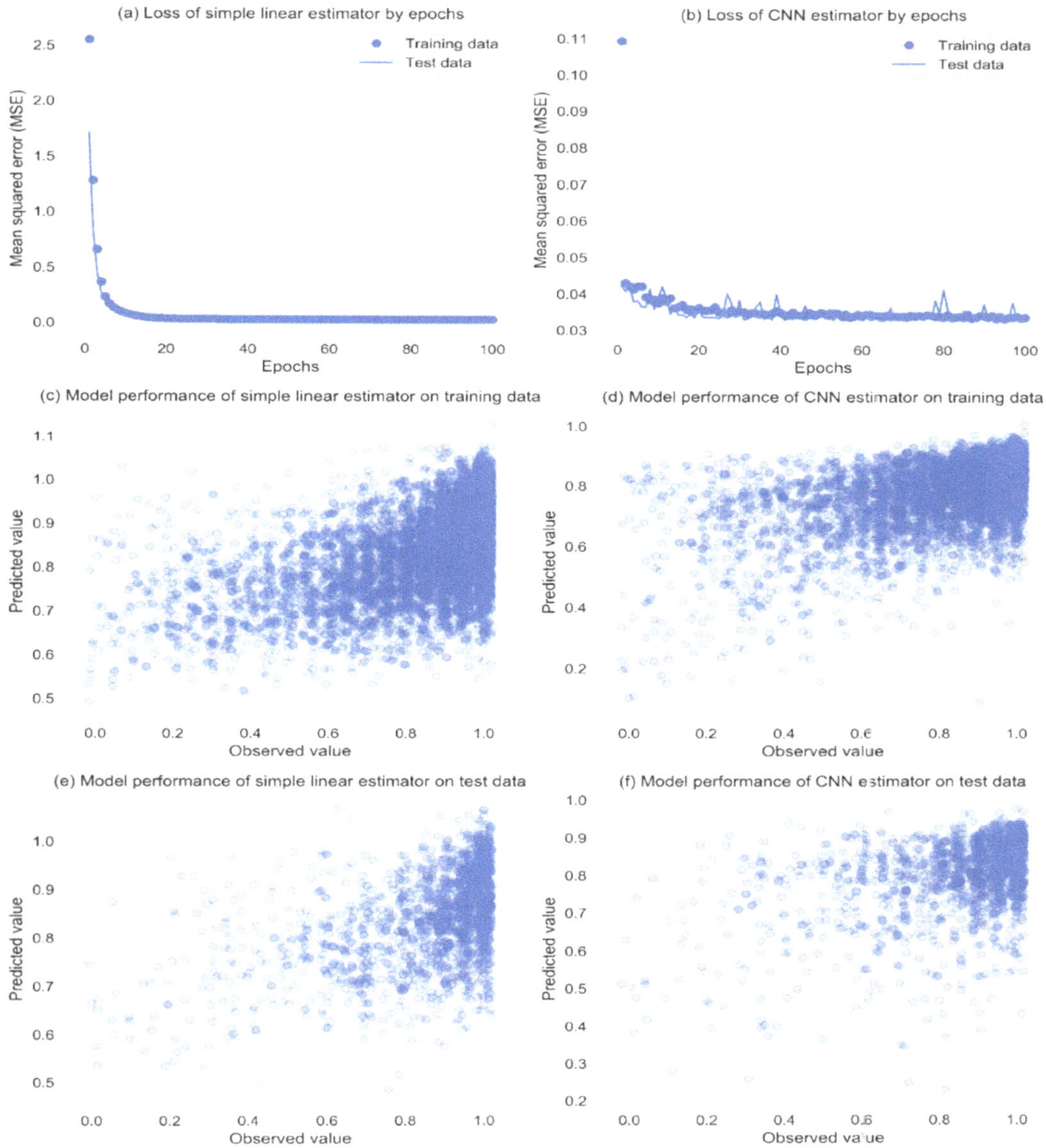

Figure 3. Model performance of the simple linear estimator and the CNN estimator. The dots in the plots (c)–(f) were jittered to avoid a heavy overlap of patients with the same coordinates. CNN, convolution neural network.

3.4. *Performance of CNN in Predicting Other HRQoL Measures*

The relationships between the baseline and the 5-year scores of other HRQoL measures in the test data are shown in Figure 4. Except for GH and VT, no clear relationship between the baseline and the observed 5-year scores is seen for the HRQoL measures (Figure 4, plots a1–j1). However, the predicted 5-year scores based on the baseline scores and the CNN model show clear correlations with the observed 5-year scores for BP, GH, VT, MH, MCS, and OP (Figure 4, plots a2–j2).

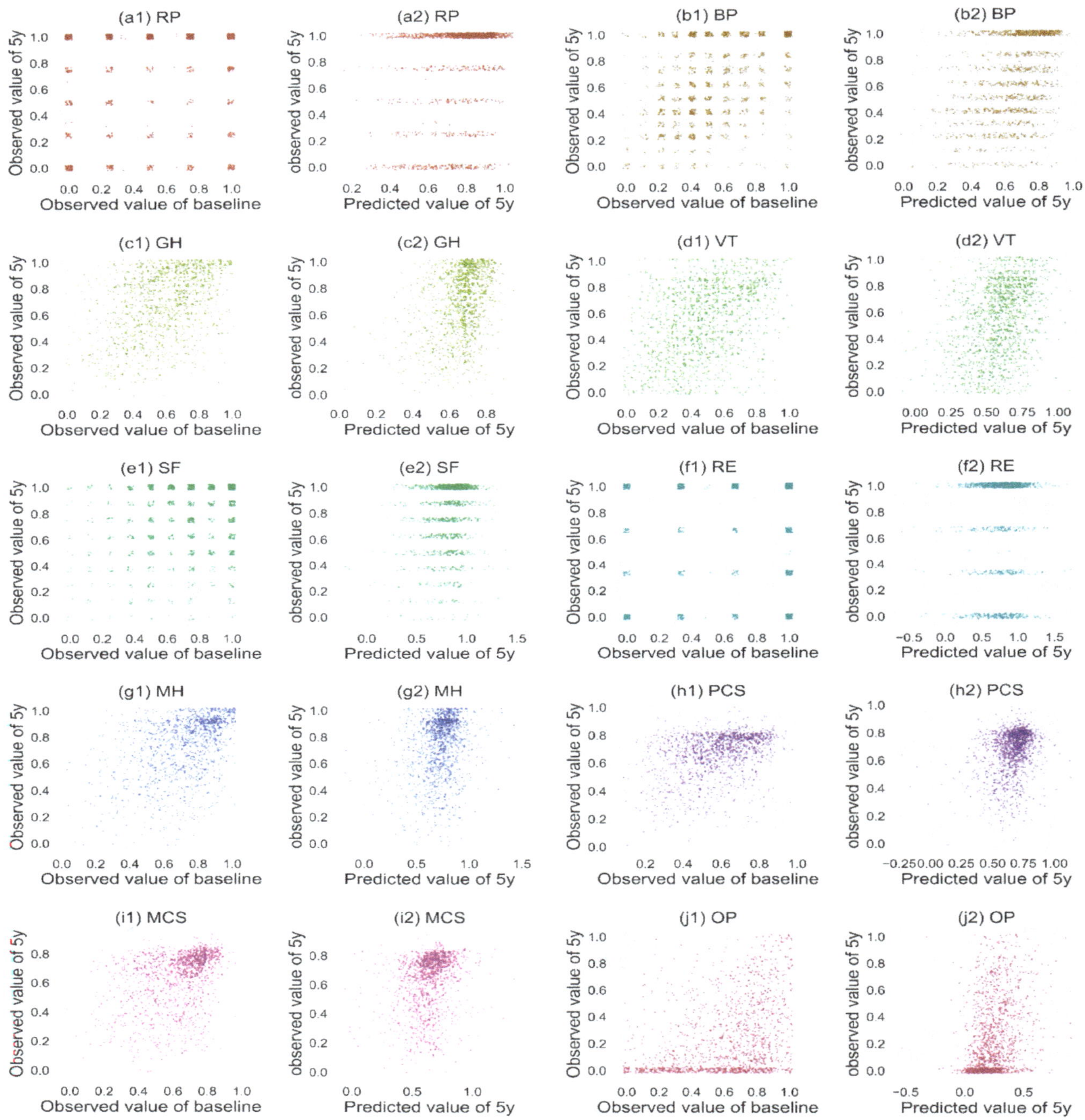

Figure 4. Correlation of the observed 5-year scores with the observed baseline scores and predicted scores for test data. The dots in the plots were jittered to avoid a heavy overlap of patients with the same coordinates. RP, role physical; BP, bodily pain; GH, general health; VT, vitality; SF, social functioning; RE, role emotional; MH, mental health; PCS, summary physical scale; MCS, summary mental scale; OP, obesity-related problems.

We compared the performance of the CNN model and the linear regression model for all the HRQoL measures in both the training data and the test data. The CNN model showed an overwhelming advantage in predicting all the HRQoL measures. The MSEs of the CNN model for the training data were 8% to 80% smaller than those of the linear regression model (Table 2). The overfitting was also apparent in the CNN model, i.e., the MSEs of the CNN model for the test data were all greater than those of the linear regression model (Table 2).

Table 2. Mean squared errors (MSEs) of the CNN model and the multivariate linear regression model.

HRQoL Measure	Training Data		Test Data	
	CNN Model	Linear Regression Model	CNN Model	Linear Regression Model
PF	0.0316	0.0329	0.0350	0.0343
RP	0.1078	0.1178	0.1324	0.1211
BP	0.0604	0.0763	0.0898	0.0772
GH	0.0280	0.0497	0.0618	0.0508
VT	0.0303	0.0572	0.0914	0.0625
SF	0.0213	0.0600	0.0995	0.0588
RE	0.0393	0.1275	0.2118	0.1269
MH	0.0119	0.0427	0.0807	0.0416
PCS	0.0087	0.0210	0.0333	0.0219
MCS	0.0075	0.0301	0.0584	0.0305
OP	0.0450	0.0625	0.0750	0.0608

PF, physical functioning; RP, role physical; BP, bodily pain; GH, general health; VT, vitality; SF, social functioning; RE, role emotional; MH, mental health; PCS, summary physical scale; MCS, summary mental scale; OP, obesity-related problems.

3.5. *Sensitivity Analysis and Computing Time*

We also conducted sensitivity analysis using different scalers and optimizers in data preparation and model compiling, and tuned the hyperparameters using the exhaustive grid search method [18]. Although they showed more or less influence on the models' performance, the influence was negligible when the number of epochs was large and the batch size was small. The computing time for the CNN model largely depends on the hyperparameter settings of the layers, number of epochs and the batch size for training, and the software and hardware used. In our study, with the model structures and hyperparameters shown in Figure S2, the running time ranged from 70 (epoch = 40, batch size = 10, without cross-validation) to 595 s (epoch = 400, batch size = 10, with five cross-validations) on our computer.

4. Discussion

Machine learning methods to predict HRQoL have been used in elderly with chronic diseases [19], cervical cancer patients [20], and osteoarthritis patients [21]. However, to our knowledge, they have not been used to predict the postoperative HRQoL of patients undergoing bariatric surgery. We explored the feasibility and capacity of a deep learning method, i.e., convolution neural network, to predict long-term HRQoL after bariatric surgery using a national register. The study can only be achieved based on a well-maintained and high-quality longitudinal database with long-term follow-up like SOReg [22].

Our results indicate that 5-year HRQoL after bariatric surgery may be well predicted preoperatively for some scale domains like PF, BP, GH, VT, MH, MCS, and OP. In our study, we aimed to evaluate and predict the quality of life of patients after bariatric surgery. Some patients were not "satisfied" even when they lost weight. Other factors, such as complications during follow-up and preoperative pharmacologic drug treatment, are associated with a change of the quality of life after bariatric surgery, whereas age, sex, and preoperative metabolic comorbidity may also play a role [11,23–25]. Our findings may provide important information for postoperative care and rehabilitation for this group of patients.

Our research question was about predicting continuous outcomes using supervised deep learning methods, which could be converted to a question of supervised two- or multi-class classification, i.e., to predict whether the quality of life of the patient has improved, remained unchanged, or deteriorated. Although the precision of prediction might be reduced in classification, the accuracy might be enhanced, and the method might be more applicable for clinical use. We would like to investigate the question in future studies.

There has been a warning that healthcare researchers should not be overly enthralled by the promises of deep learning methods [26]. Therefore, to avoid abusing the deep learning method in our study, we also compared the performance of the CNN model with a conventional statistical learning method for continuous variables, using a multivariate linear regression model. Although the conventional statistical methods require sometimes complex processing (feature engineering) to extract the requisite discriminative features, they may provide more interpretable results compared to the deep learning methods. In contrast, the biggest advantage of deep learning methods is that they try to learn high-level features from data in an incremental manner, which eliminates the need for domain expertise and hard-core feature extraction. However, the generalizability of deep learning models relies largely on the data they learned, and overfitting on unseen data is more apparent, as observed in our study. Although there are some ways in which we may reduce overfitting in deep learning models, the rule of thumb is to use more training data.

There are potential limitations to our study. In total, 28,293 patients underwent surgery for a primary gastric bypass between 2008 and 2012 and had a follow-up longer than 5 years when the study was initiated. However, only less than one quarter of the patients who had complete HRQoL information could be used for the machine learning. Compared to the patients who had no or incomplete HRQoL information, the patients with complete relevant data were older (42.7 ± 11.0 vs. 40.4 ± 10.8 years), had fewer males (21.2% vs. 25.1%), and lower BMI (42.3 ± 5.2 vs. 42.8 ± 5.5 kg/m^2). These factors have already been shown to influence HRQoL [27–29]. Because of these systematic differences in HRQoL between the patients with and without HRQoL measures, the generalizability of our CNN model may be questionable. The missing information needs to be imputed in the future for deep machine learning. We would also point out that the CNN built in our study was only based on features from gastric bypass patients, which cannot be generalized to other surgical procedures or health conditions. The application of CNN in predicting prognosis after surgeries still needs to be investigated using large data from the real world.

5. Conclusions

CNN can be used to predict long-term HRQoL after bariatric surgery based on the baseline features of patients. The performance of the CNN was found to be better than the traditional multivariate linear regression model; however, its overfitting on unseen data needs to be mitigated by using more features of patients or greater use of training data in the future.

Author Contributions: Data curation, M.R.; Formal analysis, Y.C.; Funding acquisition, Y.C.; Investigation, Y.C., M.R., S.M. and I.N.; Methodology, Y.C. and M.R.; Project administration, J.O. and I.N.; Resources, J.O. and I.N.; Software, Y.C.; Validation, Y.C. and S.M.; Visualization, Y.C.; Writing—original draft, Y.C., M.R. and I.N.; Writing—review and editing, Y.C., M.R., S.M., J.O. and I.N.

References

1. Kopelman, P.G.; Caterson, I.D.; Dietz, W.H. *Clinical Obesity in Adults and Children*; John Wiley & Sons: New York, NY, USA, 2009.
2. Organization, W.H. *Obesity: Preventing and Managing the Global Epidemic*; World Health Organization: Geneva, Switzerland, 2000.
3. Prospective Studies Collaboration; Whitlock, G.; Lewington, S.; Sherliker, P.; Clarke, R.; Emberson, J.; Halsey, J.; Qizilbash, N.; Collins, R.; Peto, R. Body-mass index and cause-specific mortality in 900 000 adults: Collaborative analyses of 57 prospective studies. *Lancet* **2009**, *373*, 1083–1096. [CrossRef] [PubMed]
4. Guh, D.P.; Zhang, W.; Bansback, N.; Amarsi, Z.; Birmingham, C.L.; Anis, A.H. The incidence of co-morbidities related to obesity and overweight: A systematic review and meta-analysis. *BMC Public Health* **2009**, *9*, 88. [CrossRef] [PubMed]
5. Wawok, P. Evaluation of Quality of Life of patient with obesity after surgical procedure. *Eur. J. Med. Res.* **2009**, *14*, 114.
6. Kawatkar, A.A.; Nichol, M.B. The Impact of Obesity on Medical Expenditure and Health Related Quality of Life. *Value Health* **2009**, *12*, A134. [CrossRef]
7. Kolotkin, R.L.; Williams, V.S.L.; Ervin, C.M.; Williams, N.; Meincke, H.H.; Qin, S.S.; Smith, L.V.; Fehnel, S.E. Validation of a new measure of quality of life in obesity trials: Impact of Weight on Quality of Life-Lite Clinical Trials Version. *Clin. Obes.* **2019**, *9*, e12310. [CrossRef]
8. Dreber, H.; Thorell, A.; Reynisdottir, S.; Hemmingsson, E. Health-Related Quality of Life 5Years After Roux-en-Y Gastric Bypass in Young (18-25Years) Versus Older (26Years) Adults: A Scandinavian Obesity Surgery Registry Study. *Obes. Surg.* **2019**, *29*, 434–443. [CrossRef]
9. Consensus Development Conference Panel. NIH conference. Gastrointestinal surgery for severe obesity. Consensus Development Conference Panel. *Ann. Intern. Med.* **1991**, *115*, 956–961. [CrossRef]
10. Mazer, L.M.; Azagury, D.E.; Morton, J.M. Quality of Life After Bariatric Surgery. *Curr. Obes. Rep.* **2017**, *6*, 204–210. [CrossRef] [PubMed]
11. Andersen, J.R.; Aasprang, A.; Karlsen, T.I.; Natvig, G.K.; Vage, V.; Kolotkin, R.L. Health-related quality of life after bariatric surgery: A systematic review of prospective long-term studies. *Surg. Obes. Relat. Dis.* **2015**, *11*, 466–473. [CrossRef]
12. Wimmelmann, C.L.; Dela, F.; Mortensen, E.L. Psychological predictors of mental health and health-related quality of life after bariatric surgery: A review of the recent research. *Obes. Res. Clin. Pract.* **2014**, *8*, e314–e324. [CrossRef]
13. Masheb, R.M.; White, M.A.; Toth, C.M.; Burke-Martindale, C.H.; Rothschild, B.; Grilo, C.M. The prognostic significance of depressive symptoms for predicting quality of life 12 months after gastric bypass. *Compr. Psychiatry* **2007**, *48*, 231–236. [CrossRef] [PubMed]
14. Hedenbro, J.L.; Naslund, E.; Boman, L.; Lundegardh, G.; Bylund, A.; Ekelund, M.; Laurenius, A.; Moller, P.; Olbers, T.; Sundbom, M.; et al. Formation of the Scandinavian Obesity Surgery Registry, SOReg. *Obes. Surg.* **2015**, *25*, 1893–1900. [CrossRef] [PubMed]
15. Matsugu, M.; Mori, K.; Mitari, Y.; Kaneda, Y. Subject independent facial expression recognition with robust face detection using a convolutional neural network. *Neural Netw.* **2003**, *16*, 555–559. [CrossRef]
16. Zeiler, M.D. ADADELTA: An adaptive learning rate method. *arXiv* **2012**, arXiv:1212.5701.
17. Raschka, S.; Mirjalili, V. *Python Machine Learning*; Packt Publishing Ltd.: Birmingham, UK, 2017.
18. Wilson, A.C.; Roelofs, R.; Stern, M.; Srebro, N.; Recht, B. The Marginal Value of Adaptive Gradient Methods in Machine Learning. *Adv. Neural Inf.* **2017**, *30*, 4148–4158.
19. Lee, S.K.; Son, Y.J.; Kim, J.; Kim, H.G.; Lee, J.I.; Kang, B.Y.; Cho, H.S.; Lee, S. Prediction Model for Health-Related Quality of Life of Elderly with Chronic Diseases using Machine Learning Techniques. *Healthc. Inf. Res.* **2014**, *20*, 125–134. [CrossRef]
20. Kumar, S.; Rana, M.L.; Verma, K.; Singh, N.; Sharma, A.K.; Maria, A.K.; Dhaliwal, G.S.; Khaira, H.K.; Saini, S. PrediQt-Cx: Post treatment health related quality of life prediction model for cervical cancer patients. *PLoS ONE* **2014**, *9*, e89851. [CrossRef]
21. Persson, P.-V.; Rietz, H. *Predicting and Analyzing Osteoarthritis Patient Outcomes with Machine Learning*; Lund University: Lund, Sweden, 2017.

22. Tao, W.; Holmberg, D.; Naslund, E.; Naslund, I.; Mattsson, F.; Lagergren, J.; Ljung, R. Validation of Obesity Surgery Data in the Swedish National Patient Registry and Scandinavian Obesity Registry (SOReg). *Obes. Surg.* **2016**, *26*, 1750–1756. [CrossRef]
23. Hell, E.; Miller, K.A.; Moorehead, M.K.; Norman, S. Evaluation of health status and quality of life after bariatric surgery: Comparison of standard Roux-en-Y gastric bypass, vertical banded gastroplasty and laparoscopic adjustable silicone gastric banding. *Obes. Surg.* **2000**, *10*, 214–219. [CrossRef]
24. Dymek, M.P.; Le Grange, D.; Neven, K.; Alverdy, J. Quality of life after gastric bypass surgery: A cross-sectional study. *Obes. Res.* **2002**, *10*, 1135–1142. [CrossRef]
25. Major, P.; Matlok, M.; Pedziwiatr, M.; Migaczewski, M.; Budzynski, P.; Stanek, M.; Kisielewski, M.; Natkaniec, M.; Budzynski, A. Quality of Life After Bariatric Surgery. *Obes. Surg.* **2015**, *25*, 1703–1710. [CrossRef] [PubMed]
26. Chen, D.; Liu, S.J.; Kingsbury, P.; Sohn, S.; Storlie, C.B.; Habermann, E.B.; Naessens, J.M.; Larson, D.W.; Liu, H.F. Deep learning and alternative learning strategies for retrospective real-world clinical data. *NPJ Digit. Med.* **2019**, *2*, 43. [CrossRef] [PubMed]
27. Chang, C.Y.; Hung, C.K.; Chang, Y.Y.; Tai, C.M.; Lin, J.T.; Wang, J.D. Health-related quality of life in adult patients with morbid obesity coming for bariatric surgery. *Obes. Surg.* **2010**, *20*, 1121–1127. [CrossRef] [PubMed]
28. Kolotkin, R.L.; Crosby, R.D.; Williams, G.R. Health-related quality of life varies among obese subgroups. *Obes. Res.* **2002**, *10*, 748–756. [CrossRef] [PubMed]
29. White, M.A.; O'Neil, P.M.; Kolotkin, R.L.; Byrne, T.K. Gender, race, and obesity-related quality of life at extreme levels of obesity. *Obes. Res.* **2004**, *12*, 949–955. [CrossRef]

11

Association between Serum Urate and Risk of Hypertension in Menopausal Women with XDH Gene

Jong-Han Lee [1], Tae Hwa Go [2], San-Hui Lee [3], Juwon Kim [1], Ji Hye Huh [4], Jang Young Kim [4], Dae Ryong Kang [2], Seongmun Jeong [5], Sang-Baek Koh [6] and Jung Ran Choi [7,*]

1 Department of Laboratory Medicine, Yonsei University Wonju College of Medicine, Wonju 26426, Korea; cello425@yonsei.ac.kr (J.-H.L.); juwon76@yonsei.ac.kr (J.K.)

2 Center of Biomedical Data Science, Institute of Genomic Cohort, Yonsei University Wonju College of Medicine, Wonju 26426, Korea; thgo1123@gmail.com (T.H.G.); dr.kang@yonsei.ac.kr (D.R.K.)

3 Department of Obstetrics and Gynecology, Yonsei University Wonju College of Medicine, Wonju 26426, Korea; sanaram@yonsei.ac.kr

4 Department of Internal Medicine, Yonsei University Wonju College of Medicine, Wonju 26426, Korea; png1212@yonsei.ac.kr (J.H.H.); kimjang713@gmail.com (J.Y.K.)

5 Genome Editing Research Center, Korea Research Institute of Bioscience and Biotechnology, Daejeon 34141, Korea; likemun@gmail.com

6 Department of Preventive Medicine and Institute of Occupational and Environmental Medicine, Wonju College of Medicine, Yonsei University, Wonju 26426, Korea; kohhj@yonsei.ac.kr

7 Institute of Genomic Cohort, Yonsei University Wonju College of Medicine, Wonju 26426, Korea

* Correspondence: christinae@yonsei.ac.kr

Abstract: Elevated serum urate (sUA) concentrations have been associated with an increased risk of hypertension. We aimed to examine the association of sUA concentration on the risk of hypertension in pre- and post-menopausal women and investigated the association between the polymorphism of the xanthine dehydrogenase gene and the risk of hypertension. Among 7294 women, 1415 premenopausal and 5879 postmenopausal women were recruited. Anthropometric parameters as risk factors of hypertension were identify by logistic regression models. In addition, we investigated an association between xanthine dehydrogenase gene and sUA and their combined associations on the risk of hypertension. Body mass index (BMI) and waist circumference (WC) were significantly increased in accordance to the increase of sUA levels ($p < 0.001$). Multivariate logistic regression analysis showed postmenopausal women with a high sUA and high BMI were 3.18 times more likely to have hypertension than in those with normal and lower sUA (Odds ratio: 3.18, 95% confidence interval: 2.54–3.96). Postmenopausal women with a high WC were 1.62 times more likely to have hypertension than in those with normal and lower sUA. Subjects with the AG genotype of rs206860 was found to be at lower risk of hypertension (odd ratio: 0.287, 95% confidence interval: 0.091–0.905, $p = 0.033$). This cross-sectional study indicated a high sUA is associated with a higher risk of hypertension in postmenopausal women. Further well-designed prospective studies in other populations are warranted to validate our results.

Keywords: serum urate; menopause; hypertension; xanthine dehydrogenase; cross-sectional cohort study

1. Introduction

An elevated serum urate (sUA) concentration is a common phenomenon in subjects with hypertension, insulin resistance, or obesity [1], and previous epidemiological studies have demonstrated that high sUA concentrations are associated with an increased risk of hypertension [1–5]. Although longitudinal studies showed sUA might play a role in the development of hypertension, the association between sUA and blood pressure may be affected by various factors [5–7]. However, it is not clear whether urate elevation is the cause or a consequence of hypertension [1,6,8].

Urate is the catabolic end-product of endogenous and dietary purine metabolism in human, and is mainly produced by xanthine oxidase, which is involved in the production of reactive-oxygen species (ROS) [5,9–11]. In addition, excessive sUA accumulation can cause various diseases [11,12]. Several studies using animal models and cell cultures have identified mechanisms whereby high sUA concentrations might lead to hypertension by reducing endothelial nitric oxide release and activating the renin–angiotensin system leading to smooth muscle cell proliferation [13–16]. Furthermore, associations between sUA and metabolic disorders are gender dependent. sUA concentrations tend to be lower in women than in men, partially due to the uricosuric effect of estrogens [10]. In addition, sUA concentrations seem to be increased in both physiologic and post-surgical menopause independently of other confounders [9,17], presumably due to the uricosuric effect of estrogens and hormone replacement therapy induced sUA reduction [18]. Estrogens have some indirect uricosuric effects that can contribute to modulate the urate before and after menopause. The sUA concentration is unlikely to reflect urate production, as an increased sUA production is compensated by increased excretion to maintain sUA within the normal range [19]. To the best of our knowledge, urate production has a limited influence on sUA concentration and both, urate concentration and the production, might influence blood pressure by a different underlying mechanism.

Mammalian xanthine oxidoreductase (XOR) has the characteristics of being found in two interconvertible forms: constitutively expressed in vivo NAD+-dependent xanthine dehydrogenase (XDH, EC 1.1.1.204) and post-transcriptionally modified xanthine oxidase (XO, EC 1.1.3.22) [20]. The XOR enzyme exists in XDH form, but when released into the circulation it is converted into XO. Although XDH preferentially reduces NAD+, both forms of the enzyme can also reduce molecular oxygen to form the ROS superoxide and hydrogen peroxide. Wu et al. reported the *XDH* gene might be associated with constitutional susceptibility to hypertension [21]. XDH alters xanthine oxidase by reversible sulfhydryl oxidation or by irreversible proteolytic modification, and the production of urate results from the metabolism of purines by XDH [21,22].

We examined the association between sUA and hypertension risk in post-menopausal women, and investigated the association between the polymorphism of *XDH* gene and the risk of hypertension.

2. Methods

2.1. Study Population

This study was conducted with participants from a population-based cohort within the Korean Genome and Epidemiology Study on Atherosclerosis Risk of Rural Areas in the Korean General Population (KoGES-ARIRANG) to assess the genetic and environmental etiology of common metabolic common metabolic and cardiovascular diseases in South Koreans [23,24]. The KoGES-ARIRANG cohort study contained all adults aged 40–70 years that resided in rural areas of Wonju and Pyeongchang, Gangwon-do, Republic of Korea.

In this cross-sectional study, the baseline survey was performed from November 2005 to January 2008 and contained 28,338 adults aged 40 to 70 years. Among 17,517 women, 8666 women with a sUA level were included in this study. After excluding 736 with experience of hormone therapy, 625 with no history of menopause, and 11 missing for blood pressure, a total of 1415 premenopausal and 5879 postmenopausal women comprised in this cross-sectional study (Figure 1). Subjects who were treated antihypertensive drugs were 1991 participants. Those who experienced anti-hypertensive drugs were considered having hypertension. Additionally, we excluded the participants without genotype, 3666 participants with the genetic variations in *XDH* were eligible for this cross-sectional study. The study protocol was approved by the Institutional Review Board of Wonju Severance Christian Hospital.

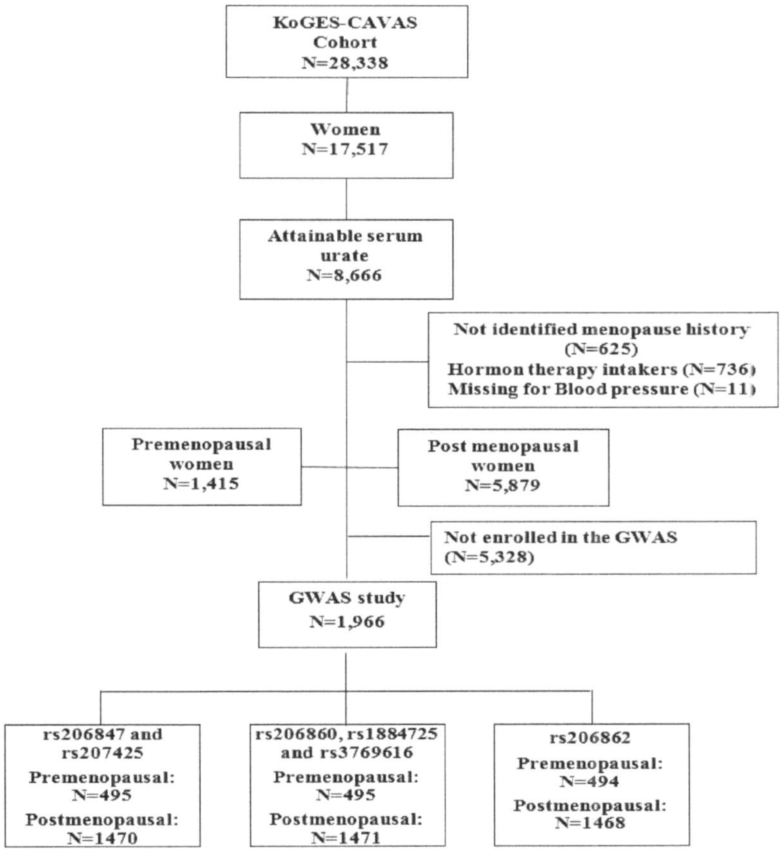

Figure 1. Flow chart of study populations in the KoGES-CAVAS cohort. Abbreviations: KoGES-CAVAS, Korean Genome and Epidemiology Study on Atherosclerosis Risk of Rural Areas in the Korean General Population; GWAS, genome wide association study.

2.2. Data Collection

At baseline examination, study participants completed a standardized medical history and lifestyle questionnaire and underwent a comprehensive health examination according to standard procedures.

Body weight and height were measured, while participants were wearing light indoor clothing without shoes. Waist circumference (WC) was measured in a horizontal plane, midway between the inferior margin of the ribs and the superior border of the iliac crest using a tape measure (SECA-200, SECA, Hamburg, Germany).

Systolic (SBP) and diastolic blood pressures (DBP) were measured twice in right arms within 5 min using a standard mercury sphygmomanometer (Baumanometer, Copiague, NY, USA). The means of the two blood pressure readings were used for the data analyses. Hypertension was defined as a SBP of ≥140 mmHg or a DBP ≥90 mmHg and/or current treatment with antihypertensive medications at the baseline survey. All the participants were examined after fasting.

A venous blood sample was drawn from study participants after fasting for >12 h or overnight. Serum aliquots were stored at −80 °C until thawed for analysis. The sUA was measured by an enzymatic coloric method that can detect the absorbance differences using uricase and peroxidase as reaction enzymes. Fasting glucose was measured using the hexokinase method. The serum concentrations of high-density lipoprotein (HDL) cholesterol, total cholesterol (TC), and triglycerides (TG) were determined using the enzymatic calorimetric method.

Alcohol and smoking habits were estimated using self-questionnaires. Individuals who had smoked ≥100 cigarettes in their lifetime were defined as current smokers, and those who had not smoked for ≥3 months were defined as ex-smokers. An interview was performed to confirm the use of medications for hypertension, and the status of regular physical exercise.

At baseline examination, study participants completed a standardized medical history and lifestyle questionnaire and underwent a comprehensive health examination according to standard procedures. At first, we estimated menopausal status using self-questionnaire. Women who had pre- and postmenopausal status were defined as "Have you always had your periods at regular 28-day intervals? Or, have you had not your periods for three months recently?" Also, an interview was performed to confirm the use of medications for hormone therapy.

2.3. Genome Wide Association Study Genotyping

Samples were analyzed using an Affymetrix Genome-Wide Human single nucleotide polymorphism (SNP) array 6.0, which contains 906,600 genome-wide SNPs and 946,000 copy number variations. Briefly, the genomic DNA was digested with two restriction enzymes (NSP I and Sty I) and processed according to the Affymetrix protocol. Digested segments were ligated to enzyme specific adaptors incorporating a universal PCR priming sequence. PCR amplification was performed using universal primers in a reaction optimized for the amplification of fragments between 200–1100 base pairs. A fragmentation step was then used to reduce the PCR products to segments of approximately 25–50 bp, which were then end-labeled using biotinylated nucleotides. The labeled products were then hybridized to a chip, washed, and detected. Images were analyzed using GeneChip Operating System software (Affymetrix, Santa Clara, CA, USA). Internal quality control measures were to ensure data fidelity, that is, a QC call rate (Dynamic Model algorithm) always was over 86% and correct identification of subject gender based on heterozygosity on the X chromosome. Genotype calling was performed using the Birdseed v2 algorithm [25].

2.4. Analysis of the XDH Genomic Polymorphism

For this study, *XDH* fragments were independently amplified by polymerase chain reaction (PCR). PCR products were purified and then sequenced using a BigDye Terminator v3.1 Cycle Sequencing Kit (Applied Biosystems, Foster City, CA, USA) and an ABI 3730 × 1 automated sequencer (Applied Biosystems). SNPs identified in the *XDH* gene by whole gene sequencing were genotyped. Genomic DNA was extracted from 5 mL of peripheral venous blood using a commercially available isolation kit (QuickGene SP Kit DNA whole blood, Fujifilm, Tokyo, Japan). Genotyping was performed using the TaqMan fluorogenic 5′ nuclease assay (Applied Biosystems) [25].

2.5. Statistical Analysis

We analyzed the study population divided in quartiles of sUA. Categorical variables were analyzed using the chi-square test and continuous variables were analyzed by ANOVA and post hoc using Scheffe's test in pre- and post-menopausal women. Interactions between drinking status, body mass index (BMI), WC, TG, and sUA on hypertension were investigated. In order to identify an association between sUA and hypertension we analyzed multivariate logistic regression which was used to evaluate the independence of associations between sUA and risk of hypertension according to menopausal status after adjusting for fasting glucose, BMI, and WC. Additionally, there might be collinearity between BMI and WC. Consequently, we demonstrated a part of odds ratio for sUA and hypertension without considering all confounding factors including age. We used SBP as confounding factors because of one of components defined participants with hypertension and without hypertension.

In additional analysis, we adjusted for age to investigate an association of sUA and clinical variables, because postmenopausal women were older than premenopausal women.

Results were expressed as ORs ratios and 95% confidence intervals (CI). All analyses were performed using SAS version 9.3 (SAS Institute, Cary, NC, USA), and SPSS version 23.0 (IBM Corp., Armonk, NY, USA). P value less than 0.05 was considered as statistically significant.

3. Results

3.1. Baseline Characteristics

The percentages of BMI, SBP, fasting glucose, and TG were significantly higher, and HDL cholesterol were significantly lower in the highest quartile of sUA (UA ≥ 5.0 mg/dL) (Table 1). BMI and WC were significantly higher in the participants with the highest quartile of sUA than those with the lowest quartile of sUA. (25.3 ± 3.4 vs. 23.6 ± 3.2; 85.2 ± 8.9 vs. 81.0 ± 9.0; respectively, $p < 0.01$) (Table 1). In the beginning of study design, we analyzed an association of sUA and hypertension with substantial confounding factors that related with sUA such as BMI and alcohol consumption. However, we did not confirm an association between sUA and hypertension after adjusted for all potential confounding factors.

Table 1. Sociodemographic characteristics of the study population.

Variable	Serum Urate (sUA)				*p*-Value	Post-Hoc *
	Quartile 1 (<3.7 mg/dL)	Quartile 2 (3.7 ≤ 4.3 mg/dL)	Quartile 3 (4.3 ≤ 5.0 mg/dL)	Quartile 4 (≥5.0 mg/dL)		
Women						
Premenopausal	411 (24.3)	385 (23.4)	381 (20.0)	238 (11.6)	<0.01	
Postmenopausal	1282 (75.7)	1258 (76.6)	1524 (80.0)	1815 (88.4)		
Age	60.5 ± 10.6	60.2 ± 10.5	60.4 ± 10.3	62.6 ± 9.6	<0.01	a, b, c < d
Smoking status						
Non, ex-smoker	1039 (96.9)	978 (96.4)	1140 (96.9)	1116 (35.1)	0.2	
Current smoker	22 (3.1)	36 (3.6)	37 (3.1)	58 (4.9)		
Alcohol						
Yes	458 (27.1)	447 (27.3)	573 (30.1)	602 (29.3)	0.11	
No	1235 (72.9)	1193 (72.7)	1330 (69.9)	1451 (70.7)		
Weight (kg)	54.6 ± 8.5	56.1 ± 8.2	57.4 ± 8.7	58.8 ± 9.5	<0.01	a < b < c < d
Height (cm)	152.0 ± 6.2	152.6 ± 6.2	152.5 ± 5.9	152.1 ± 6.0	0.02	
BMI (kg/m^2)	23.6 ± 3.2	24.1 ± 3.0	24.7 ± 3.2	25.3 ± 3.4	<0.01	a < b < c < d
WC (cm)	81.0 ± 9.0	81.9 ± 8.8	83.4 ± 9.0	85.2 ± 8.9	<0.01	a < b < c < d
HC (cm)	91.7 ± 6.3	92.5 ± 6.2	93.3 ± 6.8	94.0 ± 6.9	<0.01	a < b < c < d
Creatinine (mg/dL)	0.8 ± 0.1	0.8 ± 0.1	0.9 ± 0.1	0.9 ± 0.3	<0.01	a < b < c < d
HDL-C (mg/dL)	47.9 ± 11.2	46.9 ± 10.9	45.8 ± 11.2	43.7 ± 10.4	<0.01	a, b > c > d
Fasting glucose (mg/dL)	97.9 ± 24.5	95.9 ± 19.3	98.0 ± 19.2	100.4 ± 21.1	<0.01	a < d, b < c < d
Total cholesterol (mg/dL)	199.0 ± 36.0	200.6 ± 34.7	203.7 ± 36.2	208.8 ± 38.6	<0.01	a < c < d, b < d
Triglycerides (mg/dL)	126.4 ± 67.2	130.7 ± 72.2	146.1 ± 83.4	171.8 ± 104.0	<0.01	a, b < c < d
Total protein (g/dL)	7.3 ± 0.4	7.3 ± 0.4	7.4 ± 0.4	7.5 ± 0.4	<0.01	a < c < d, b < d
Albumin (g/dL)	4.4 ± 0.2	4.4 ± 0.2	4.5 ± 0.2	4.5 ± 0.2	<0.01	a, b < c, d
GGT (I/U)	17.2 ± 15.7	17.8 ± 21.7	20.4 ± 28.2	24.8 ± 30.8	<0.01	a, b < c < d
SBP (mmHg)	122.3 ± 18.1	122.3 ± 17.7	123.6 ± 18.4	126.4 ± 18.0	<0.01	a, b, c < d
DBP (mmHg)	75.8 ± 10.3	75.9 ± 10.4	76.5 ± 10.4	77.7 ± 10.4	<0.01	a, b, c < d
Hypertension	545 (32.2)	569 (34.6)	748 (39.3)	1103 (53.7)	<0.01	a, b < c < d

Abbreviations: sUA, serum urate; WC, waist circumference; HC, hip circumference; BMI, body mass index; HDL-C, high-density lipoprotein cholesterol; lipoprotein cholesterol; GGT, gamma-glutamyl transferase; SBP, systolic blood pressure; DBP, diastolic blood pressure. * post-hoc analysis was conducted using Scheffe's test, a: quartile 1, b: quartile 2, c: quartile 3, d: quartile 4.

3.2. Anthropometric Characteristics of Premenopausal and Postmenopausal Women with Hypertension

In postmenopausal women, the mean sUA values were higher in the participants in whom hypertension development was observed than in those who did not develop hypertension (4.72 ± 1.25 vs. 4.35 ± 1.03, $p < 0.001$). In the premenopausal women who developed hypertension, the baseline SBP and TC were 136.00 ± 16.44 mg/dL and 197.40 ± 33.90 mg/dL, respectively, and these parameters were higher than in those who did not develop hypertension ($p < 0.001$ vs. $p = 0.002$). There were no differences in smoking habits and the regular exercise status, between the pre- and postmenopausal women (Table 2).

Table 2. Anthropometric characteristics of premenopausal and postmenopausal women with hypertension.

Variables	Premenopausal Women (N = 1415)			Postmenopausal Women (N = 5879)		
	Without Hypertension (N = 1142)	With Hypertension (N = 273)	p *	Without Hypertension (N = 3187)	With Hypertension (N = 2692)	p *
sUA (mg/dL)	4.08 ± 0.87	4.42 ± 1.06	<0.01	4.35 ± 1.03	4.72 ± 1.25	<0.01
Age (year)	46.65 ± 3.98	48.57 ± 4.27	<0.01	63.08 ± 8.44	65.84 ± 7.82	<0.01
BMI (kg/m^2)	24.10 ± 2.96	26.19 ± 3.55	<0.01	23.94 ± 3.15	25.06 ± 3.33	<0.01
WC (cm)	79.25 ± 8.18	84.26 ± 8.65	<0.01	82.35 ± 8.96	85.25 ± 8.98	<0.01
HC (cm)	93.45 ± 6.31	96.14 ± 6.39	<0.01	92.06 ± 6.48	93.54 ± 6.83	<0.01
SBP (mmHg)	111.00 ± 11.22	136.00 ± 16.44	<0.01	116.30 ± 12.00	136.90 ± 17.92	<0.01
DBP (mmHg)	72.43 ± 8.41	88.61 ± 9.81	<0.01	73.14 ± 7.97	81.14 ± 11.08	<0.01
TC (mg/dL)	190.40 ± 32.36	197.40 ± 33.90	0.002	205.48 ± 36.26	206.94 ± 37.99	0.14
TG (mg/dL)	114.80 ± 70.17	146.30 ± 94.17	<0.01	141.50 ± 78.67	162.50 ± 95.14	<0.01
HDL (mg/dL)	47.55 ± 11.10	46.49 ± 11.40	0.16	46.48 ± 11.10	44.55 ± 10.74	<0.01
Total protein (g/dL)	7.34 ± 0.38	7.43 ± 0.42	0.01	7.35 ± 0.40	7.42 ± 0.42	<0.01
Albumin (g/dL)	4.42 ± 0.22	4.44 ± 0.26	0.22	4.43 ± 0.23	4.48 ± 0.24	<0.01
GGT (I/U)	18.34 ± 27.48	22.56 ± 27.39	0.03	19.06 ± 20.14	22.38 ± 29.59	<0.01
Fasting glucose (mg/dL)	92.93 ± 15.41	98.30 ± 23.20	<0.01	97.10 ± 20.58	101.70 ± 23.00	<0.01
Creatinine (mg/dL)	0.85 ± 0.08	0.85 ± 0.11	0.88	0.86 ± 0.10	0.90 ± 0.25	<0.01
Current smoking (%)	7 (1.2)	2 (1.4)	0.93	90 (2.8)	66 (2.5)	0.53
Current drinker (%)	448 (39.2)	108 (39.6)	0.89	886 (27.8)	638 (23.7)	0.001
Regular exercise (%)	459 (40.2)	107 (39.2)	0.76	849 (26.6)	785 (29.2)	0.11

Abbreviations: sUA, serum urate; BMI, body mass index; WC, waist circumference; HC, hip circumference; SBP, systolic blood pressure; DBP, diastolic blood pressure; TC, total cholesterol; TG, triglyceride; HDL, high-density lipoprotein; GGT, gamma-glutamyl transferase. *, p-value was calculated by t-test.

3.3. Univariate and Multivariate Logistic Regression Analyses

In univariate logistic regression analysis, we investigated that postmenopausal women with a high sUA and high BMI were 3.13 times more likely to have hypertension than those with a normal BMI and a lower sUA (OR 3.13, 95% CI 2.67–3.66 vs. OR 1.85, 95% CI 1.63–2.11, respectively) (Table 3). A higher sUA level and TG were positively and significantly associated with the development of hypertension in postmenopausal women (OR 2.63, 95% CI 2.25–3.08) (Table 3). Pre-menopausal women with high sUA and high BMI showed 5.20 times more likely to have hypertension than those with normal BMI and a lower sUA (OR 5.20, 95% CI 3.48–7.78) (Table 3).

Multivariate logistic analysis after adjusting for age, SBP and BMI showed that a higher sUA and a high WC was found to be significantly associated with a 1.62-fold increased risk of hypertension in postmenopausal women (Table 3). After adjusting for age, SBP and BMI showed that a high sUA and a high TG were found to be significantly associated with a 2.08-fold increased risk of hypertension in postmenopausal women (OR 2.08, 95% CI 1.72–2.53) (Table 3).

Table 3. Effect of interactions between anthropometric parameters on hypertension in premenopausal and postmenopausal women.

Variables	Crude Odds Ratio (95% CI)		Adjusted Odds Ratio (95% CI)	
	Premenopausal (N = 1415)	Postmenopausal (N = 5879)	Premenopausal (N = 1415)	Postmenopausal (N = 5879)
Drinking status × sUA †				
Never, past drinker and sUA < 5 mg/dL	1.00 (reference)	1.00 (reference)	1.00 (reference)	1.00 (reference)
Current drinker and sUA < 5 mg/dL	0.95 (0.69–1.30)	0.82 (0.71–0.95)	0.92 (0.60–1.42)	0.79 (0.66–0.95)
Never, past drinker and sUA ≥ 5 mg/dL	**2.16 (1.44–3.24)**	**1.96 (1.71–2.23)**	1.57 (0.88–2.77)	**1.91 (1.62–2.25)**
Current drinker and sUA ≥ 5 mg/dL	**2.66 (1.67–4.23)**	**1.42 (1.17–1.71)**	**2.09 (1.10–4.00)**	**1.44 (1.14–1.81)**
BMI × urate ‡				
Normal and sUA < 5 mg/dL	1.00 (reference)	1.00 (reference)	1.00 (reference)	1.00 (reference)
Obesity and sUA < 5 mg/dL	**3.11 (2.27–4.25)**	**1.85 (1.63–2.11)**	1.15 (0.69–1.92)	**1.61 (1.33–1.94)**
Normal and sUA ≥ 5 mg/dL	**2.32 (1.34–4.00)**	**1.82 (1.56–2.12)**	1.93 (0.92–4.06)	**1.86 (1.53–2.25)**
Obesity and sUA ≥ 5 mg/dL	**5.20 (3.48–7.78)**	**3.13 (2.67–3.66)**	**2.13 (1.14–3.99)**	**3.18 (2.54–3.96)**
Waist circumference × urate †				
Normal and sUA < 5 mg/dL	1.00 (reference)	1.00 (reference)	1.00 (reference)	1.00 (reference)
Abdominal obesity and sUA < 5 mg/dL	**2.58 (1.87–3.56)**	**1.60 (1.41–1.82)**	0.77 (0.43–1.27)	0.86 (0.71–1.03)
Normal and sUA ≥ 5 mg/dL	**2.27 (1.46–3.53)**	**1.87 (1.59–2.18)**	**1.97 (1.08–3.60)**	**1.84 (1.51–2.24)**
Abdominal obesity and sUA ≥ 5 mg/dL	**4.59 (2.98–7.06)**	**2.74 (2.35–3.20)**	1.27 (0.64–2.52)	**1.62 (1.30–2.01)**
Triglyceride × sUA †				
Normal and sUA < 5 mg/dL	1.00 (reference)	1.00 (reference)	1.00 (reference)	1.00 (reference)
Hypertriglyceridemia and sUA < 5 mg/dL	**2.03 (1.43–2.88)**	**1.50 (1.32–1.72)**	1.26 (0.78–2.06)	1.14 (0.96–1.34)
Normal and sUA ≥ 5 mg/dL	**2.19 (1.45–3.31)**	**1.78 (1.53–2.07)**	1.65 (0.92–2.96)	**1.82 (1.51–2.20)**
Hypertriglyceridemia and sUA ≥ 5 mg/dL	**3.88 (2.49–6.04)**	**2.63 (2.25–3.08)**	**2.38 (1.28–4.43)**	**2.08 (1.72–2.53)**

Abbreviations: sUA, serum urate; BMI, body mass index. † Adjusted for age, systolic blood pressure and BMI. ‡ Adjusted for age, systolic blood pressure and waist circumference. Statistically significant results were presented by bold type.

3.4. *Hypertension Risk of Participants according to Genotypes of Xanthine Dehydrogenase (XDH)*

We found that participants with *XDH* rs206847 CC genotype had a risk of hypertension with statistical significance (OR=3.63). Multivariate logistic regression analysis showed a significantly lower risk of hypertension in women with rs206860AG genotypes than those with the wild type (AA) (OR = 0.26, 95% CI 0.08–0.89, p = 0.03) (Table 4). After adjusting for age, smoking status, alcohol consumption, and regular exercise, rs206826 AC genotype was associated with a decreased risk of hypertension (OR = 0.28 95 % CI 0.08–0.98). However, women with rs206847 CC and rs207425 GA genotypes had an elevated risk of hypertension.

Table 4. Association of *XDH* genetic variants and risk of hypertension.

SNP Number	SNP Type	Crude	p	Model 1	p	Model 2	p
rs206847	AA	1.000 (ref)		1.000 (ref)		1.000 (ref)	
	AC	2.467 (0.677–8.997)	0.17	2.519 (0.690–9.202)	0.16	3.174 (0.807–12.491)	0.1
	CC	3.631 (0.863–15.287)	0.08	3.755 (0.887–15.900)	0.07	5.076 (1.044–24.682)	**0.04**
rs206860	AA	1.000 (ref)		1.000 (ref)		1.000 (ref)	
	AG	0.287 (0.091–0.905)	0.03	0.282 (0.089–0.893)	0.03	0.263 (0.078–0.888)	**0.03**
	GG	0.661 (0.183–2.386)	0.53	0.646 (0.178–2.342)	0.51	0.451 (0.109–1.866)	0.27
rs207425	GG	1.000 (ref)		1.000 (ref)		1.000 (ref)	
	GA	2.065 (0.770–5.537)	0.15	2.044 (0.758–5.509)	0.16	3.160 (1.015–9.841)	**0.05**
	AA	-	0.99	-	0.99	-	0.99
rs1884725	GG	1.000 (ref)		1.000 (ref)		1.000 (ref)	
	GA	1.052 (0.338–3.279)	0.93	1.011 (0.323–3.162)	0.99	0.957 (0.282–3.244)	0.94
	AA	3.668 (0.805–16.725)	0.09	3.935 (0.854–18.127)	0.08	11.162 (1.525–81.706)	**0.02**

Table 4. *Cont.*

SNP Number	SNP Type	Crude	*p*	Model 1	*p*	Model 2	*p*
rs3769616	GG	1.000 (ref)		1.000 (ref)		1.000 (ref)	
	GA	-	0.99	-	0.99	-	0.99
	AA	1.580 (0.207–12.037)	0.66	1.562 (0.203–12.013)	0.67	9.732 (0.972–97.400)	0.05
rs206826	AA	1.000 (ref)		1.000 (ref)		1.000 (ref)	
	AC	0.351 (0.110–1.123)	0.08	0.355 (0.110–1.139)	0.08	0.282 (0.081–0.979)	**0.05**
	CC	0.907 (0.283–2.913)	0.87	0.905 (0.280–2.918)	0.87	0.588 (0.158–2.180)	0.43

Abbreviations: SNP, single nucleotide polymorphism; A, adenine, C, cytosine, G, guanine. Model 1 was adjusted for age, smoking status, alcohol consumption, regular exercise. Model 2 was adjusted for Model 1 and additionally adjusted for systolic blood pressure, total cholesterol and baseline body mass index. Statistically significant results were presented by bold type.

4. Discussion

In the present study, an elevated sUA was observed to be positively associated with an increased risk of hypertension and postmenopausal women with high sUA and BMI were 3.13 times more likely to have hypertension than those who had low sUA and BMI. Furthermore, *XDH* rs206860 AG genotype was found to be associated with the decreased risk of hypertension.

The present study showed that hyperuricemia was significantly associated with elevated risk of hypertension after adjusting for known confounders. Several potential mechanisms might explain the association between sUA and hypertension [5,26]. The first involves insulin resistance. Elevated insulin levels cause low urinary ammonium levels and predispose the precipitation of sUA [5,26]. Furthermore, insulin resistance is known to contribute to the developments of several metabolic disorders that influence the development of coronary artery disease [5,27], and to increase postmenopausal sUA concentrations. The second involves the detrimental effect of an elevated sUA concentration on renal function. Hyperuricemia leads to hypertension and renal injury via a crystal-independent mechanism by stimulating the renin–angiotensin system and inhibiting neuronal nitric oxide synthase [5,28]. Also, as sUA in rats induces sodium excretion to decrease by the epithelial sodium channel, it therefore contributes hypertension [29]. The third mechanism involves endothelial dysfunction. Experimental evidence suggests a potentially causal role for urate in the pathogenesis of hypertension and atherosclerosis [28]. It was reported that sUA concentrations are higher in postmenopausal than in premenopausal women [30]. As far as we know, in postmenopausal women who did not receive estrogen hormone therapy, sUA concentration tended to increase due to a shortage of the uricosuric effect of estrogen.

Although the association between sUA and hypertension has been already demonstrated in epidemiological and clinical studies, the nature of the interaction between sUA and hypertension remains debatable. The sUA might not be an independent risk factor of hypertension after controlling for other risk factors, but some studies have reported sUA is predictive of hypertension and renal disease development after controlling for associated risk factors. However, a recent meta-analysis including 25 studies of 97,824 participants has shown that high sUA significantly predicts systemic hypertension [16].

In fact, urate found to have several beneficial and potentially detrimental biologic effects [31]. Our results suggest hyperuricemia dose-dependently predicts higher risks of hypertension as proportions of subjects with hypertension increased significantly with sUA quartile, which is consistent with the findings of previous studies. Interestingly, we found genetic variations of the rs206860 polymorphism of *XDH* gene might lower the risk of hypertension. To the best of our knowledge, the association between polymorphism of rs206860 and hypertension was not widely reported. rs206860 was investigated in the studies of advanced liver disease [32] and anti-tuberculosis drug-induced hepatotoxicity [33]. As far as we know, other SNPs were not directly reported regarding association between heterogeneity of SNPs and hypertension.

Other SNPs of *XDH* gene associated with hypertension were also reported. Recently, Scheepers et al. reported that mean arterial pressure and DBP increased approximately 1 mmHg less in carriers of minor alleles of *XDH* rs2043013 in a European population [19]. Yang J et al. reported multivariate logistic regression analysis showed a significant association between the three SNPs of *XDH* at rs2043013 and hypertension in men: 47686C>T and 69901A>C in the recessive model, and 67873A>C (N1109T) in the dominant model [34]. Wu B et al. showed the *XDH* gene polymorphisms rs1042039, rs1054889, and rs2073316 might be associated with hypertension in the rural Han Chinese population [21].

The present study has some limitations that warrant considerations. First, subjects were not analyzed over a follow-up period, and therefore, we could not individually evaluate whether the association between sUA concentration and new-onset hypertension was relevant over a longer period. Second, the genome wide association study (GWAS) population included a smaller number of postmenopausal women with hypertension than our basic subjects for each parameter analysis. Third, our findings might be differently applied to other populations, especially younger age groups of different ethnicities. As far as we know, *XDH* rs206860 and its associations with hypertension have not been studied. rs206860 of *XDH* is unknown genetic variant so far and further studies in gene discovery and function needs to be verified. Also, cross-sectional nature of study has limited power to make conclusions about causality.

In order to investigate an association between genetic variants in *XDH* and risk of hypertension, we examined confounding factors in multivariate logistic regression analysis gradually. We identified the optimal model adjusted for age, smoking status, alcohol consumption, regular exercise, systolic blood pressure, total cholesterol, and baseline body mass index. However, we recognized that women with hypertension were few and have very wide confidence intervals because some women do not have the genotype of *XDH*. Also, it is not possible to identify whether high urate leads to hypertension or not from a cross-sectional study

However, this study showed a significant association between sUA and hypertension risk in postmenopausal women. sUA might be a useful marker to predict disease modality and progression of chronic metabolic diseases such as hypertension in clinical practice.

5. Conclusions

This study suggests that sUA concentrations might be associated with an increased risk of hypertension in postmenopausal women and that the rs206860 polymorphism of the *XDH* gene might be associated with a low risk of hypertension in Koreans. It seems that sUA may be a cost-effective, applicable parameter to evaluate hypertension risk of postmenopausal women. Further well-designed, large-scale studies in other populations are warranted to validate our results.

Author Contributions: Conceptualization, J.-H.L. and J.R.C.; methodology, J.-H.L., T.H.G. and J.R.C.; software, T.H.G. and S.J.; validation, J.-H.L., T.H.G. and J.R.C.; formal analysis, J.-H.L., T.H.G and J.R.C.; investigation, J.-H.L. and J.R.C.; resources, J.-H.L. and J.R.C.; data curation, J.-H.L., T.H.G. and J.R.C.; writing—original draft preparation, J.-H.L.; writing—review and editing, J.-H.L. and J.R.C.; visualization, J.-H.L., T.H.G. and J.R.C.; supervision, S.-H.L., J.K., J.H.H., J.Y.K., D.R.K. and S.-B.K.; project administration, J.-H.L.; funding acquisition, J.R.C. and S.-B.K.

Acknowledgments: The authors would like to express their gratitude to members of the Institute of Genomic Cohort in Wonju Severance Christian Hospital for helpful discussions.

Abbreviations

sUA: serum urate; BMI, body mass index; WC, waist circumference; HC, hip circumference; HDL-C, high density lipoprotein cholesterol; GGT, gamma-glutamyl transferase; SBP, systolic blood pressure; DBP, diastolic blood pressure.

References

1. Chang, C.C.; Wu, C.H.; Liu, L.K.; Chou, R.H.; Kuo, C.S.; Huang, P.H.; Chen, L.K.; Lin, S.J. Association between serum uric acid and cardiovascular risk in nonhypertensive and nondiabetic individuals: The Taiwan I-Lan Longitudinal Aging Study. *Sci. Rep.* **2018**, *8*, 5234. [CrossRef]
2. Orlando, A.; Cazzaniga, E.; Giussani, M.; Palestini, P.; Genovesi, S. Hypertension in Children: Role of Obesity, Simple Carbohydrates, and Uric Acid. *Front. Public Health* **2018**, *6*, 129. [CrossRef]
3. Krishnan, E.; Kwoh, C.K.; Schumacher, H.R.; Kuller, L. Hyperuricemia and incidence of hypertension among men without metabolic syndrome. *Hypertension (Dallas Tex. 1979)* **2007**, *49*, 298–303. [CrossRef]
4. Jossa, F.; Farinaro, E.; Panico, S.; Krogh, V.; Celentano, E.; Galasso, R.; Mancini, M.; Trevisan, M. Serum uric acid and hypertension: The Olivetti heart study. *J. Hum. Hypertens.* **1994**, *8*, 677–681. [PubMed]
5. Chen, Q.; Yin, Y.J.; Chen, W.Y.; Wu, J.N.; Huang, X. Assessment of the association between serum uric acid levels and the incidence of hypertension in nonmetabolic syndrome subjects: A prospective observational study. *Medicine* **2018**, *97*, e9765. [CrossRef] [PubMed]
6. Wei, F.; Sun, N.; Cai, C.; Feng, S.; Tian, J.; Shi, W.; Xu, W.; Wang, Y.; Yang, X.; Li, W.D. Associations between serum uric acid and the incidence of hypertension: A Chinese senior dynamic cohort study. *J. Transl. Med.* **2016**, *14*, 110. [CrossRef]
7. Amos, C.I.; Wu, X.; Broderick, P.; Gorlov, I.P.; Gu, J.; Eisen, T.; Dong, Q.; Zhang, Q.; Gu, X.; Vijayakrishnan, J.; et al. Genome-wide association scan of tag SNPs identifies a susceptibility locus for lung cancer at 15q25.1. *Nat. Genet.* **2008**, *40*, 616–622. [CrossRef]
8. Nieto, F.J.; Iribarren, C.; Gross, M.D.; Comstock, G.W.; Cutler, R.G. Uric acid and serum antioxidant capacity: A reaction to atherosclerosis? *Atherosclerosis* **2000**, *148*, 131–139. [CrossRef]
9. Sciacqua, A.; Perticone, M.; Tassone, E.J.; Cimellaro, A.; Miceli, S.; Maio, R.; Sesti, G.; Perticone, F. Uric acid is an independent predictor of cardiovascular events in post-menopausal women. *Int. J. Cardiol.* **2015**, *197*, 271–275. [CrossRef] [PubMed]
10. Cheng, D.; Du, R.; Wu, X.Y.; Lin, L.; Peng, K.; Ma, L.N.; Xu, Y.; Xu, M.; Chen, Y.H.; Bi, Y.F.; et al. Serum Uric Acid is Associated with the Predicted Risk of Prevalent Cardiovascular Disease in a Community-dwelling Population without Diabetes. *Biomed. Environ. Sci.* **2018**, *31*, 106–114. [CrossRef]
11. Kawamoto, R.; Ninomiya, D.; Senzaki, K.; Kumagi, T. Interaction between body mass index and serum uric acid in relation to blood pressure in community-dwelling Japanese men. *Clin. Hypertens.* **2018**, *24*, 1. [CrossRef] [PubMed]
12. Jin, M.; Yang, F.; Yang, I.; Yin, Y.; Luo, J.J.; Wang, H.; Yang, X.F. Uric acid, hyperuricemia and vascular diseases. *Front. Biosci. (Landmark Ed.)* **2012**, *17*, 656–669. [CrossRef]
13. Corry, D.B.; Eslami, P.; Yamamoto, K.; Nyby, M.D.; Makino, H.; Tuck, M.L. Uric acid stimulates vascular smooth muscle cell proliferation and oxidative stress via the vascular renin-angiotensin system. *J. Hypertens.* **2008**, *26*, 269–275. [CrossRef]
14. Kang, D.H.; Park, S.K.; Lee, I.K.; Johnson, R.J. Uric acid-induced C-reactive protein expression: Implication on cell proliferation and nitric oxide production of human vascular cells. *J. Am. Soc. Nephrol. JASN* **2005**, *16*, 3553–3562. [CrossRef]
15. Mazzali, M.; Hughes, J.; Kim, Y.G.; Jefferson, J.A.; Kang, D.H.; Gordon, K.L.; Lan, H.Y.; Kivlighn, S.; Johnson, R.J. Elevated uric acid increases blood pressure in the rat by a novel crystal-independent mechanism. *Hypertension (Dallas Tex. 1979)* **2001**, *38*, 1101–1106. [CrossRef]
16. Wang, J.; Qin, T.; Chen, J.; Li, Y.; Wang, L.; Huang, H.; Li, J. Hyperuricemia and risk of incident hypertension: A systematic review and meta-analysis of observational studies. *PLoS ONE* **2014**, *9*, e114259. [CrossRef]
17. Hak, A.E.; Choi, H.K. Menopause, postmenopausal hormone use and serum uric acid levels in US women–the Third National Health and Nutrition Examination Survey. *Arthritis Res. Ther.* **2008**, *10*, R116. [CrossRef] [PubMed]

18. Sumino, H.; Ichikawa, S.; Kanda, T.; Nakamura, T.; Sakamaki, T. Reduction of serum uric acid by hormone replacement therapy in postmenopausal women with hyperuricaemia. *Lancet (Lond. Engl.)* **1999**, *354*, 650. [CrossRef]
19. Scheepers, L.E.; Wei, F.F.; Stolarz-Skrzypek, K.; Malyutina, S.; Tikhonoff, V.; Thijs, L.; Salvi, E.; Barlassina, C.; Filipovsky, J.; Casiglia, E.; et al. Xanthine oxidase gene variants and their association with blood pressure and incident hypertension: A population study. *J. Hypertens.* **2016**, *34*, 2147–2154. [CrossRef]
20. Battelli, M.G.; Bolognesi, A.; Polito, L. Pathophysiology of circulating xanthine oxidoreductase: New emerging roles for a multi-tasking enzyme. *Biochim. Biophys. Acta* **2014**, *1842*, 1502–1517. [CrossRef]
21. Wu, B.; Hao, Y.; Shi, J.; Geng, N.; Li, T.; Chen, Y.; Sun, Z.; Zheng, L.; Li, H.; Li, N.; et al. Association between xanthine dehydrogenase tag single nucleotide polymorphisms and essential hypertension. *Mol. Med. Rep.* **2015**, *12*, 5685–5690. [CrossRef]
22. Verdecchia, P.; Schillaci, G.; Reboldi, G.; Santeusanio, F.; Porcellati, C.; Brunetti, P. Relation between serum uric acid and risk of cardiovascular disease in essential hypertension. The PIUMA study. *Hypertension (Dallas Tex. 1979)* **2000**, *36*, 1072–1078. [CrossRef]
23. Choi, J.R.; Ahn, S.V.; Kim, J.Y.; Koh, S.B.; Choi, E.H.; Lee, G.Y.; Jang, Y.E. Comparison of various anthropometric indices for the identification of a predictor of incident hypertension: The ARIRANG study. *J. Hum. Hypertens.* **2018**, *32*, 294–300. [CrossRef]
24. Kim, J.; Yoon, D.W.; Lee, S.K.; Lee, S.; Choi, K.M.; Robert, T.J.; Shin, C. Concurrent presence of inflammation and obstructive sleep apnea exacerbates the risk of metabolic syndrome: A KoGES 6-year follow-up study. *Medicine* **2017**, *96*, e4488. [CrossRef] [PubMed]
25. Choi, J.R.; Jang, Y.; Kim Yoon, S.; Park, J.K.; Sorn, S.R.; Park, M.Y.; Lee, M. The Impact of CDH13 Polymorphism and Statin Administration on TG/HDL Ratio in Cardiovascular Patients. *Yonsei Med. J.* **2015**, *56*, 1604–1612. [CrossRef] [PubMed]
26. Bonora, E.; Capaldo, B.; Perin, P.C.; Del Prato, S.; De Mattia, G.; Frittitta, L.; Frontoni, S.; Leonetti, F.; Luzi, L.; Marchesini, G.; et al. Hyperinsulinemia and insulin resistance are independently associated with plasma lipids, uric acid and blood pressure in non-diabetic subjects. The GISIR database. *Nutr. Metab. Cardiovasc. Dis. NMCD* **2008**, *18*, 624–631. [CrossRef] [PubMed]
27. Ninomiya, T.; Kubo, M.; Doi, Y.; Yonemoto, K.; Tanizaki, Y.; Rahman, M.; Arima, H.; Tsuryuya, K.; Iida, M.; Kiyohara, Y. Impact of metabolic syndrome on the development of cardiovascular disease in a general Japanese population: The Hisayama study. *Stroke* **2007**, *38*, 2063–2069. [CrossRef]
28. Kanellis, J.; Kang, D.H. Uric acid as a mediator of endothelial dysfunction, inflammation, and vascular disease. *Semin. Nephrol.* **2005**, *25*, 39–42. [CrossRef]
29. Xu, J.; Lloyd, D.J.; Hale, C.; Stanislaus, S.; Chen, M.; Sivits, G.; Vonderfecht, S.; Hecht, R.; Li, Y.S.; Lindberg, R.A.; et al. Fibroblast growth factor 21 reverses hepatic steatosis, increases energy expenditure, and improves insulin sensitivity in diet-induced obese mice. *Diabetes* **2009**, *58*, 250–259. [CrossRef]
30. Techatraisak, K.; Kongkaew, T. The association of hyperuricemia and metabolic syndrome in Thai postmenopausal women. *Climacteric J. Int. Menopause Soc.* **2017**, *20*, 552–557. [CrossRef]
31. Johnson, R.J.; Kang, D.H.; Feig, D.; Kivlighn, S.; Kanellis, J.; Watanabe, S.; Tuttle, K.R.; Rodriguez-Iturbe, B.; Herrera-Acosta, J.; Mazzali, M. Is there a pathogenetic role for uric acid in hypertension and cardiovascular and renal disease? *Hypertension (Dallas Tex. 1979)* **2003**, *41*, 1183–1190. [CrossRef] [PubMed]
32. Roberts, K.E.; Kawut, S.M.; Krowka, M.J.; Brown, R.S., Jr.; Trotter, J.F.; Shah, V.; Peter, I.; Tighiouart, H.; Mitra, N.; Handorf, E.; et al. Genetic risk factors for hepatopulmonary syndrome in patients with advanced liver disease. *Gastroenterology* **2010**, *139*, 130–139.e24. [CrossRef]
33. Li, Y.; Tang, H.; Qi, H.; Shen, C.; Sun, L.; Li, J.; Xu, F.; Jiao, W.; Yang, X.; Shen, A. rs1800796 of the IL6 gene is associated with increased risk for anti-tuberculosis drug-induced hepatotoxicity in Chinese Han children. *Tuberculosis* **2018**, *111*, 71–77. [CrossRef] [PubMed]
34. Yang, J.; Kamide, K.; Kokubo, Y.; Takiuchi, S.; Horio, T.; Matayoshi, T.; Yasuda, H.; Miwa, Y.; Yoshii, M.; Yoshihara, F.; et al. Associations of hypertension and its complications with variations in the xanthine dehydrogenase gene. *Hypertens. Res. Off. J. Jpn. Soc. Hypertens.* **2008**, *31*, 931–940. [CrossRef] [PubMed]

12

Seasonal Variation in Physical Activity among Preoperative Patients with Lung Cancer Determined Using a Wearable Device

Sunga Kong [1,2,†], Hye Yun Park [3,†], Danbee Kang [1,4], Jae Kyung Lee [2], Genehee Lee [2], O Jung Kwon [3], Young Mog Shim [5], Jae Ill Zo [5,*] and Juhee Cho [1,4,6,*]

1 Department of Clinical Research Design and Evaluation, SAIHST, Sungkyunkwan University, Seoul 06351, Korea; sunga00kong@gmail.com (S.K.); dbee.kang@gmail.com (D.K.)
2 Patient-Centered Outcomes Research Institute, Samsung Medical Center, Seoul 06351, Korea; roemgirls1230@gmail.com (J.K.L.); genehee@gmail.com (G.L.)
3 Division of Pulmonary and Critical Care Medicine, Department of Medicine, Samsung Medical Center, Sungkyunkwan University School of Medicine, Seoul 06351, Korea; hyeyunpark@skku.edu (H.Y.P.); ojung.kwon@samsung.com (O.J.K.)
4 Center for Clinical Epidemiology, Samsung Medical Center, Sungkyunkwan University School of Medicine, Seoul 06351, Korea
5 Department of Thoracic and Cardiovascular Surgery, Samsung Medical Center, Sungkyunkwan University School of Medicine, Seoul 06351, Korea; youngmog.shim@samsung.com
6 Departments of Epidemiology and Health, Behavior and Society, Johns Hopkins Bloomberg School of Public Health, Baltimore, MD 21205, USA
* Correspondence: jayl.zo@samsung.com (J.I.Z.); jcho@skku.edu (J.C.);

† S.K. and H.Y.P. contributed equally as joint first authors.

Abstract: We aim to examine how season and temperature levels affect physical activity using a wearable device among patients scheduled to undergo surgical resection of lung cancer. Physical activity (PA) data from the wearable device were analyzed by seasons for 555 preoperative lung cancer patients from the CATCH-LUNG cohort study. The seasons were divided into spring, summer, autumn, and winter using the study enrollment date before surgery. The overall mean (SD) age was 61.1 (8.9) years, and the mean (SD) daily steps at each season were 11,438 (5922), 11,147 (5065), 10,404 (4403), and 8548 (4293), respectively. In the fully-adjusted models, patients in the winter season had 27.04% fewer daily steps (95% CI = −36.68%, −15.93%) and 35.22% less time spent performing moderate to vigorous physical activity (MVPA) compared to patients in the spring. The proportion of participants with over 8000 steps and duration of MVPA were significantly lower in the winter than the spring. In particular, daily steps had a negative linear association with wind chill temperature in patients who lived in Seoul. In conclusion, PA was significantly lower in the winter and it was more robust in patients who had a low cardiorespiratory function.

Keywords: lung cancer; physical activity; season; preoperative; wearable

---

1. Introduction

Lung cancer is the leading cause of cancer-related death worldwide, contributing to 1.6 million deaths annually [1]. Surgical resection remains the best curative treatment option in patients with early-stage non-small cell lung cancer (NSCLC), and a patient's preoperative status is important to assess the feasibility of undergoing surgical lung resection under general anesthesia. In particular, patients with poor pulmonary function and cardiorespiratory fitness are considered inoperable due to increased morbidity and mortality after surgical resection [2]. Both cardiopulmonary fitness and functional capacity are widely recognized as strong predictors of postoperative complications, specifically mortality and long-term survival, in NSCLC [3].

Cardiorespiratory fitness (CRF) and functional capacity are affected by physical activity (PA) [4]. Numerous studies have conducted PA or exercise programs to improve physical fitness and functions before thoracic surgery [2,5]. Adopting and sustaining a more physically active lifestyle has been shown to reduce the risk of complications and mortality and improve health-related quality of life in patients who underwent thoracic surgery [6]. However, promoting long-term PA has been challenging due to various factors such as lack of motivation, access to facilities for physical activities, and inclement weather [7]. Studies reported that seasonal weather conditions could promote or deter PA [8]. Furthermore, most studies were conducted with a small number of participants (<50) and only included limited populations such as children [9] or the elderly [10]. In addition, few quantitative assessments have been focused on seasonal variation in PA among preoperative lung cancer patients. Studies have attempted to measure daily PA with quantitative assessments using simple and non-expensive devices during the perioperative periods of lung cancer surgery [11–13]. They found that that daily walk distance predicted maximum oxygen consumption per minute in patients undergoing lung resection [11], and the time and the quality of the daily ambulatory activity of the patients decreased during the first postoperative month [12]. Thus, our study aims to use a wearable device (Fitbit) to examine how the season and temperature level affect PA among patients who are scheduled to undergo surgical resection for lung cancer.

2. Methods

2.1. Subjects and Data Sources

Patients with lung cancer in this study were selected from the Coordinate Approach to Cancer patients' Health for Lung Cancer (CATCH-LUNG) cohort of preoperative lung cancer patients between March 2016 and October 2018 at the Samsung Medical Center in Seoul, Korea. Inclusion criteria for CATCH-LUNG cohort were (1) patients who were expected to undergo curative lung cancer surgery for suspected or histologically confirmed NSCLC, (2) patients who were able to walk and keep a normal life with the Eastern Cooperative Oncology Group Performance Status (ECOG PS $\leq$1), and (3) patients understood the purpose of this study and agreed to participate in the study. Exclusion criteria were (1) patients who had undergone neoadjuvant treatment before surgery, (2) patients free of NSCLC after pathological exams, (3) patients whose surgery was canceled, or (4) patients who withdrew consent before baseline data collection. Among patients who met these criteria, we furthermore excluded patients who had either pathologically confirmed stage IV cancer after surgery (n = 2) and 63 patients who were excluded due to lack of Fitbit data (28 patients wore their Fitbit less than one day and 35 patients had either hardware or software failures of Fitbit). The final study sample included 555 patients. The study protocol was approved by the Institutional Review Board of Samsung Medical Center (no. 2015-11-025). Written informed consent was obtained from all participants.

2.2. Grouping and Weather Data Collection

The main exposure variable was the season, which was divided into spring (March to May), summer (June to August), autumn (September to November), and winter (December to February) using the study enrollment date before surgery. For preoperative patients living in the metropolitan Seoul area, the weather-related factor of wind chill temperature was obtained from the Korea Meteorological Administration (https://data.kma.go.kr).

2.3. Physical Activity and other Variable

The main outcome was PA, which was assessed using a reliable wearable activity tracker [14]. The Flex tracker (Fitbit, San Francisco, CA, USA) was used to quantify the PA intensity, time, activity type, and steps per day. We asked participants to wear a Fitbit activity tracker 24 h per day for 7 consecutive days. We determined that patients did not wear the Fitbit if there was no movement (0 steps) for more than 4 consecutive hours during daytime (9:00 a.m. to 4:00 p.m.). Physical activity time, frequency, and intensity data were automatically measured and saved by an internal sensor. We then calculated activity level by combining the Fitbit data with age, gender, height, and weight data recorded at registration. Activities were classified into four categories: (1) sleeping or sedentary activity (1 MET), (2) light physical activity (1~2.9 METs), (3) moderate physical activity (3~5.9 METs), and (4) vigorous physical activity (more than 6 METs). The calculated values were averaged to define daily activity level.

The tracker was worn on the wrist. To reduce bias, the device had no screen so that patients could not see their recorded level of PA. In addition, there was no specific education or guidelines for patients regarding PA and patients were recommended to maintain PA prior to surgery, as usual.

CRF was measured using the 6-min walk test (6MWT), which was performed according to ATS guidelines [15]. Each participant was asked to walk (not run) back and forth along the corridor as far as possible for 6 min and was given standardized verbal encouragement every minute. The test has been widely used for preoperative and postoperative evaluations of CRF. In some clinical situations, the 6MWT provides a better index of the patient's ability to perform daily activities compared to peak oxygen uptake [16]. In addition, the 6MWT is a sub-maximal test of CRF, as opposed to cardiopulmonary exercise testing (CPET). While it is well known that the incremental shuttle walk test (ISWT) has a higher correlation with CPET than 6MWT, we could not use the ISWT because it was not available in Korea. In fact, 6MWT has been widely used in real-world clinics for cardiopulmonary evaluation in patients with chronic obstructive pulmonary disease (COPD) [17]. To obtain quality data, trained researchers provided study participants detailed instructions about 6MWT, and asked patients to do a pilot walk (for 15~20 s) before the actual test.

Spirometry and DLco measurements were performed using a Vmax 22 respiratory analyzer (SensorMedics, OH, USA) according to the American Thoracic Society/European Respiratory Society criteria [18,19]. Absolute values of forced expiratory volume in 1 s (FEV_1), forced vital capacity (FVC), and DLco were obtained, and the percentage of predicted values (% predicted) for FEV_1, FVC, and DLco were calculated using a representative Korean sample [20,21] as a reference. Sociodemographic and behavioral information, including age, smoking status, and comorbidities, were recorded before surgery using a questionnaire. Treatment information regarding pathological stage and pulmonary function were collected after surgery.

2.4. Statistical Analysis

Continuous and categorical variables were compared among the seasons using analysis of variance (ANOVA) and the $\chi 2$ test, respectively.

For the main analyses, we used linear regression to compare the daily number of steps and the moderate-to-vigorous physical activity (MVPA) time by season. Since steps per day and MVPA minutes are markedly right skewed (p-values based on Shapiro–Wilk and Shapiro–Francia tests for normality were <0.001), we used log-transformed daily number of steps and MVPA time as the outcomes. The average difference (as a percent difference with 95% confidence interval (CI)) was estimated comparing patients enrolled in the summer, autumn, or winter to those patients enrolled in the spring.

Using daily number of steps and MVPA duration, we developed a dichotomized outcome to evaluate the proportion of participants who were physically active. Being physically active was defined as either taking more than 8000 steps per day or performing more than 60 min of MVPA. We chose 8000 steps per day based on a reference that adults usually take 5000 steps per day and perform daily activities such as house errands, walking, or shopping [22]. We then added 3000 steps per day to account for 30 min of MVPA (10 min of MVPA is around 1000 steps [23,24]). From this, we equated 8000 steps to 60 min of MVPA.

Logistic regression was conducted to compare the odds of being physically active by season with adjustments made for age, sex, smoking status, FEV_1% pred, any pulmonary comorbidities (COPD, asthma, or ILD), and any extra-pulmonary comorbidities (cardiovascular diseases or diabetes mellitus). In addition, we performed stratified analyses to evaluate differences in PA associated with the season in prespecified subgroups of age (<65 vs. ≥65 years) [25] and CRF (<500 vs. ≥500 m in 6MWD) [26].

To determine factors leading to the differences in PA according to season, we conducted an additional analysis for patients (n = 85) living in the Seoul metropolitan area because we considered the bias of area environment and topography in Korea. To find an association between weather and daily steps, we modeled wind chill temperature as a continuous variable using restricted cubic splines with knots at the 5th, 35th, 65th, and 95th percentiles of the sample distribution to provide a flexible estimate of the dose-response relationship between weather factors and daily steps.

For all analyses, a p-value of <0.05 was considered statistically significant. All analyses were performed using STATA software, version 14 (Stata Corp LP, College Station, TX, USA).

3. Results

The characteristics of 555 patients are described in Table 1. The mean (SD) age and daily steps of study participants were 61.1 (8.9) years and 10,603 (5200) (range, 425–32,143), respectively. Among the participants, Fitbit data from 30.8% (n = 171), 32.1% (n = 178), 17.8% (n = 99), and 19.3% (n = 107) of the study subjects were collected in the spring, summer, autumn, and winter seasons, respectively. Although patients in the winter season were likely to be younger and have better pulmonary function than patients in other seasons, the clinical characteristics, including sex, BMI, smoking status, comorbidities, pathologic stage, and cardiorespiratory fitness, were not different across the seasons (Table 1).

Table 1. Characteristics of study participants by season (n = 555).

Characteristics	Spring (n = 171)	Summer (n = 178)	Autumn (n = 99)	Winter (n = 107)	p
Mean age	60.6 (8.9)	62.6 (8.3)	60.6 (9.0)	59.9 (9.4)	0.05
Age categories					0.04
<65	118 (69.0)	104 (58.4)	66 (66.7)	79 (73.8)	
≥65	53 (31.0)	74 (41.6)	33 (33.3)	28 (26.2)	
Sex, male	97 (56.7)	101 (56.7)	57 (57.6)	57 (53.3)	0.92
Body mass index, kg/m^2	24.1 (2.9)	24.3 (2.7)	24.1 (2.7)	24.5 (3.2)	0.67
Smoking status					0.32
Never-smoker	78 (45.6)	89 (50.0)	48 (48.5)	57 (53.3)	
Ex-smoker	59 (34.5)	34 (19.1)	27 (27.3)	16 (15.0)	
Current smoker	34 (19.9)	55 (30.9)	24 (24.2)	34 (31.8)	
Marital status					0.64
Married	151 (88.3)	159 (89.3)	91 (91.9)	91 (85.1)	
Single/divorced/widowed	19 (11.1)	19 (10.7)	7 (7.1)	15 (14.0)	
Unknown	1 (0.6)	0	1 (1.0)	1 (0.9)	
Employment status					0.46
Current work	98 (57.3)	81 (45.5)	49 (49.5)	58 (54.2)	
No work	72 (42.1)	96 (53.9)	49 (49.5)	48 (44.9)	
Unknown	1 (0.6)	1 (0.6)	1 (1.0)	1 (0.9)	
Monthly family income					0.19
<$3.000	54 (31.6)	51 (28.7)	23 (23.2)	31 (29.0)	
≥$3.000	87 (50.9)	93 (52.3)	54 (54.6)	66 (61.7)	
Unknown	30 (17.5)	34 (19.1)	22 (22.2)	10 (9.4)	
Comorbidities					
Pulmonary comorbidities					
COPD	40 (23.4)	43 (24.2)	26 (26.3)	19 (17.8)	0.49
Asthma	3 (1.8)	8 (4.5)	1 (1.0)	3 (2.8)	0.34
ILD	1 (0.6)	2 (1.1)	1 (1.0)	2 (1.9)	0.86

Table 1. *Cont.*

Characteristics	Spring (n = 171)	Summer (n = 178)	Autumn (n = 99)	Winter (n = 107)	p
Extra-pulmonary comorbidities					
Hypertension	52 (30.4)	72 (40.5)	28 (28.3)	35 (32.7)	0.12
Diabetes mellitus	22 (12.9)	27 (15.2)	11 (11.1)	7 (6.5)	0.18
Cardiovascular disease	12 (7.0)	20 (11.2)	9 (9.1)	9 (8.4)	0.58
Pathologic stage					0.81
I	128 (74.9)	130 (73.0)	75 (75.8)	75 (70.1)	
II	25 (14.6)	31 (17.4)	13 (13.1)	16 (15.0)	
III	18 (10.5)	17 (9.6)	11 (11.1)	16 (15.0)	
Pulmonary function test					
FVC, L	3.6 (0.9)	3.4 (0.8)	3.7 (0.9)	3.7 (0.8)	0.02
FVC, % predicted	93.4 (11.5)	89.8 (12.9)	94.3 (12.7)	96.4 (12.1)	< 0.01
FEV_1, L	2.7 (0.7)	2.5 (0.6)	2.7 (0.6)	2.8 (0.6)	< 0.01
FEV_1, % predicted	90.0 (13.2)	87.5 (15.5)	90.2 (14.9)	95.0 (13.5)	< 0.01
FEV_1/FVC	73.8 (8.2)	73.6 (8.6)	72.6 (8.6)	75.1 (8.3)	0.21
DLco, %	91.6 (16.0)	89.2 (17.3)	89.7 (15.2)	91.3 (13.7)	0.47
Cardiorespiratory fitness					
6 min walk distance (m)	520.1(85.7)	506.9(89.1)	515.0(66.8)	508.1(80.7)	0.46
6 min walk distance					0.69
Short distance (<500 m)	68 (39.9)	77 (43.3)	37 (37.4)	49 (45.8)	
Long distance (≥500 m)	102 (59.7)	97 (54.5)	60 (60.1)	56 (52.3)	
Unknown	1 (0.6)	4 (2.3)	2 (2.1)	2 (1.9)	

Values are presented as either n (%) or mean (SD). COPD, chronic obstructive pulmonary disease; ILD, interstitial lung disease; FVC, forced vital capacity; FEV_1, forced expiratory volume in 1 s; DLco, diffusing capacity of carbon monoxide.

The mean (SD) daily steps were 11,438 (5922), 11,147 (5065), 10,404 (4403), and 8548 (4293) in patients who participated in this study in the spring, summer, autumn, and winter seasons, respectively. The proportion of patients who had 8000 or more steps per day was 71%, 72%, 71%, and 54% in participants who received surgery in the spring, summer, autumn, and winter seasons, respectively (Figure 1).

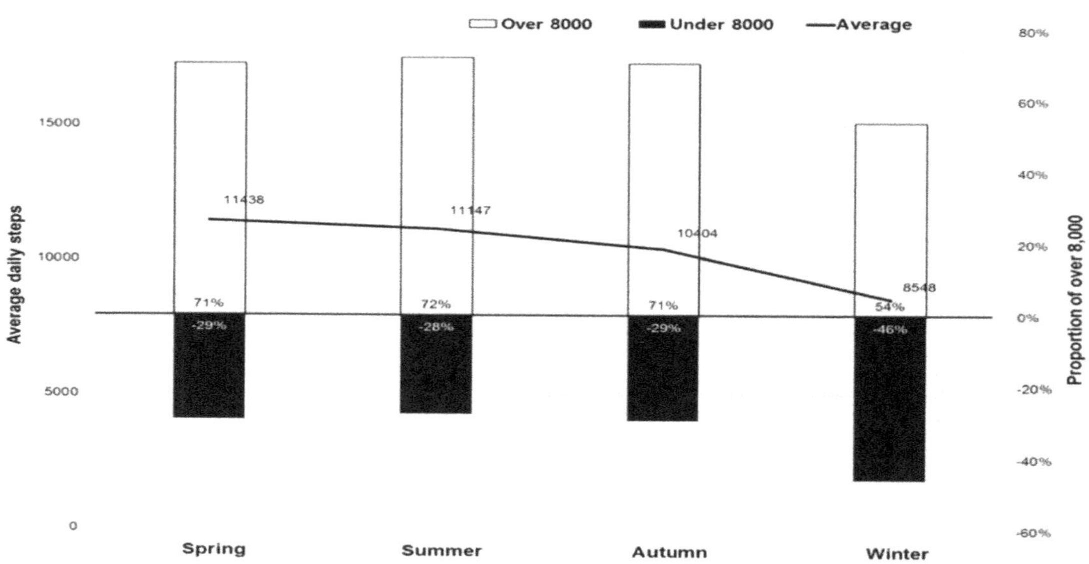

Figure 1. Mean daily steps and the proportion of participants who had more than 8000 steps in each season.

In the fully-adjusted models, patients in the winter season had a significantly lower number of daily steps, with a low of 27.04% (95% CI = −36.68%, −15.93%) compared to the daily steps of patients in the spring season. In comparing the mean (SD) MVPA time, patients in the winter season had the lowest MVPA among subjects (spring, 60.3 (57.2) min/d; summer, 58.5 (46.4) min/d; autumn, 51.0 (35.6) min/d; and winter, 35.0 (36.3) min/d). In the fully-adjusted models, compared to patients in the spring season, the MVPA time was significantly shorter by 35.22% (95% CI = −49.18%, −17.43%) for patients in the winter season. The number of steps and duration of MVPA were significantly lower in the winter season compared to spring season irrespective of age and 6MWD (Table 2).

Table 2. Differences in physical activity by season.

	Spring	Summer	Autumn	Winter
Difference in steps per day (%)				
Overall	Reference	−0.86 (−12.38, 12.18)	−6.24 (−18.86, 8.33)	−27.04 (−36.68, −15.93)
Age				
<65 years	Reference	−8.08 (−21.25, 7.30)	−10.27 (−24.74, 6.98)	−25.21 (−36.65, −11.70)
≥65 years	Reference	11.91 (−9.08, 37.74)	2.36 (−20.65, 32.02)	−32.16 (−48.31, −10.97)
p for interaction		0.14	0.40	0.55
Cardiorespiratory fitness (6MWD)				
<500 m	Reference	−1.21 (−18.1, 19.18)	7.07 (−14.97, 34.83)	−27.63 (−41.48, −10.50)
≥500 m	Reference	−0.75 (−15.53, 16.62)	−12.95 (−27.52, 4.55)	−20.97 (−34.54, −4.59)
p for interaction		0.97	0.17	0.54
Difference in MVPA minutes per day (%)				
Overall	Reference	5.06 (−14.6, 29.24)	−2.11(−23.13, 24.67)	−35.22 (−49.18, −17.43)
Age				
<65 years	Reference	5.13 (−19.26, 36.89)	−1.43 (−26.71, 32.57)	−33.03 (−49.63, −10.95)
≥65 years	Reference	4.05 (−26.37, 47.04)	−3.75 (−37.24, 47.60)	−40.72 (−62.76, −5.62)
p for interaction		0.96	0.93	0.66
Cardiorespiratory fitness (6MWD)				
<500 m	Reference	−4.25 (−30.56, 32.04)	20.57 (−18.5, 78.39)	−38.65 (−57.62, −11.18)
≥500 m	Reference	11.12 (−15.17, 45.55)	−10.57 (−34.3, 21.73)	−26.01 (−46.46, 2.25)
p for interaction		0.48	0.24	0.03

Models were adjusted for age, sex, smoking status, FEV_1% pred, any pulmonary comorbidities, and any extra-pulmonary comorbidities. Pulmonary comorbidities include chronic obstructive pulmonary disease, asthma, or interstitial lung disease, and extra-pulmonary comorbidities include cardiovascular diseases or diabetes mellitus. 6MWD, 6-min walk distance. MVPA, moderate-to-vigorous physical activity.

In the fully-adjusted models, the OR for 8000 or more steps per day was 0.46 (95% CI 0.28, 0.77) for patients in the winter compared to those in the spring. The proportion of patients who had 60 min or more MVPA per day was also similar (spring, 30.4%; summer, 42.7%; autumn, 32.3%; winter, 18.7%). In the fully-adjusted models, the OR for MVPA ≥ 60 min/day was 0.52 (95% CI = 0.29, 0.94) for patients in the winter compared to those in the spring. In particular, the OR for low CRF (<500 m) was 0.30 (95% CI 0.10, 0.87) for patients in the winter compared to those in the spring (Table 3).

Table 3. Odds ratios (95% CI) for physical activity by season.

	Spring	Summer	Autumn	Winter
Steps ≥8000/day				
Overall	Reference	1.11 (0.69, 1.79)	0.98 (0.57, 1.70)	0.46 (0.28, 0.77)
Age				
<65 years	Reference	0.79 (0.43, 1.44)	0.73 (0.37, 1.45)	0.38 (0.20, 0.71)
≥65 years	Reference	2.00 (0.93, 4.31)	1.75 (0.67, 4.56)	0.67 (0.26, 1.74)
p for interaction		0.06	0.15	0.32
Cardiorespiratory fitness (6MWD)				
<500 m	Reference	0.94 (0.48, 1.82)	1.75 (0.73, 4.20)	0.45 (0.21, 0.96)
≥500 m	Reference	1.35 (0.67, 2.74)	0.74 (0.36, 1.55)	0.58 (0.28, 1.22)
p for interaction		0.46	0.14	0.63
MVPA ≥60 min/day				
Overall	Reference	1.73 (1.10, 2.71)	1.07 (0.62, 1.83)	0.52 (0.29, 0.94)
Age				
<65 years	Reference	1.59 (0.91, 2.79)	1.19 (0.62, 2.27)	0.59 (0.30, 1.15)
≥65 years	Reference	2.11 (0.96, 4.61)	0.92 (0.34, 2.50)	0.29 (0.07, 1.13)
P for interaction		0.50	0.72	0.42
Cardiorespiratory fitness (6MWD)				
<500 m	Reference	1.26 (0.61, 2.58)	1.24 (0.52, 2.98)	0.30 (0.10, 0.87)
≥500 m	Reference	1.97 (1.10, 3.55)	1.03 (0.52, 2.05)	0.77 (0.37, 1.61)
p for interaction		0.34	0.75	0.15

Models were adjusted for age, sex, smoking status, FEV_1% pred, any pulmonary comorbidities, and any extra-pulmonary comorbidities. Pulmonary comorbidities include chronic obstructive pulmonary disease, asthma, or interstitial lung disease, and extra-pulmonary comorbidities include cardiovascular diseases or diabetes mellitus. 6MWD, 6-min walk distance. MVPA, moderate-to-vigorous physical activity.

In the spline regression models, the relationship between wind chill temperature and daily steps was linear below 25° wind chill temperature, with lower daily steps corresponding to colder temperatures (Figure 2). The association between winter and the decline in PA was consistent across all the subgroups.

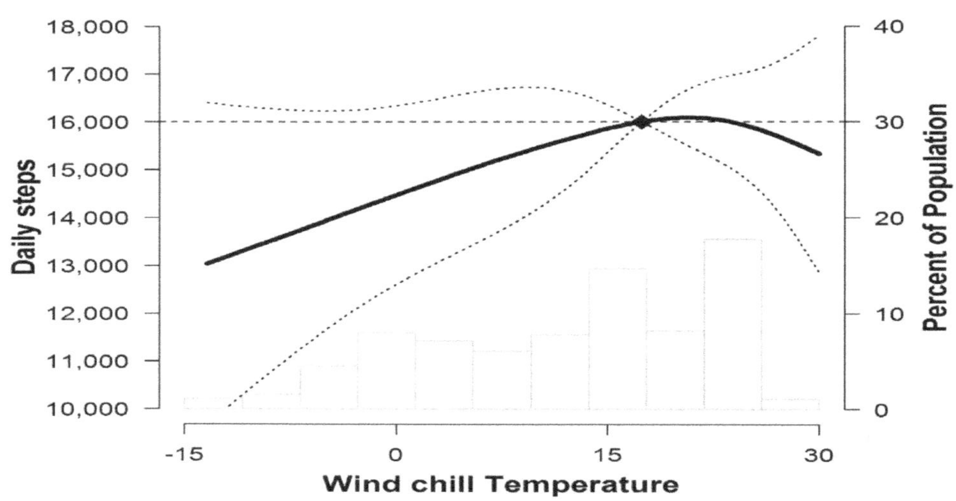

Figure 2. Mean daily steps (95% CI) by wind chill temperature. The curves represent daily step (solid line) and their 95% confidence intervals (dashed lines) based on restricted cubic splines for wind chill temperature with knots at the 5th, 35th, 65th, and 95th percentiles of their sample distributions. The reference value (diamond dot) was set at the 90th percentile.

4. Discussion

We found that preoperative PA was significantly lower in the winter season compared to other seasons, irrespective of age and CRF. In particular, the low MVPA in the winter season was more robust in patients who had low CRF, but the effect was not statistically significant. In terms of weather factors, wind chill temperature was inversely associated with PA. These results demonstrate that the PA of preoperative lung cancer patients is significantly affected by the season and temperature levels.

Our study showed that daily step was lower by 27% in the winter season compared with the spring season. These findings are consistent with previous studies that showed the association between daily PA and the season [8,27–30]. Those studies observed that PA decreased during the winter season in healthy adults [8] and elderly subjects [29]. This phenomenon was profoundly observed in patients with lung and heart diseases. In COPD patients, the daily step count reduced by 43.3 steps/day/°C in the winter season [27], and in heart failure patients, there was a significant seasonal variation in activity between summer and winter ranging from 13.78% to 20.69% [30]. In addition, the odds of walking more than 8000 steps or having more than 60 min MVPA per day in winter is around 0.5 compared to those in spring. It means that only about 50% of patients in the winter season had similar levels of PA as those of patients in spring time. It would be important for clinicians and researchers to evaluate PA in different seasons, especially in winter and provide more tailored educations for PA depending on season. In fact, the cold and snow of winter weather can significantly affect participation in outdoor activity. In particular, influenza during the winter season is an important contributor to the winter burden among older adults and lung-disease patients [31]. Furthermore, slippery roads and a high risk of falling can affect the decline in PA [32]. When outdoor activities are complicated by weather conditions, indoor activity equipment such as treadmills and stationary bicycles offer a helpful alternative. A recent study found that preoperative exercise was effective in reducing postoperative complications and length of hospital stay in patients with lung cancer [6], suggesting the importance of maintaining PA before lung cancer surgery. Another study found that that pulmonary rehabilitation programs using treadmills and bicycles were a valid preoperative strategy to improve physical performance in patients with both NSCLC and COPD [33]. It would be worthwhile to develop a PA intervention program for winter and evaluate its impact on postoperative pulmonary complications.

We found that a few patients achieving MVPA $\geq$ 60 min/day were more robust in patients with low CRF ($\leq$500 m of 6MWD) compared to those with high CRF (>500 m of 6MWD). Lower exercise tolerance assessed through the 6MWD is associated with poorer postoperative outcomes after lung resection [34]. However, a 7-day intensive preoperative program of PA combined with inspiratory muscle training increased the 6MWD in lung cancer patients in a previous study [35]. Increasing PA has positive effects on CRF and muscle power, such as health-related physical function, leading to improved postoperative recovery in early-stage NSCLC patients. In a previous study, structured and planned preoperative PA reduced postoperative complications (from 45% to 67%) and the length of hospital stay (by 4–5 days) in patients with lung cancer [3,6], suggesting that preoperative PA is an effective strategy for lung cancer patients who will undergo surgical resection. Thus, a strategic PA program should be recommended to maintain and promote PA even in the winter season, especially for low-CRF patients and older adults, for whom it is feasible to receive surgery for lung cancer.

However, seasons are a crude measure when it comes to understanding the effects of weather on PA [36]. Previous studies have observed the effects of several factors related to the season on daily activities. In a healthy population, there was a 2.9% decrease in steps per day for every 10 °C drop in temperature [37]. In addition to temperature, day length and daylight hours account for 73% of the monthly differences in daily activity level, and these three parameters are independent predictors of daily activities [38]. To analyze the climate conditions affecting PA in our study, we conducted a subgroup analysis to identify the relationship between climate conditions and activity for 85 people living in the capital city of South Korea. We found that wind chill temperature significantly affected the steps per day of preoperative patients. In the spline regression models, the relationship between wind chill temperature and daily steps was linear below 25 °C wind chill temperature, with lower daily steps corresponding to colder temperatures. This is similar to the previous findings [30,39]. The wind chill temperature used in our study is likely to be more closely related to patients' PA behavior compared to absolute temperature, as the wind chill temperature is a quantitative measure of the heat or cold that the human body feels, calculated based on air temperature and wind velocity [40]. While it is not possible to change the weather conditions, a better understanding of how weather influences PA might be helpful when developing strategies to ameliorate the impact of adverse weather conditions on future PA interventions in low-CRF patients and older adults.

There are several limitations to this study. Firstly, this was a cross-sectional study and we were not able to observe the change of PA of the same patient group in different seasons. In addition, due to enrollment periods, a limited number of patients were observed in the winter season. These factors limited our ability to observe the magnitude of seasonal variation in PA among patients. Despite these limitations, our study indicates little variability in PA by season. In fact, patients in the winter season were younger and had better lung function than patients in other season and we still see the different levels of PA depending on season. Secondly, patients who were motivated to perform PA might be more likely to participate in the study. The mean daily step figures were higher in this study compared to data reported in earlier studies [11]. This might be due to our recruitment of patients with ECOG 0 or 1 as they would be healthier and more physically active than general cancer patients. However, mean 6MWD was similar to that reported in the previous study [26], suggesting our study participants had similar CRF to other lung cancer patients. Thirdly, the physical activity device used only counts the steps and the time spent on all those steps, but it does not differentiate whether the steps are outside or inside the house. Therefore we have a limitation in assuming that patients in the winter season were less active due to decreased outdoor PA. Lastly, the results of this study might not be generalizable as it was conducted with patients at a tertiary cancer center in Seoul, Korea. Additional studies would be necessary to confirm the findings with different populations and in different settings.

5. Conclusions

In this study, we found that season and temperature levels affect PA among preoperative lung cancer patients. Patients were much less physically active in the winter season than other seasons and patients in the winter season had lower cardiorespiratory function. Health professionals need to be aware of these seasonal differences and recommend indoor physical activities that preoperative patients with lung cancer can do in winter.

Author Contributions: Conceptualization: S.K., H.Y.P., J.I.Z., and J.C.; study design: S.K., H.Y.P., J.I.Z., and J.C.; data collection: S.K., J.K.L., G.L., O.J.K., Y.M.S., and J.I.Z.; data and statistical analysis: S.K., D.K., and J.C.; drafting the manuscript: S.K., H.Y.P., J.I.Z., and J.C.; revising the manuscript: S.K., H.Y.P., D.K., J.K.L., G.L., O.J.K., Y.M.S., J.I.Z., and J.C. All authors have read and agreed to the published version of the manuscript.

References

1. Fitzmaurice, C.; Allen, C.; Barber, R.M.; Barregard, L.; Bhutta, Z.A.; Brenner, H.; Dicker, D.J.; Chimed-Orchir, O.; Dandona, R.; Dandona, L.; et al. Global, Regional, and National Cancer Incidence, Mortality, Years of Life Lost, Years Lived With Disability, and Disability-Adjusted Life-years for 32 Cancer Groups, 1990 to 2015: A Systematic Analysis for the Global Burden of Disease Study. *JAMA Oncol.* **2017**, *3*, 524–548. [PubMed]
2. Sebio Garcia, R.; Yanez Brage, M.I.; Gimenez Moolhuyzen, E.; Granger, C.L.; Denehy, L. Functional and postoperative outcomes after preoperative exercise training in patients with lung cancer: A systematic review and meta-analysis. Interact. Cardiovasc. *Thorac. Surg.* **2016**, *23*, 486–497. [CrossRef] [PubMed]
3. Bade, B.C.; Thomas, D.D.; Scott, J.B.; Silvestri, G.A. Increasing physical activity and exercise in lung cancer: Reviewing safety, benefits, and application. *J. Thorac. Oncol.* **2015**, *10*, 861–871. [CrossRef]

4. Vainshelboim, B.; Muller, J.; Lima, R.M.; Nead, K.T.; Chester, C.; Chan, K.; Kokkinos, P.; Myers, J. Cardiorespiratory fitness, physical activity and cancer mortality in men. *Prev. Med.* **2017**, *100*, 89–94. [CrossRef]
5. Kehler, D.S.; Stammers, A.N.; Tangri, N.; Hiebert, B.; Fransoo, R.; Schultz, A.S.H.; Macdonald, K.; Giacomontonio, N.; Hassan, A.; Legare, J.F.; et al. Systematic review of preoperative physical activity and its impact on postcardiac surgical outcomes. *BMJ Open* **2017**, *7*, e015712. [CrossRef]
6. Steffens, D.; Beckenkamp, P.R.; Hancock, M.; Solomon, M.; Young, J. Preoperative exercise halves the postoperative complication rate in patients with lung cancer: A systematic review of the effect of exercise on complications, length of stay and quality of life in patients with cancer. *Br. J. Sports Med.* **2018**, *52*, 344. [CrossRef]
7. Chen, Y.M. Perceived barriers to physical activity among older adults residing in long-term care institutions. *J. Clin. Nurs.* **2010**, *19*, 432–439. [CrossRef] [PubMed]
8. Tucker, P.; Gilliland, J. The effect of season and weather on physical activity: A systematic review. *Public Health* **2007**, *121*, 909–922. [CrossRef] [PubMed]
9. Ridgers, N.D.; Salmon, J.; Timperio, A. Seasonal changes in physical activity during school recess and lunchtime among Australian children. *J. Sports Sci.* **2018**, *36*, 1508–1514. [CrossRef]
10. Wu, Y.T.; Luben, R.; Wareham, N.; Griffin, S.; Jones, A.P. Weather, day length and physical activity in older adults: Cross-sectional results from the European Prospective Investigation into Cancer and Nutrition (EPIC) Norfolk Cohort. *PLoS ONE* **2017**, *12*, e0177767. [CrossRef]
11. Novoa, N.M.; Varela, G.; Jimenez, M.F.; Ramos, J. Value of the average basal daily walked distance measured using a pedometer to predict maximum oxygen consumption per minute in patients undergoing lung resection. *Eur J Cardiothorac Surg.* **2011**, *39*, 756–762. [CrossRef] [PubMed]
12. Novoa, N.; Varela, G.; Jimenez, M.F.; Aranda, J.L. Influence of major pulmonary resection on postoperative daily ambulatory activity of the patients. *Interact. Cardiovasc. Thorac. Surg.* **2009**, *9*, 934–938. [CrossRef] [PubMed]
13. Granger, C.L.; McDonald, C.F.; Irving, L.; Clark, R.A.; Gough, K.; Murnane, A.; Mileshkin, L.; Krishnasamy, M.; Denehy, L. Low physical activity levels and functional decline in individuals with lung cancer. *Lung Cancer* **2014**, *83*, 292–299. [CrossRef] [PubMed]
14. Sushames, A.; Edwards, A.; Thompson, F.; McDermott, R.; Gebel, K. Validity and Reliability of Fitbit Flex for Step Count, Moderate to Vigorous Physical Activity and Activity Energy Expenditure. *PLoS ONE* **2016**, *11*, e0161224. [CrossRef]
15. ATS Committee on Proficiency Standards for Clinical Pulmonary Function Laboratories. ATS statement: Guidelines for the six-minute walk test. *Am. J. Respir. Crit. Care Med.* **2002**, *166*, 111–117. [CrossRef]
16. Guyatt, G.H.; Thompson, P.J.; Berman, L.B.; Sullivan, M.J.; Townsend, M.; Jones, N.L.; Pugsley, S.O. How should we measure function in patients with chronic heart and lung disease? *J. Chronic Dis.* **1985**, *38*, 517–524. [CrossRef]
17. Celli, B.; Tetzlaff, K.; Criner, G.; Polkey, M.I.; Sciurba, F.; Casaburi, R.; Tal-Singer, R.; Kawata, A.; Merrill, D.; Rennard, S. The 6-Minute-Walk Distance Test as a Chronic Obstructive Pulmonary Disease Stratification Tool. Insights from the COPD Biomarker Qualification Consortium. *Am. J. Respir. Crit. Care Med.* **2016**, *194*, 1483–1493. [CrossRef]
18. Miller, M. ATS/ERS task force: Standardisation of spirometry. *Eur. Respir. J.* **2005**, *26*, 319–338. [CrossRef]
19. American Thoracic Society. Single-breath carbon monoxide diffusing capacity (transfer factor). Recommendations for a standard technique—1995 update. *Am. J. Respir. Crit. Care Med.* **1995**, *152*, 2185–2198. [CrossRef]
20. Choi, J.K.; Paek, D.; Lee, J.O. Normal predictive values of spirometry in Korean population. *Tuberc. Respir. Dis.* **2005**, *58*, 230–242. [CrossRef]
21. Park, J.; Choi, I.; Park, K. Normal predicted standards of single breath carbon monoxide diffusing capacity of lung in healthy nonsmoking adults. *J. Korean J. Intern. Med.* **1985**, *28*, 176–183.
22. Tudor-Locke, C.; Craig, C.L.; Aoyagi, Y.; Bell, R.C.; Croteau, K.A.; De Bourdeaudhuij, I.; Ewald, B.; Gardner, A.W.; Hatano, Y.; Lutes, L.D.; et al. How many steps/day are enough? For older adults and special populations. *Int. J. Behav. Nutr. Phys. Act.* **2011**, *8*, 80. [CrossRef] [PubMed]

23. Tudor-Locke, C.; Jones, R.; Myers, A.M.; Paterson, D.H.; Ecclestone, N.A. Contribution of structured exercise class participation and informal walking for exercise to daily physical activity in community-dwelling older adults. *Res. Q. Exerc. Sport* **2002**, *73*, 350–356. [CrossRef] [PubMed]
24. American College of Sports Medicine Position Stand. The recommended quantity and quality of exercise for developing and maintaining cardiorespiratory and muscular fitness, and flexibility in healthy adults. *Med. Sci. Sports Exerc.* **1998**, *30*, 975–991.
25. World Health Organization (WHO). Definition of an Older or Elderly Person. *World Health Organization.* 2016. Available online: http://www.who.int/healthinfo/survey/ageingdefnolder/en/ (accessed on 3 August 2017).
26. Marjanski, T.; Wnuk, D.; Bosakowski, D.; Szmuda, T.; Sawicka, W.; Rzyman, W. Patients who do not reach a distance of 500 m during the 6-min walk test have an increased risk of postoperative complications and prolonged hospital stay after lobectomy. *Eur. J. Cardiothorac. Surg.* **2015**, *47*, e213–e219. [CrossRef]
27. Alahmari, A.D.; Mackay, A.J.; Patel, A.R.; Kowlessar, B.S.; Singh, R.; Brill, S.E.; Allinson, J.P.; Wedzicha, J.A.; Donaldson, G.C. Influence of weather and atmospheric pollution on physical activity in patients with COPD. *Respir. Res.* **2015**, *16*, 71. [CrossRef]
28. Merchant, A.T.; Dehghan, M.; Akhtar-Danesh, N. Seasonal variation in leisure-time physical activity among Canadians. *Can. J. Public Health* **2007**, *98*, 203–208. [CrossRef]
29. Klenk, J.; Buchele, G.; Rapp, K.; Franke, S.; Peter, R. Walking on sunshine: Effect of weather conditions on physical activity in older people. *J. Epidemiol. Community Health* **2012**, *66*, 474–476. [CrossRef]
30. Shoemaker, M.J.; Roper, S.E.; Calkins, T.N. Seasonal variation of daily physical activity in individuals with heart failure. *Heart Int.* **2016**, *11*, e25–e31. [CrossRef]
31. Elliot, A.J.; Cross, K.W.; Fleming, D.M. Acute respiratory infections and winter pressures on hospital admissions in England and Wales 1990–2005. *J. Public Health* **2008**, *30*, 91–98. [CrossRef]
32. Hasegawa, J.; Suzuki, H.; Yamauchi, T. Impact of season on the association between muscle strength/volume and physical activity among community-dwelling elderly people living in snowy-cold regions. *J. Physiol. Anthr.* **2018**, *37*, 25. [CrossRef] [PubMed]
33. Stefanelli, F.; Meoli, I.; Cobuccio, R.; Curcio, C.; Amore, D.; Casazza, D.; Tracey, M.; Rocco, G. High-intensity training and cardiopulmonary exercise testing in patients with chronic obstructive pulmonary disease and non-small-cell lung cancer undergoing lobectomy. *Eur. J. Cardiothorac. Surg.* **2013**, *44*, e260–e265. [CrossRef] [PubMed]
34. Hattori, K.; Matsuda, T.; Takagi, Y.; Nagaya, M.; Inoue, T.; Nishida, Y.; Hasegawa, Y.; Kawaguchi, K.; Fukui, T.; Ozeki, N.; et al. Preoperative six-minute walk distance is associated with pneumonia after lung resection. *Interact. Cardiovasc. Thorac. Surg.* **2018**, *26*, 277–283. [CrossRef] [PubMed]
35. Lai, Y.; Huang, J.; Yang, M.; Su, J.; Liu, J.; Che, G. Seven-day intensive preoperative rehabilitation for elderly patients with lung cancer: A randomized controlled trial. *J. Surg. Res.* **2017**, *209*, 30–36. [CrossRef]
36. Aspvik, N.P.; Viken, H.; Ingebrigtsen, J.E.; Zisko, N.; Mehus, I.; Wisloff, U.; Stensvold, D. Do weather changes influence physical activity level among older adults?—The Generation 100 study. *PLoS ONE* **2018**, *13*, e0199463. [CrossRef]
37. Chan, C.B.; Ryan, D.A.; Tudor-Locke, C. Relationship between objective measures of physical activity and weather: A longitudinal study. *Int. J. Behav. Nutr. Phys. Act.* **2006**, *3*, 21. [CrossRef]
38. Kimura, T.; Kobayashi, H.; Nakayama, E.; Kakihana, W. Seasonality in physical activity and walking of healthy older adults. *J. Physiol. Anthr.* **2015**, *34*, 33. [CrossRef]
39. Togo, F.; Watanabe, E.; Park, H.; Shephard, R.J.; Aoyagi, Y. Meteorology and the physical activity of the elderly: The Nakanojo Study. *Int. J. Biometeorol.* **2005**, *50*, 83–89. [CrossRef]
40. Bluestein, M. An evaluation of the wind chill factor: Its development and applicability. *J. Biomech. Eng.* **1998**, *120*, 255–258. [CrossRef]

13

Two-Dimensional Laser-Align Device for Ultrasound-Guided Injection

Eric Chiwei Shiao [1] and Po-Ling Kuo [1,2,*]

1 Graduate Institute of Biomedical Electronics and Bioinformatics, National Taiwan University, Taipei 10617, Taiwan
2 Department of Electrical Engineering, Department of Physical Medicine and Rehabilitation, College of Medicine, Health Science and Wellness Center, National Taiwan University, Taipei 10617, Taiwan
* Correspondence: poling@ntu.edu.tw

Abstract: Ultrasound-guided injection is a widely used technique, however, it takes substantial amounts of time for novices to master the skill. The most critical issue to improve the accuracy of the injection is to align the needle with the scan plane of the ultrasound beam and orient the needle angle after piercing skin to aim at the targeted tissue. In the present study, we developed a two-dimensional laser align device to assist physicians to accurately position the needle in the scan plane and advance it at an angle correctly pointing to the target. The device is inexpensive, light-weighted, and easy to fabricate and accommodate for any types of ultrasound probe. Statistical analysis revealed that the assistance with our device significantly reduced the successful targeting time and times of retargeting in comparison with the traditional freehand approach or only with in-plane assistance for inexperience subjects. Our results indicate that the device exhibits great potential in effectively reducing the learning time to master the skill and speeding up the procedure for ultrasound-guided injection.

Keywords: ultrasound-guided injection; laser assisted; long-axis injection

1. Introduction

As point-of-care has gained increasing attention, ultrasound-guided injection becomes an important and popular technique for physician. The real-time feature of ultrasonography allows clinicians to target tissue for treatment more accurately and efficiently. However, it takes substantial amounts of time for novices to master the skill. For example, the in-plane approach requires well-trained coordination between hand and eyes to accurately position the needle in the scan plane and advance it at an angle correctly pointing to the target. It is of great importance to develop tools that assist the novices in accessing the target more easily and hence to improve their learning curve.

Several devices have been developed to assist clinicians in aiming the target more quickly and precisely [1]. However, limitations still exist. For examples, the Infiniti Plus™ needle guidance system (CIVCO Medical Solutions, Kalona, IA, USA) lacks the flexibility for direct adjustment of needle angle once the needle is inserted into the tissue [2]; the electromagnetic tracking system [3], optical tracking system [4,5], and robotic assistance system [6] are too large and expensive to be used in regular clinics. In contrast, laser assisting approaches are relatively inexpensive and compact-sized. However, most of the recently developed laser-based systems for needle guidance [7–9] only focus on the assistance in positioning the needle in the scan plane, without aiding its insertion angle.

In this research, we developed a novel two-dimensional (2D) laser-align (LA) device to help clinicians position the needle in the scan plane and at the right angle to precisely access the targeted tissue in ultrasound-guided injection. The device is inexpensive, light-weighted, and easy to fabricate and accommodate for any types of transducer. The device is switchable among three modes: 2DLA assisting, one-dimensional (1D) in-plane LA assisting without guidance for the inserting angle of the needle, and no LA assisting, namely the traditional freehand approach. We further compared the changes in the performance of ultrasound-guided targeting for novices and experienced physicians when assisted by different modes.

2. Materials and Methods

2.1. Device Fabrication

The 2DLA device consisted of a 5 V power module containing two coin batteries, a laser module, a clip, and a transparent film printed with slanting lines corresponding to various angles for needle advancement. The laser module included two laser units and on-off and brightness were independently controlled by two sets of switch and variable resistor, respectively. This design allowed users to switch the device function among the 2D, 1D, or no LA assisting mode. The variable resistors let the user change the brightness of lasers in an environment of various darkness.

The 2DLA assistance was accomplished by composing the laser module with two miniature laser diodes and their associated lenses, such that a laser line and a laser point were projected along and on a line aligned with the scan plane of the ultrasound beam, respectively. The pointing laser unit was used to guide the needle angle when entering the tissue. This was done by matching the projected laser point with a particular mark on the surface of the syringe body, while the marks corresponding to various needle angle were determined using the method described below. The lining laser unit was converted from a pointing laser unit with a half cylinder shaped lens, which refracted a point light source into a line one. It emitted a sector plane which aligned with the scan plane of the ultrasound beam. The sector plane projected a line on the skin surface next to the transducer and the point where the line began indicated the point where the needle tip was expected to enter the skin.

The clip was custom-made by 3D printing to fit a 10 MHz ultrasonic probe (BenQ, Taipei, Taiwan). It firmly mounted the laser units onto the probe at a specific angle, such that the pointing laser always projected on the syringe surface whatever the needle angle was and provided sharp laser contrast for needle and syringe positioning. The angle was determined as follows. Given a syringe of body length L and its attached needle of length l, the syringe body should be confined within the region between the interior and exterior of two concentric circles of radius L and l, respectively, as the needle angle to the skin changes. It is assumed that the circles are centered at point p, where the needle tip was placed, as shown in Figure 1a. To ensure that the spot emitted from the pointing laser unit always projects on the syringe body as the needle angle changes, the unit could be positioned either at position a or b as shown in Figure 1a, both of which are close to the two ends of the syringe body when the needle angle was 90° to the skin, respectively, and the laser emitted from both positions is tangent to the inner circle. These setups allowed the projection to cover the whole syringe body and hence provided better spatial resolution for angle guidance.

Let the angle of the laser light with respect to the line vertical to the skin, and that of the needle to the skin be φ and θ, respectively, and the distance from the needle tip to the point where the laser light projected on the syringe body be x (Figure 1b), we have

$$\varphi_a = \sin^{-1}(l/\overline{pa}) = \sin^{-1}(l/L), \tag{1}$$

$$\varphi_b = \cos^{-1}(l/L), \tag{2}$$

$$\overline{pb} = L \times \cot\varphi = l \times L/\sqrt{(L^2 - l^2)}, \tag{3}$$

$$x = h(\sin\theta + \tan(\varphi - \theta)\cos\theta) = h\sin\varphi\sec(\varphi - \theta), \tag{4}$$

$$x' \equiv dx/d\theta = -\mathrm{h} \times \sin\varphi\tan(\varphi - \theta)\sec(\varphi - \theta), \tag{5}$$

where φ_a and φ_b represents the angle φ when the unit was set at position a and b, respectively, h denotes $\overline{pa}$ or $\overline{pb}$ in each condition, and x' is the slope of x against various θ.

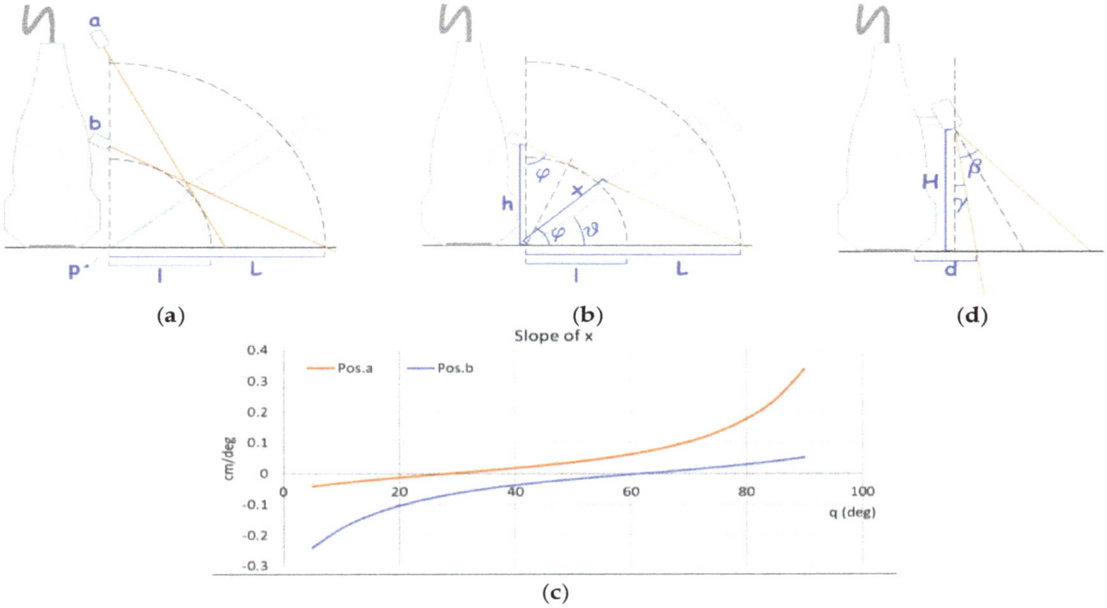

Figure 1. Geometric representation of the proposed positioning of the laser units. (**a**) Proposed setups of the pointing laser unit. (**b**) Geometric characteristics of the setup. (**c**) Profiles of slope of x against various needle angles. (**d**) Geometric layout of the lining laser unit.

Figure 1c depicts the change in x' as the needle angle varied. Note that larger x' offered finer spatial resolution for the guided points projected on the syringe body. Thus, the laser emitted from position a were projected on a wider range at larger needle angle, while that of position b was opposite. Since the needle angle is usually smaller than 45° in regular clinical practice, we chose position b to setup the pointing laser unit. The projected range of the pointing laser calculated using Equation (2) and Equation (3) would be the widest as the needle angle varied from 0° to 30°, if φ and $\overline{pb}$ were set to be 61.5° and 5.42 cm, respectively. An array of marks corresponding to various θ was determined using Equation (4) and labeled on the syringe. Thus, the needle was expected to enter the skin at a specific angle if the emitted laser spot was aligned with the mark corresponding to the angle.

The lining laser unit was set close to the pointing one to save the device size. Figure 1d demonstrates the geometric layout of the setup. The emitting angle of the laser sector plane is denoted by β, while the plane was aligned with the scan plane of the ultrasound beam and projected as a line on the surface of the skin or the syringe. The vertical distance between the unit and the skin surface is H, and d represents the distance between the end of the probe and the beginning of the projected line, which corresponds to point p in Figure 1a. Note that d is usually about 1 cm in clinical setting. Hence, the unit had to be tilted and γ represents the angle between the vertical line through the emitting point of the laser and the boundary of the sector plane, and we have

$$\gamma = \tan^{-1}(d/H). \quad (6)$$

Note that the unit was tilted by an angle of $\gamma + 0.5\beta$. We set β and γ as 52.7° and 9.46°, respectively, and $H = 6$ cm, such that the two units were separated by 0.58 cm to reduce the device size.

A transparent film printed with slanting lines was attached to the ultrasound monitor. Each line represented a particular angle for needle entering and had the corresponding mark labeled on the syringe. The labels included marks for various angles and a line aligned with the long axis of the syringe. One was expected to enter the needle in the scan plane at correct angle to the target; once the syringe was aligned with the projected laser line and the pointing laser was pointed to the right mark that matching the angle determined by the slanting lines. Figure 2 illustrates the device prototype and the typical procedure of needle entering with the 2DLA assistance was demonstrated in Figure 3.

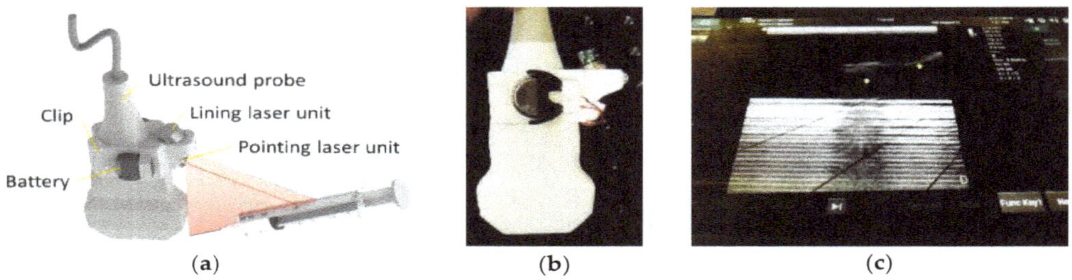

Figure 2. Schematic and photographs of the 2DLA device. (**a**) Diagram simulating the device in work. (**b**) A device assembled with an ultrasound probe. (**c**) The transparent film printed with the slanting lines for various needle entering angle and attached to an ultrasound screen.

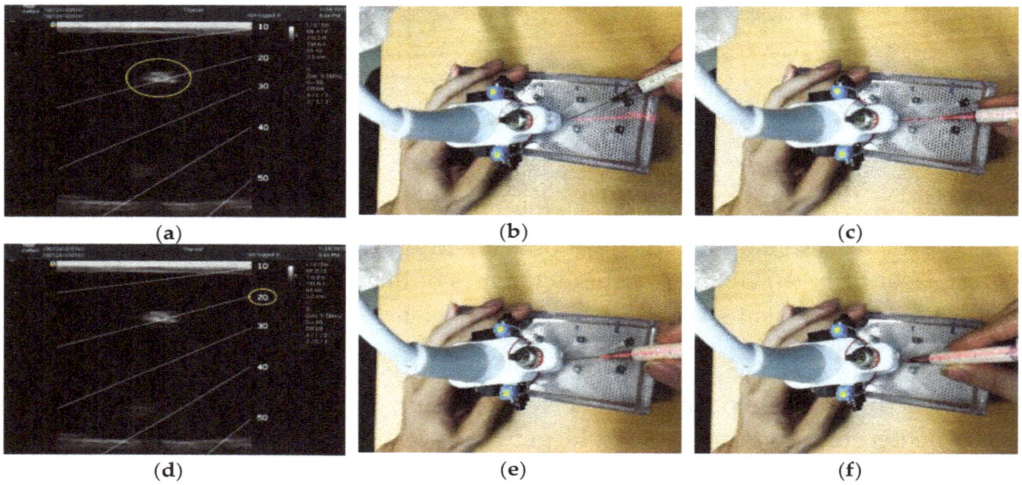

Figure 3. Procedure of needle entering guided with the 2DLA mode. (**a**) Position the probe to clearly visualize the target (highlighted by the yellow circle) on the screen. (**b**) Turn on the lasers and place the needle tip right at the beginning point of the projected laser line (the end of the laser line close to the probe). (**c**) Reorient the needle to match the projected laser line with the straight line attached on the syringe surface, which indicates the long axis of the needle. (**d**) Determine the insertion angle (highlighted by the yellow circle) using the slanting lines attached on the screen. (**e**) Adjust the entering angle to match the laser spot projected by the pointing laser unit with the mark labeled on the syringe surface corresponding to the insertion angle determined in (**d**). (**f**) Enter the needle into the phantom with persistent needle orientation until the needle tip touches the target on the screen.

2.2. *Device Performance*

To evaluate the effectiveness of our device, twenty subjects were enrolled to perform ultrasound-guided targeting in phantoms. Six of the subjects were physicians experienced in ultrasound-guided injection and the other fourteen subjects had little experience in ultrasound imaging before this study.

The phantoms were mainly composed of liquid paraffin and thermoplastic styrene-butadiene rubber which allowed the phantoms being formed and reshaped easily. The thermal-cured phantoms were transparent, excellent for ultrasound transmission, and possessed elasticity similar to that of soft tissues. The transparency of the phantoms allowed direct visualization of the needle advancement during practice and the performance test. Blocks made of poly (dimethylsiloxane) and iron powders with high echogenicity were embedded in the phantoms to simulate targets. There were two types of phantoms used in this study (Figure 4a,b); one was for practicing and had targets embedded at the same distance to the phantom surface; and the other was made for the performance test and the distance of the simulated targets to the phantom surface varied from 1 to 2 cm.

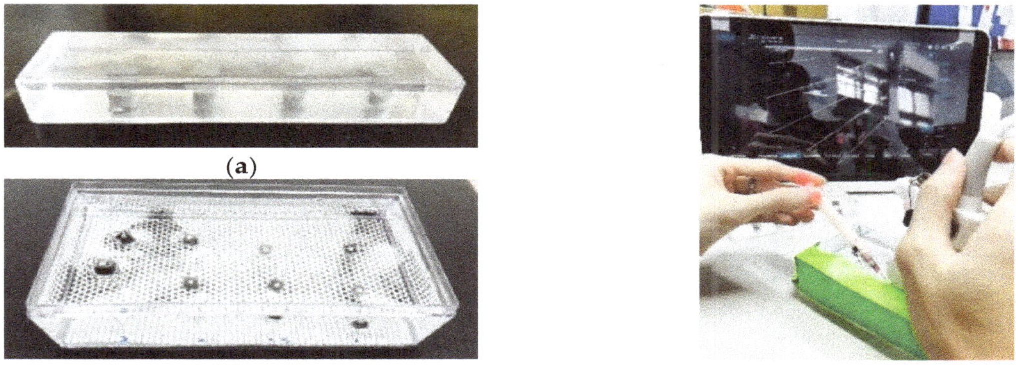

(a)

(b)

(c)

Figure 4. Photographs of the two types of phantom and its use in the performance test. Phantoms for (**a**) practicing, (**b**) performance test for ultrasound-guided targeting and (**c**) A subject performed ultrasound-guided targeting with a masked phantom.

The performance test was conducted by asking all participants to needle three targets of different depths and each needling was guided with one of the three assisting modes in randomized order. The order of the target depths was randomized as well and the variation of target depth was to prevent subjects from being familiar with the target depth from the preceding needling. In the 2DLA mode, both the lining and pointing lasers were turned on; the subject was instructed to locate the target for injection on the B-mode image, place the needle tip at the beginning end of the projected laser line, align the needle and overlap the long-axis line labeled on the syringe body with the laser line, estimate the needle angle to the target using the slanting lines on the transparent film, match the mark on the syringe body corresponding to the angle with the laser point, and advance the needle until the tip touched the target and complete the task. The procedure in the 1DLA condition was similar except that the pointing laser was turned off and the subjects had to estimate the needle angle by themselves, while the laser units were completely turned off in the no LA assisting, freehand (FH) condition. Before the performance test, the participants had unlimited time to practice targeting in the three modes. In the performance test, the phantom was masked on the side facing the subject to prevent direct visualization of the needle advancement by the subject, while the opposite side of the phantom remained transparent for video recording (Figure 4c). For each assigned target, the subject was allowed to withdraw the needle unlimited times to adjust the needle angle until successful targeting, which was considered as the needle tip penetrated the target with the presence of the entire inserted needle on the screen. Performance was evaluated by the total duration spent from entering the needle to the phantom to the moment when a successful targeting was achieved; the number of needle withdrawals until successful targeting; and the last duration, defined as the time spent from the last withdrawal to the successful targeting, which was equal to the total time if there was no needle withdrawal.

2.3. Statistics

Statistical analysis was performed using IBM SPSS Statistics 25. The differences of the three performance variables grouped with respect to different subjects, task order, and target depths were analyzed with Kruskal-Wallis one-way ANOVA test. The differences of the performance conducted in the three modes were examined using Mann-Whitney U test. Significance was set as $p < 0.05$.

3. Results

We first asked whether the performance of individuals of the same experience level was significantly different, and whether the performance was affected by the task order and the target depths. Table 1 summarized the statistical results of the performance data (Table A1) grouped against different subjects, task order, and target depths, while the data were categorized based on the level of experience. Given the subjects of the same experience level, it appears that there was no significant difference between the averaged total durations they spent to finish the three tasks, the number of needle withdrawals, and the last durations to achieve successful targeting. Likewise, the performance was not significantly different whether the task was the first or last conducted, or the target was positioned more superficially or deeper. Detailed data were listed in the Appendix A.

Table 1. Significances of differences between the means of the performance data categorized with respect to different subjects, task orders, and target depths. * $p < 0.05$.

	Group	Subjects	Orders	Target depths
Total Duration	Inexperienced	35.83 ± 22.18, $p = 0.133$	35.83 ± 10.90, $p = 0.134$	35.83 ± 3.71, $p = 0.779$
	Experienced	25.56 ± 16.34, $p = 0.471$	25.56 ± 5.99, $p = 0.535$	25.56 ± 8.20, $p = 0.385$
Withdrawals	Inexperienced	3.31 ± 1.90, $p = 0.281$	3.31 ± 0.85, $p = 0.234$	3.31 ± 0.36, $p = 0.975$
	Experienced	1.67 ± 0.43, $p = 0.206$	1.67 ± 0.36, $p = 0.076$	1.67 ± 0.24, $p = 0.331$
Last Duration	Inexperienced	9.43 ± 3.72, $p = 0.120$	9.43 ± 0.78, $p = 0.582$	9.43 ± 0.53, $p = 0.883$
	Experienced	13.44 ± 4.75, $p = 0.925$	13.44 ± 2.12, $p = 0.804$	13.44 ± 5.69, $p = 0.162$

We next examined the performance differences in various assisting conditions. Figure 5 depicts the performance of the inexperienced and experienced subjects and the data were detailed in Table 2. As for the inexperienced subjects, they less frequently withdrew the needle for retargeting as more assistance was provided, while the last duration for successful targeting followed an opposite trend. As expected, they also spent significantly longer total duration in the FH condition than in the other two conditions. In contrast, the experienced subjects spent the shortest total duration and last duration in the FH condition than in the other two conditions. Detail p-values of comparisons between conditions were summarized in Table 3. As one may expect, the inexperienced subjects took significantly longer total duration and more frequent needle withdrawals than the experienced subjects in the FH condition. However, their performances were not significantly different when the LA assistances were employed, except that the experienced subjects spent significantly longer time in the last duration than the inexperienced ones in the 2DLA condition. Detail data of the two subject groups and the p-values of comparisons between them were summarized in Table 2.

Table 2. Means and standard deviations of inexperienced group and experienced group in FH, 1DLA, and 2DLA conditions with significance level of relation between two groups. * $p < 0.05$.

	Group	FH		1DLA		2DLA	
Total Duration	Inexperienced	56.21 ± 48.67	$p = 0.012$ *	29.36 ± 19.90	$p = 0.968$	21.93 ± 10.91	$p = 0.207$
	Experienced	9.33 ± 6.60		29.50 ± 23.24		37.83 ± 25.90	
Withdrawals	Inexperienced	5.79 ± 4.36	$p = 0.026$ *	2.64 ± 1.39	$p = 0.274$	1.50 ± 0.63	$p = 0.718$
	Experienced	1.83 ± 0.69		1.83 ± 0.69		1.33 ± 0.47	
Last Duration	Inexperienced	5.86 ± 3.60	$p = 0.179$	9.14 ± 4.73	$p = 0.312$	13.29 ± 5.23	$p = 0.050$ *
	Experienced	3.33 ± 1.25		13.50 ± 7.46		23.50 ± 11.54	

Table 3. Significance of difference in the performance of the inexperienced and experienced subjects compared between various assistance conditions. * $p < 0.05$, ** $p < 0.01$.

	Group	FH–1DLA	FH–2DLA	1DLA–2DLA
Total Duration	Inexperienced	$p = 0.210$	$p = 0.039$ *	$p = 0.541$
	Experienced	$p = 0.026$ *	$p = 0.015$ *	$p = 0.485$
Withdrawals	Inexperienced	$p = 0.019$ *	$p = 0.001$ **	$p = 0.039$ *
	Experienced	$p = 1.000$	$p = 0.310$	$p = 0.310$
Last Duration	Inexperienced	$p = 0.039$ *	$p < 0.001$ **	$p = 0.044$ *
	Experienced	$p = 0.002$ **	$p = 0.002$ **	$p = 0.093$

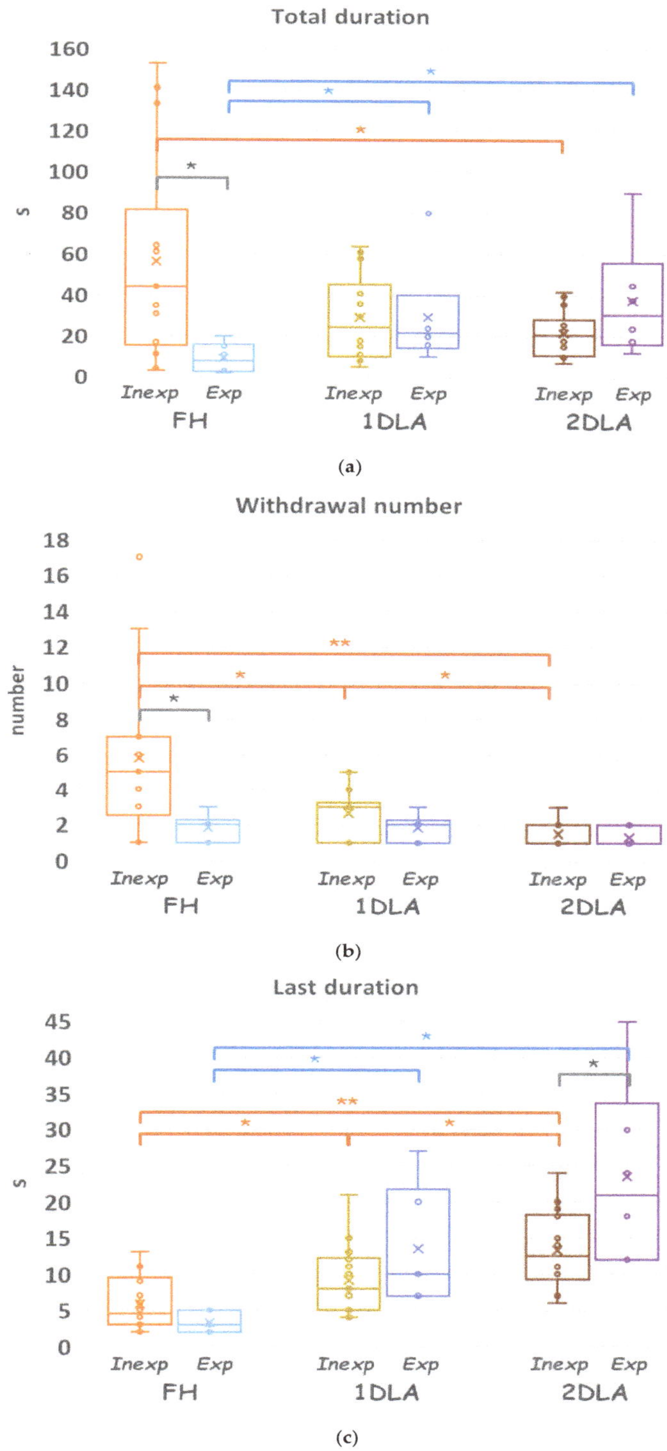

Figure 5. Comparisons of the performance of the subjects assisted by the three different modes. Data of (**a**) total duration, (**b**) withdrawal number, and (**c**) last duration of the inexperienced and experienced subjects performing in the freehand (FH), assisted with the lining laser (1DLA), and assisted with lining plus pointing laser (2DLA) condition. * $p < 0.05$, ** $p < 0.01$.

4. Discussion

In the present work, we showed that for people new to ultrasound-guided injection, our novel device did help their performance in reducing the spent time and number of needle withdrawals for successful targeting. These results agree well with those reported previously [7–9], and we further demonstrated that our novel 2DLA design significantly helped the inexperienced operators to perform better than in the traditional freehand condition or simply assisted by a lining laser. By following the guidance provided by the pointing laser and the marks on the syringe, most of the inexperienced participants could pierce the target in one shot. This is reasonable since the 2DLA mode provided a vast amount of information for needle operation such that the subject's expertise in ultrasound-guided injection had a minor role. This may explain the fact that most of the performance of the inexperienced and experienced subjects was not significantly distinguishable when assisted in the two LA modes. Indeed, the experienced subjects even spent much longer time to achieve the successful targeting in the two LA modes than that in the FH condition, since they already had good eye-hand coordination and individual tempo for injection and may have been confused with the laser assistance. Furthermore, it may be cumbersome to check many parameters before needle advancement in the 2DLA mode, which may explain why it took longer time for the last successful targeting in both inexperienced and experienced groups. However, we believe this drawback can be overcome as the operators become familiar with the device. Nevertheless, this mode still improved the efficacy of the inexperienced operators as the total time was less, owing to the much fewer withdrawals. The results shown in Table 1 indicate that the randomly assigned targets of different depths were successful to prevent the participants from predicting the needle angle using the experience learned in preceding tests. Furthermore, these results suggest that the task difficulty perceived by the participants was not dependent on the target depth, nor the task order. Collectively, our results indicate that the 2DLA device has a high potential to speed up the learning curve of novices in ultrasound-guided injection.

With 5.5 × 5.0 × 2.8 cm in size, 32 g in weight, and a price of about $20, our 2DLA device was compact, lightweight, inexpensive, easy to mount onto the probe, and provided immediate guidance if the operators need to change the target suddenly. Unlike the device designed by Daehee et al. [10], there is no direct contact between our device and patients' skin or needle, which reduced the risk of infection. These features render our device competitive in clinical use or medial training when compared with commercially available products. For example, although the Infiniti Plus™ needle guidance system provided by the CIVCO company has very affordable price (~$10 for each set), it prohibits repeated adjustment of the needle orientation for injection of multiple targets, or immediate replacement of syringe of various size in conditions such as the combined operation of ultrasound-guided aspiration and injection [11]. The eTRAX needle tip tracking guidance system, which is also from the CIVCO, embeds an electromagnetic sensor in the needle tip to provide needle tracking, but it costs more than 2 thousand dollars and is roughly forty times larger than ours in volume [12]. The SCENERGY system from the Clear Guide Medical attaches stereocameras to the ultrasound probe and integrates the ultrasound image with the CT/MRI image to improve needle navigation, but the assistive device is much larger than ours, and it requires attachment of labels on the subject's skin for recognition, which may increase the risk of infection [13].

However, there are limitations in the present study. Although nonparametric tests were applied to make our results statistically stricter, the enrollment size was small. Furthermore, the marks labeled on the syringe for guidance of injection angle were calculated based on a flat skin surface, which may well approximate conditions when the radius of curvature of the skin is much larger than the probe size, such as scanning along the long axis of an arm. However, the guidance will be erroneous when entering the needle through skin surface with smaller radius of curvature, holding the ultrasound probe askew or using a curvilinear array probe. Additional calculation is required to fix the scale distortion arising in these conditions. For example, when our device is applied to a curvilinear probe, the slanting lines printed on the transparent film should be curved to match the sector image generated by the probe. Likewise, since the needle entering point is usually out of the image view when the probe is applied on a curved surface with a large curvature, such as scanning along the transverse plane of an arm, it is hard to predict the needle orientation unless the geometric condition between the probe and the entering point is given.

5. Conclusions

In summary, we developed a novel 2DLA device that provided guidance for needle orientation both for the image plane and the angle for entering. Statistical analysis revealed that the 2DLA mode significantly reduced the time for successful targeting and frequency of retargeting in comparison with the FH and 1DLA mode. Injecting quickly and accurately is one of the most challenging tasks during the training for ultrasound-guided injection. Our device exhibits great potential in effectively reducing the learning time to master the skill and speeding up the procedure.

Author Contributions: Conceptualization, E.C.S. and P.L.K.; methodology, E.C.S.; validation, P.L.K.; formal analysis, E.C.S.; investigation, E.C.S.; data curation, E.C.S.; writing—original draft preparation, E.C.S.; writing—review and editing, P.L.K.; visualization, E.C.S. and P.L.K.; supervision, P.L.K.; project administration, P.L.K.; funding acquisition, P.L.K.

Acknowledgments: The authors are grateful for the valuable input about the tips of ultrasound-guided injection in clinical practices by Chueh-Hung Wu, Ming-Yen Hsiao, Shaw-Gang Shyu, and Yi-Chian Wang in National Taiwan University Hospital, Taipei, Taiwan.

Appendix A

Table A1. Data of each subject in inexperienced group and experienced group.

	Subject	Task	Order	Target Depth (cm)	Total Duration (s)	Withdraw Times (#)	Duration of Last Insertion (s)
Inexperienced Group	1	FH	I	1	64	4	7
		1DLA	II	1.5	15	1	15
		2DLA	III	2	10	1	10
	2	FH	I	2	61	7	11
		1DLA	II	1.5	58	5	13
		2DLA	III	1	42	2	14
	3	FH	III	2	31	3	9
		1DLA	II	1	8	1	8
		2DLA	I	1.5	26	2	11
	4	FH	III	1	44	7	2
		1DLA	I	2	36	3	5
		2DLA	II	1.5	23	2	6
	5	FH	II	2	17	5	3
		1DLA	I	1	19	3	4
		2DLA	III	1.5	11	1	11
	6	FH	I	1.5	35	6	3
		1DLA	III	1	18	3	5
		2DLA	II	2	7	1	7
	7	FH	II	1	46	4	6
		1DLA	III	1.5	5	1	5
		2DLA	I	2	10	1	10
	8	FH	II	1.5	3	1	3
		1DLA	I	2	11	1	11
		2DLA	III	1	19	1	19
	9	FH	III	1.5	4	1	4
		1DLA	II	2	37	3	7
		2DLA	I	1	15	1	15
	10	FH	II	1	11	1	11
		1DLA	III	2	8	1	8
		2DLA	I	1.5	40	2	20
	11	FH	III	1.5	133	13	5
		1DLA	I	1	64	5	21
		2DLA	II	2	24	1	24
	12	FH	I	2	141	17	2
		1DLA	III	1.5	30	4	4
		2DLA	II	1	36	3	7
	13	FH	I	2	153	7	13
		1DLA	II	1.5	61	3	12
		2DLA	III	1	18	1	18
	14	FH	III	1	44	5	3
		1DLA	I	1.5	41	3	10
		2DLA	II	2	26	2	14

Table A1. *Cont.*

	Subject	Task	Order	Target Depth (cm)	Total Duration (s)	Withdraw Times (#)	Duration of Last Insertion (s)
Experienced Group	1	FH	III	1.5	11	2	3
		1DLA	II	2	80	3	20
		2DLA	I	1	90	2	30
	2	FH	I	1.5	15	2	5
		1DLA	II	1	24	2	10
		2DLA	III	2	12	1	12
	3	FH	II	2	20	3	5
		1DLA	III	1.5	16	2	7
		2DLA	I	1	45	1	45
	4	FH	I	1	3	1	3
		1DLA	II	1.5	20	2	7
		2DLA	III	2	38	2	12
	5	FH	II	2	2	1	2
		1DLA	I	1	10	1	10
		2DLA	III	1.5	18	1	18
	6	FH	III	1.5	5	2	2
		1DLA	II	1	27	1	27
		2DLA	I	2	24	1	24

References

1. Scholten, H.; Pourtaherian, A.; Mihajlovic, N.; Korsten, H.; Bouwman, R.A. Improving needle tip identification during ultrasound-guided procedures in anaesthetic practice. *Anaesthesia* **2017**, *72*, 889–904. [CrossRef] [PubMed]
2. Infiniti Plus™. In-Plane Ultrasound Needle Guides. Available online: https://www.civco.com/catalog/ultrasound-needle-guides/infiniti-plus-ultrasound-needle-guides/ (accessed on 16 July 2019).
3. Ungi, T.; Sargent, D.; Moult, E.; Lasso, A.; Pinter, C.; McGraw, R.C.; Fichtinger, G. Perk tutor: An open-source training platform for ultrasound-guided needle insertions. *IEEE Trans. Biomed. Eng.* **2012**, *59*, 3475–3481. [CrossRef] [PubMed]
4. Najafi, M.; Abolmaesumi, P.; Rohling, R. Single-camera closed-form real-time needle tracking for ultrasound-guided needle insertion. *Ultrasoun. Med. Biol.* **2015**, *41*, 2663–2676. [CrossRef] [PubMed]
5. Hoßbach, M.; Noll, M.; Wesarg, S. Simplified stereo-optical ultrasound plane calibration. *Int. Soc. Opt. Photonics* **2013**. [CrossRef]
6. Hemmerling, T.M.; Taddei, R.; Wehbe, M.; Cyr, S.; Zaouter, C.; Morse, J. Technical communication: First robotic ultrasound-guided nerve blocks in humans using the Magellan system. *Anesth. Analg.* **2013**, *116*, 491–494. [CrossRef] [PubMed]
7. Collins, G.B.; Fanou, E.-M.; Young, J.; Bhogal, P. A comparison of free-hand vs laser-guided long-axis ultrasound techniques in novice users. *Br. J. Radiol.* **2013**, *86*, 20130026. [CrossRef] [PubMed]
8. Tsui, B.C.H. Facilitating needle alignment in-plane to an ultrasound beam using a portable laser unit. *Reg. Anesth. Pain Med.* **2007**, *32*, 84–88. [CrossRef] [PubMed]
9. Liu, S.-Y.; Liao, M.-Y.; Wei, T.-S.; Yang, C.-P.; Chen, L.-W.; Lin, S.-J.; Ding, Y.-S.; Chang, Y.-J. Laser assisted ultrasound guided aspiration improves procedure time and reduces number of withdrawals. *Ultrasonics* **2008**, *48*, 647–651. [CrossRef] [PubMed]
10. Daehee, H.; Lan Seo, Y.; Choi, C.S.; Chul Kim, H.; Yoon, D.Y.; Bae, S.; Moon, J.; Kim, S.H.; Soo Kim, S.; Han, H. A steerable guiding device: The new method in ultrasound guidance. *Investig. Radiol.* **2002**, *37*, 626–631. [CrossRef]
11. Infiniti Plus™. Disposable Needle Guide Replacement Kits. Available online: https://www.civco.com/catalog/ultrasound-needle-guides/infiniti-plus-disposable-needle-guide-replacement-kits/ (accessed on 25 June 2019).
12. eTRAX. Needle Tip Tracking Guidance System—12GA. Available online: https://www.civco.com/catalog/fusion-tracking-technology/etrax-needle-tip-tracking-guidance-12ga/ (accessed on 25 June 2019).
13. Clear Guide Scenergy. Available online: https://clearguidemedical.com/ (accessed on 25 June 2019).

14

Decision Support for the Optimization of Provider Staffing for Hospital Emergency Departments with a Queue-Based Approach

Fuu-Cheng Jiang [1,†], Cheng-Min Shih [2,4,†], Yun-Ming Wang [2], Chao-Tung Yang [1,*], Yi-Ju Chiang [3] and Cheng-Hung Lee [4,5]

1. Department of Computer Science, Tunghai University, No. 1727, Section 4, Taiwan Boulevard, Taichung 40704, Taiwan; admor@thu.edu.tw
2. Department of Biological Science and Technology, National Chiao Tung University, No. 1001, Daxue Rd., Hsinchu 30010, Taiwan; 10chengmin@gmail.com (C.-M.S.); ymwang@mail.nctu.edu.tw (Y.-M.W.)
3. Information and Communication Research Division, National Chung-Shan Institute of Science & Technology, Taoyuan 32546, Taiwan; yjchiang0320@gmail.com
4. Department of Orthopedics, Taichung Veterans General Hospital, No. 1650, Section 4, Taiwan Boulevard, Taichung 40705, Taiwan; leechenghung0115@gmail.com
5. Department of Food Science and Technology, Hung Kuang University, No. 1018, Section 6, Taiwan Boulevard, Taichung 43302, Taiwan

* Correspondence: ctyang@thu.edu.tw

† These authors contributed equally.

Abstract: Deployment or distribution of valuable medical resources has emerged as an increasing challenge to hospital administrators and health policy makers. The hospital emergency department (HED) census and workload can be highly variable. Improvement of emergency services is an important stage in the development of the healthcare system and research on the optimal deployment of medical resources appears to be an important issue for HED long-term management. HED performance, in terms of patient flow and available resources, can be studied using the queue-based approach. The kernel point of this research is to approach the optimal cost on logistics using queuing theory. To model the proposed approach for a qualitative profile, a generic HED system is mapped into the M/M/R/N queue-based model, which assumes an R-server queuing system with Poisson arrivals, exponentially distributed service times and a system capacity of N. A comprehensive quantitative mathematical analysis on the cost pattern was done, while relevant simulations were also conducted to validate the proposed optimization model. The design illustration is presented in this paper to demonstrate the application scenario in a HED platform. Hence, the proposed approach provides a feasibly cost-oriented decision support framework to adapt a HED management requirement.

Keywords: hospital emergency department; queuing theory; decision support; cost optimization

1. Introduction

1.1. Background

Hospitals play an important role in the healthcare system of society. They have changed rapidly in parallel with improvements in medical instruments and medicine. Administrators of hospital institutions should have spared no effort in developing strategies that enable the provision of high-quality services, while operating with increased costs and pressure from competition [1]. One of the most demanding departments in terms of economic resource consumption and programming is the hospital emergency department (HED). To this extent its operational profile should be monitored and optimized in order to provide the optimal quality of medical service subject to the budget constraint.

HEDs must be operational 24 h, and, moreover, should respond to multiple demands requiring sophisticated technical equipment and the manpower to operate them, all of which imply higher costs. Large HEDs have even higher costs because they offer a wide range of services that would be unavailable in a small rural HED [2]. Emergency Departments have traditionally been a crucial issue in the hospitals' cost containment and management. The optimization of patient flow and bottleneck elimination in key departments could be a viable way for policy makers to decrease operational costs and boost quality of care [3]. In the interest of improving patient throughput and resource utilization, appropriate key performance measures are selected, like the size of staffing providers, HED patient arrival patterns, service rate of staffing providers, waiting time, etc. To explore the tradeoff among them, the proposed queue-based optimization technique on cost may provide hospital management with a decision support for deploying staffing providers under the constraints of the kernel performance parameters.

An M/M/R/N queuing model was adopted to explore the cost profile from analyzing the relationships among relevant performance parameters in a HED, such as the number of staffing providers (i.e., servers) needed during each staffing interval. This model assumes a single queue with a limited system capacity of N that feeds into R identical medical servers (i.e., staffing providers). The fourth symbol "N" of the notation M/M/R/N indicates the restriction on the system capacity of the HED. The value of (N−R) gives the number of waiting rooms for incoming patients when all staffing providers in the HED are busy. Arrivals occur according to a time-homogeneous Poisson process with a constant rate, and the service duration (e.g., provider time associated with a patient) has an exponential distribution. In the language of queuing theory [4,5], these two assumptions are often called Markovian, hence the use of the two "M's" in the notation used for the model. One advantage of adopting the M/M/R/N model is that given an arrival rate, an average service duration, and the number of servers, formulae for performance measures such as the cost profile, the average number of patients, or the average waiting time can be easily obtained.

1.2. Contribution Profile

This novel idea in this work originated from the theory of an M/M/R/N queuing system (QS), which is used to estimate the optimal number of providers needed during each staffing interval [4,5]. At some pre-configured period (say a shift, or a day), a finite quantity of staffing providers exists to provide medical services for patients under limited waiting rooms in HEDs. On application modeling, such a finite quantity of staffing providers (i.e., R) can be regarded as the term "server" in the M/M/R/N model of queuing theory. The quantity of (N−R) can be considered to be the rather limited waiting rooms in HEDs regulated by each hospital.

The research goal for this work is to explore whether, with cost-based deployment, how many sets of staffing providers in the HED schedule would be optimal if a certain level of the server availability is kept? To explore the tradeoff between them, the proposed optimization technique may provide the HED management with decision support on the number of staffing providers. The key contributions of this paper are threefold: (1) This work provides HED administrators with an efficient deployment of staffing providers for the HED platform to optimize the cost improvement. In regards to management, the proposed system can be adopted as a decision-making methodology approaching predictive management, rather than reactive or chaotic management. (2) For quantitative analysis, the M/M/R/N queue model was applied and derived, and then the relevant system metrics were established in a brand-new manner. The mathematical expression of the cost function was established for the evaluation requirement. (3) In regards to verification, relevant experimental results were obtained in terms of configurations on cost optimization and average waiting time. The simulated results indicate that the proposed approach may provide a feasible decision support for deployment on quantities of standby servers.

The rest of the paper is organized as follows: Section 2 describes related work and the motivation behind this research. To demonstrate the framework qualitatively, an M/M/R/N model of queuing theory is adopted and the mapping profile is demonstrated in Section 3. Quantitative work is presented in Section 4, where the mathematical analysis is conducted in detail and the relevant system performance measures, such as the expected number of online servers, the expected number of spares, etc., are derived. Following this, in Section 5, the queue-based model is further addressed in terms of cost function, and the simulations of the feasibility of the proposed scheme are conducted. Finally, some concluding remarks are made in Section 6.

2. Related Work

HED crowding represents an important issue that may affect the quality and access of health care. Accordingly, the optimization of average waiting times has become a focus across many mainstream hospitals. As defined by the Canadian Association of Emergency Physicians [6], HED overcrowding is a situation in which the demand for services exceeds the ability of health care professionals to provide care within a reasonable length of time. As stated in [7], significant variation in HED patient arrival rates necessitates the adjustment of staffing patterns to optimize the timely care of patients. Green et al. [7] collected detailed HED arrival data from an urban hospital and used a queue-based analysis to gain insights on how to change provider staffing to decrease the proportion of patients who leave without being seen. However, no optimization materials in terms of mathematical theory were addressed at all in these studies [8–10].

Finamore et al. [6] described an innovative use of a satellite clinic to prevent patients returning to HED for care on a scheduled basis. Their strategy allows patients returning for follow-up diagnostics or treatment to bypass the main HED. The proposed HED satellite clinic may shorten the waiting times in multiple ways, such as increasing the capacity to remove returning patients from the pool of patients requiring care in the HED, and creating a separate registration area and a separated staffed treatment area. The visit data in the HED were used to measure crowding and completion of waiting room time, treatment time, and boarding time for all patients treated and released or admitted to a single HED during 2010. In [11], the authors conducted a relevant statistical analysis and concluded that a HED census at arrival demonstrated variation in crowding exposure over time. In the work of Wiler et al. [12], the authors developed an agent-based simulation model for the evaluation of the FTS (fast track strategies) scheme applied in the HED to reduce patient waiting time. By and large, the issues regarding cost optimization on the HED management cost are not a concern for these open studies [5,11,12].

Vass and Szabo [13] evaluated 2195 questionnaires in the HED situated in Mures County, Romania, for a period three years (2010–2013). Their research reported that long waiting times were the most important complaint in patient's satisfaction surveys. To perceive the waiting times, only a specific M/M/3 queuing model was considered in their work to demonstrate the computation details. The work of [13] has motivated us to consider whether it is possible to provide an effective and feasible approach to decision support for the optimization of provider staffing under cost constraints for the HEDs with more elaborative queue-based frameworks. This research generalizes the queuing model of [13] into the M/M/R/N queuing framework in terms of three practical aspects: (1) Numbers of medical servers (provider staffing) can be configured to one of the system parameters instead of a fixed quantity. Such a dynamic staffing level enables a hospital to quantify the cost patterns and the alleviation of HED waiting times. (2) The space available in the HED would be limited for every hospital management. The fourth factor (N) in the notation of the M/M/R/N model symbolizes the fact that only N patients can be allowed to enter the waiting rooms of the HED in order not to exacerbate the issue of overcrowding. (3) The exact mathematical expressions would be derived in an elaborative manner and the relevant cost formulation would be used to provide the generic decision support for the hospital administrators.

3. The Proposed Model of Medical Emergency Services

3.1. The Generic Platform of Medical Emergency Services

This research explores feasible decision support that is proposed to optimize running costs under the constraint of the waiting time at a HED using queue-based models. The exemplified HED is in a metropolitan hospital (Taichung Veterans General Hospital or TVGH) located in central Taiwan. It began offering medical services on 16 September 1982. Since 1991, it has been accredited as a "Medical Center and First-Class Teaching Hospital" by the Department of Health, Taiwan. Taichung Veterans General Hospital is a 1500-bed hospital with up to 3900 employees. According to the latest statistical average data of registration accessed in TVGH, it offers a capacity of about 7000 outpatients and 190 patients in the emergency room daily [14]. As a public medical center, it provides safe, high-quality medical services with advanced facilities and training programs, as well as outstanding research and development programs.

The HED building, with eight floors at the TVGH (TVGH-ED), provides comprehensive emergency services 24 h a day. The functional deployment on the ground floor of the TVGH-ED building, as shown in Figure 1, is composed of different zones, including the Registration and Triage Area, Resuscitation Areas, Internal Medicine Areas, the Pediatric Treatment Area, Waiting Areas, Clinic Areas, Monitor Rooms and the Fever Screen Center, and relevant auxiliary service units such as the X-ray service and nursing stations. As this HED is a rather complicated service system due to random arrivals, various disease chains, uncertain service times of care, and randomness in human decision-making, it is difficult to model the whole HED with a single operational model. From the perspective of the model attribute [15], a generic operational model is defined as a formal description of operations performed to deliver a health service that is applicable over a wide range of health service delivery settings. For the sake of simplicity, this research concentrates the optimization issue on a specific platform of medical service, which is used hereafter to model staffing providers for a single disease chain.

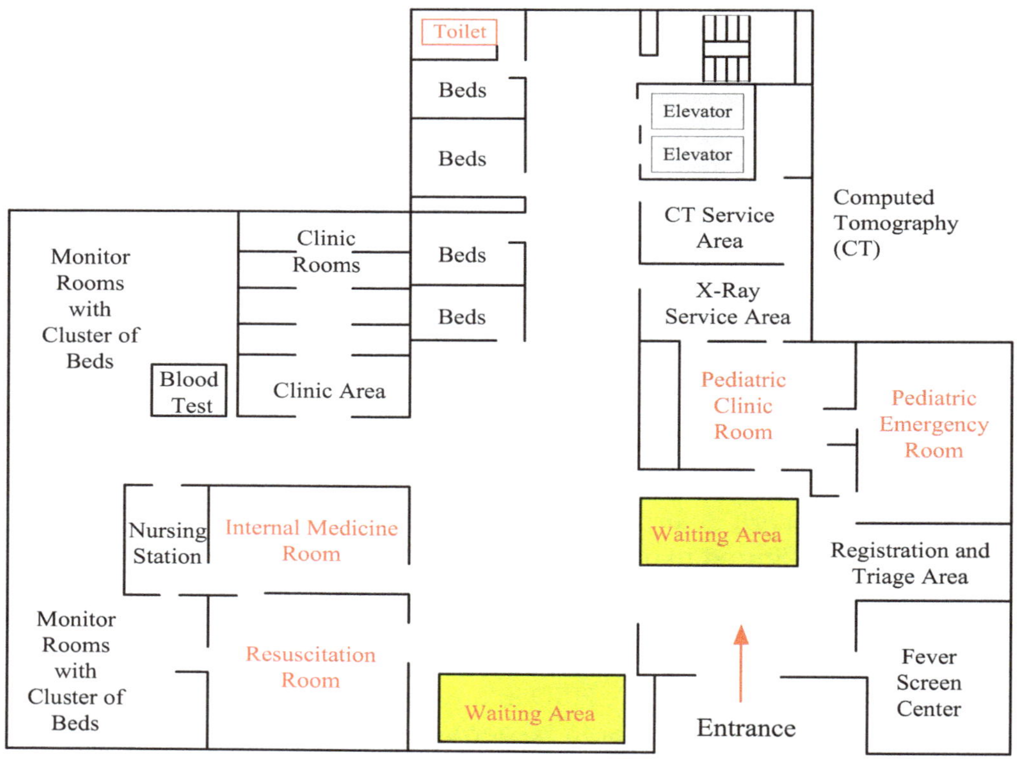

Figure 1. The functional deployment on the ground floor of the TVGH-ED building. TVGH-ED, Taichung Veterans General Hospital - Emergency Department.

3.2. *Mapping Profile between the HED Service Platform and the M/M/R/N Queuing System*

The proposed generic framework on the HED service platform is considered to be modeled as an M/M/R/N queuing system (QS), which is used to estimate the optimal number of providers needed during each staffing interval. An input-throughput-output framework of HED operations is used as the prototype shown in Figure 2 for a generic profile [16]. The ambulance icon symbolizes the arrivals of HED patients. Practically, patient arrivals are hard to schedule, or even control significantly. Arrivals may surge in some unpredictable time windows due to a short-term disaster, car accidents, and seasonal influences [17]. In modeling language, the busy and regular time windows can be associated with high and normal arrival rates, respectively. Patient arrivals in the proposed model are assumed to be Poisson processes [18], with average hourly rates that are forecasted for each future hour in question (say a shift, or a day) [19].

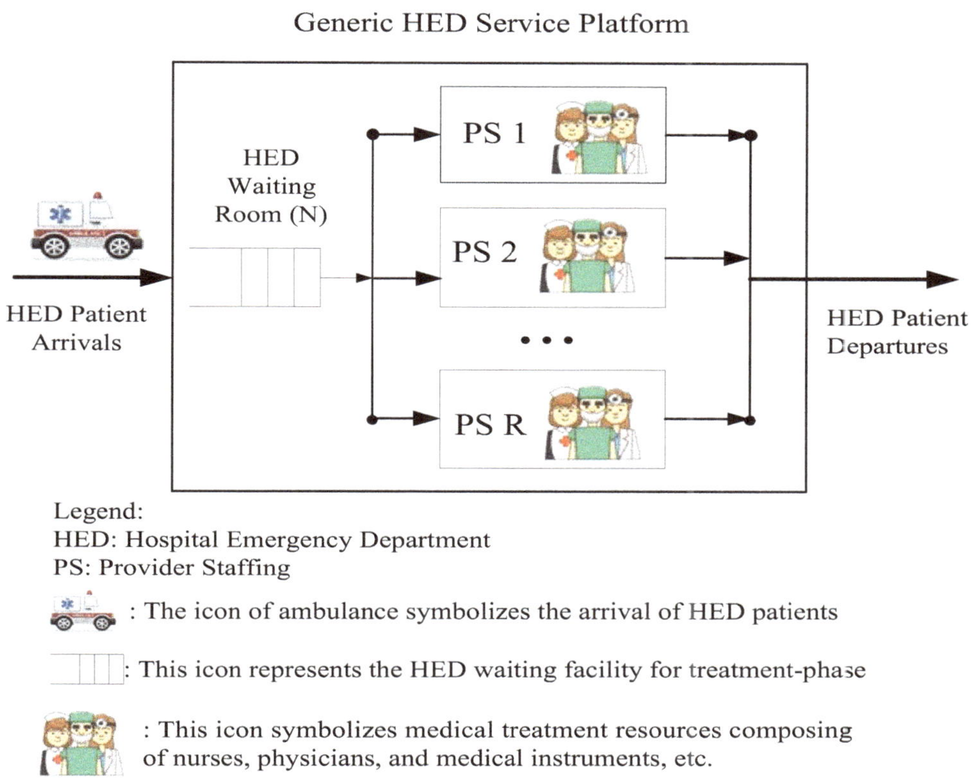

Figure 2. The generic service platform of an emergency department.

The itinerary for HED patients from arrival to exit can conceptually be divided into three phases [12]. The first phase, named "Waiting for treatment phase (*waiting phase*)", is symbolized by the icon HED Waiting Rooms in Figure 2. In the waiting phase, the patient goes through some standard processes that assist the HED to grasp the record of patients and their current medical condition. These are termed the Registration and Triage process, respectively. Registration guarantees administratively that patient demographics are captured accurately for billing and maintaining the record. Triage is the first assessment conducted by a healthcare professional after the patient arrives in the HED. The second phase (*treatment phase*) begins when the patient is placed in bed. For simplicity, the treatment phase is represented by the icons of provider staffing (medical servers) in Figure 3 for a generic profile. The whole medical service largely depends on patient acuity and physician activities. In modeling language, the duration of treatment can be regarded mathematically as the service rate of (medical) servers. The treatment phase is followed by the post-treatment phase, which is represented by the expression HED patient departures in Figure 3. Exiting from the treatment area of the HED is reasonably assumed to mean that the patients are discharged, either as an outpatient or into the hospital [16].

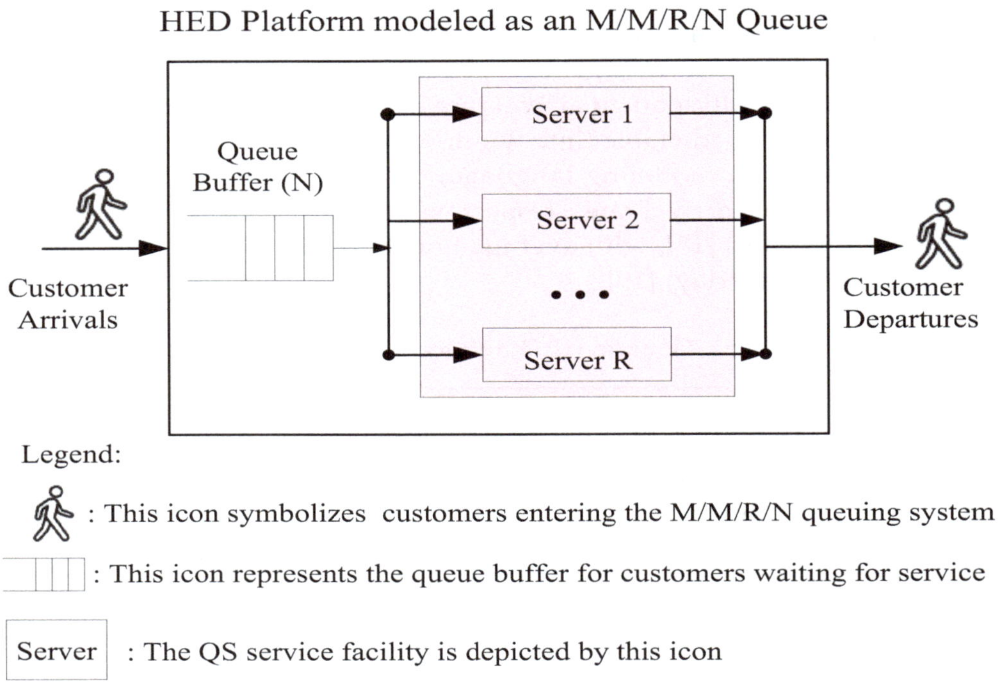

Figure 3. An M/M/R/N queue system mapped by the HED service platform.

The mapping scenarios for the theoretical approach are illustrated in Figures 2 and 3. An M/M/R/N queuing model was used to estimate the number of providers needed during each staffing time window. In Figure 3, the proposed model assumes a single queue with regulated and finite waiting rooms that feed into R identical servers with blue highlights, which is mapped to providers in the HED. The walking-man (customers) icons symbolize HED patient arrivals. Based on the proposed queuing model, relevant system metrics, such as average waiting times, expected number of customers in the queue buffer, and the probability that all servers are busy, can be analyzed and derived mathematically [7]. For instance, a patient's total length-of-stay from arrival to departure from the HED platform is termed as the patient throughput time, which is equivalent to the waiting time in the QS. Patient throughput time has a significant impact on operational and economic efficiency as well as overall patient satisfaction, which is a measure of medical service quality [20].

Generally, the performance metric on average waiting times may provide the HED administrator with decision support on how to alleviate patients' complaints. To avoid the deterioration of average patient throughput time (i.e., the average wait times in the QS), the optimization approach on the average waiting times, under some constraints such as a limited number of servers in the QS (i.e., mapped counterpart: level of staffing in the HED platform), is explored further in this article. The metric is the probability that all servers can be used to reveal the possibility and scenario in which notorious HED crowding may occur. The question is how to reduce this HED crowding phenomenon in some specific time windows. Such a metric can provide decision support for the administrator in order to properly configure or deploy hospital resources.

4. Quantitative Modeling and System Measures for the HED Platform

4.1. Theoretical Analysis

The service-oriented model on the HED platform in Figure 3 is considered to have R servers with an adequate level of staffing and a finite size (N) of waiting rooms for HED arrivals. The birth-and-death process is adopted to derive analytic steady-state solutions to the M/M/R/N queuing system (QS). Let the states n ($n = 0, 1, 2, \ldots, N$) represent the number of customers in the QS. McManus et al. [18] studied all admissions to the medical–surgical intensive care unit (ICU) of a large, urban children's hospital during a 2-year period. Their statistical analysis confirmed that the arrival rate of patients to ICUs follows a Poisson distribution, and the durations of stay (service times) were found to follow an exponential distribution. Hence, it is reasonably assumed that the customers arrive according to a Poisson process with mean arrival rate $\lambda_n = \lambda$ if $0 \le n \le N$ and $\lambda_n = 0$ if $n > N$ due to a finite system capacity. The QS has R servers, each having an exponential distribution of service times with an identical service rate $\mu_n = \mu$. The service volume can be classified into two parts as follows:

Mean Service Rate:

$$\mu_n = \begin{cases} n\,\mu, & \text{if } 1 \le n \le R \\ R\mu, & \text{if } (R+1) \le n \le N \end{cases} \tag{1}$$

To approach analytic steady-state results for the proposed model, we first construct the state-transition-rate diagram depicted in Figure 4. The number inside the circle represents the number of customers (patients) in the system. Each circle in Figure 4 shows the steady-state probability scenario that may occur during the service period in the system. For each circle except the first one (n = 0) and the last one (n = N), there are four arrows marked with the corresponding values of the state-transition rate. The quantity marked along each arrow gives either the flow-in probability into that state or the flow-out probability off that state.

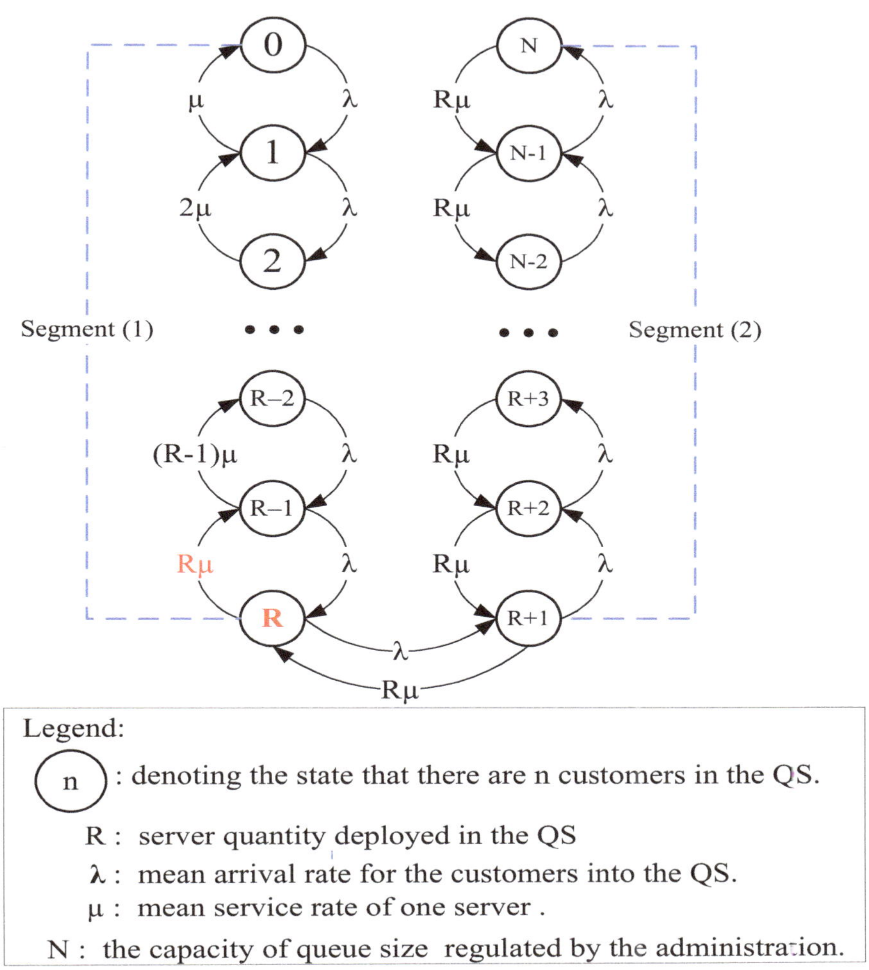

Figure 4. State-transition-rate diagram for the proposed model.

Let the notation P(n) = the probability that there are n customers in the system, where $n = 0, 1, 2, \ldots, N$. Hence, for a steady-state case, the state probability functions P(n) can be obtained from the birth-and-death formula [5] in association with the state-transition-rate diagram shown in Figure 4. We define notation $\rho = \lambda/\mu$ for the server utilization and $\rho_S = \rho/R = \lambda/(R\mu)$ for the system utilization. According to the value n (number of customers in the QS that may be present), two segments are defined by the vector: (Segment 1, Segment 2) = ($1 \le n \le R$, $(R+1) \le n \le N$). The state probability functions P(n) can then be derived in terms of two segments as follows:

(A) Segment (1): $1 \le n \le R$

$$P(n) = \frac{\lambda_0 \cdot \lambda_1 \cdot \lambda_2 \cdots \lambda_{n-1}}{\mu_1 \cdot \mu_2 \cdot \mu_3 \cdots \mu_n} P(0) = \frac{\lambda^n}{\mu\,(2\mu)(3\mu)\cdots(n\mu)} P(0) = \frac{\lambda^n}{\mu^n\, n!} P(0) = \frac{\rho^n}{n!} P(0) \tag{2}$$

(B) Segment (2): $(R+1) \le n \le N$,

$$\begin{aligned} P(n) &= \frac{\lambda_0 \cdot \lambda_1 \cdot \lambda_2 \cdots \lambda_{n-1}}{(\mu_1 \cdot \mu_2 \cdots \mu_R)(\mu_{R+1} \cdots \mu_n)} P(0) = \frac{\lambda^n}{[\mu \cdot (2\mu) \cdots (R\mu)](R\mu \cdots R\mu)} P(0) = \\ &= \frac{\lambda^n}{R!\ \mu^R\ (R\mu)^{n-R}} P(0) = \frac{\rho^n}{R!\ (R)^{n-R}} P(0) \end{aligned} \tag{3}$$

There are (n–R) terms of Rμ in the parenthesis (Rμ. Rμ) of the above denominator. Equations (2) and (3) are the closed-forms for the state probability functions P(n) in terms of two segments in which the number of customers may be present. To obtain P(0), we substitute expressions (2) and (3) in the normalizing equation $\sum_{n=0}^{N} P(n) = 1$, which yields:

$$\sum_{n=0}^{R} \frac{\rho^n}{n!} P(0) + \sum_{n=R+1}^{N} \left(\frac{\rho^n}{R!\ R^{n-R}} \right) P(0) = 1$$

$$P(0) = \left[\sum_{n=0}^{R} \frac{\rho^n}{n!} + \sum_{n=R+1}^{N} \left(\frac{\rho^n}{R!\ R^{n-R}} \right)\right]^{-1} = \left[\sum_{n=0}^{R} \frac{\rho^n}{n!} + \frac{\rho^R\left(1 - \rho_s^{N-R+1}\right)}{R!\ (1-\rho_s)}\right]^{-1} \tag{4}$$

4.2. System Performance Measures

Mathematical expectations are crucially important for the long-run theoretical average values of relevant parameters in the system. To formulate the expressions of the system performance metrics, it is necessary to construct average-based functions, such as the expected number of customers in the queue, expected number of busy servers in the system, etc. The following mathematical analyses are all necessary for the system performance measures of an M/M/R/N QS.

Let

Ls = expected number of customers in the system,
Lq = expected number of customers in the queue buffer,
E[I] = expected number of idle servers,
E[B] = expected number of busy servers,
P_B = Probability that all servers are busy,
Ws = average waiting times in the system,
Wq = average waiting times in the queue buffer.

With steady-state probability functions (2) and (3), it yields

$$L_s = \sum_{n=0}^{N} n\, P(n) \tag{5}$$

$$L_q = \sum_{n=R}^{N} (n-R)\, P(n) \tag{6}$$

$$E[I] = \sum_{n=0}^{R-1} (R-n)\, P(n) \tag{7}$$

$$E[B] = R - E[I] \tag{8}$$

$$P_B = \sum_{n=R}^{N} P(n) \tag{9}$$

To express the above parameters in terms of (R, N, ρ, ρ_S, P_0), the system performance measures can be derived as follows:

$$\begin{aligned} L_s &= \sum_{n=0}^{N} n\, P(n) = \sum_{n=0}^{R-1} n\, P(n) + \sum_{n=R}^{N} n\, P(n) = \sum_{n=0}^{R-1} n\cdot\tfrac{\rho^n}{n!} P(0) + \sum_{n=R}^{N} (n-R+R) P(n) = \\ &= \sum_{n=0}^{R-1} n\cdot\tfrac{\rho^n}{n!} P(0) + \sum_{n=R}^{N} (n-R) P(n) + R \sum_{n=R}^{N} P(n) = \sum_{n=0}^{R-1} n\cdot\tfrac{\rho^n}{n!} P(0) + L_q + R\, P_B \end{aligned} \tag{10}$$

$$P_B = \sum_{n=R}^{N} P(n) = \sum_{n=R}^{N} \frac{\rho^n}{R!\, R^{n-R}} P(0) = \frac{\rho^R}{R!} \frac{\left[1-(\rho_s)^{N-R+1}\right]}{(1-\rho_s)} P(0) \tag{11}$$

By changing the indices of **j = n—R** so that n = R is changed to j = 0, and n = N is changed to j = N—R,

$$L_q = \sum_{n=R}^{N} (n-R)\, P(n) = \sum_{n=R}^{N} (n-R) \frac{\rho^n}{R!\, R^{n-R}} P(0) = \frac{\rho^R P(0)}{R!} \sum_{j=0}^{N-R} \left[j\cdot(\rho_s)^j\right] \tag{12}$$

The average waiting times in the system and in the queue buffer (Ws, Wq) can be derived by applying Little's formula, which gives $W_s = \frac{L_s}{\lambda}$ and $W_q = \frac{L_q}{\lambda}$, respectively.

4.3. An Illustrative Example with Computation Details

To gain prompt perception on the theoretical implication of the quantitative modeling, an example is given by a detailed calculation. Let (R, N) = (4, 5) and (λ, μ) = (2, 1), then the server utilization ρ = λ/μ= 2 and the system utilization ρ_S = ρ/R= 0.5, which is less than unity for the stable system.

(1) $0 \le n \le (R-1) = 3$, $P(n) = \frac{\rho^n}{n!} P(0) = \frac{2^n}{n!} P(0)$

$$P(1) = \frac{2^1}{1!} P(0) = 2P(0);\ P(2) = \frac{2^2}{2!} P(0) = 2P(0);\ P(3) = \frac{2^3}{3!} P(0) = (1.33)P(0) \tag{13}$$

(2) $R \le n \le N$, i.e., For $4 \le n \le 5$, $P(n) = \frac{\rho^n}{R!\, R^{n-R}} P(0)$

$$P(4) = \frac{2^4}{4!\, 4^{4-4}} P(0) = 0.667\, P(0);\ P(5) = \frac{2^5}{4!\, 4^{5-4}} P(0) = 0.333\, P(0) \tag{14}$$

$$\Rightarrow [P(1), P(2), P(3), P(4), P(5)] = = [2, 2, 1.333, 0.667, 0.333]\ P(0). \tag{15}$$

The complete five state probabilities are assembled and expressed in terms of P(0) as follows: Using the normalization condition, $\sum_{n=0}^{N} P(n) = 1 \Rightarrow \sum_{n=0}^{5} P(n) = (7.33)P(0)$

$$\Rightarrow P(0) = 0.136\ \# \tag{16}$$

And from Equations (5)–(9), the system metrics can be computed sequentially as follows:

$$L_s = \sum_{n=0}^{N} n\, P(n) = P(1) + 2P(2) + 3P(3) + 4P(4) + 5P(5) = (14.333)\cdot(0.136) = 1.949 \tag{17}$$

$$L_q = \sum_{n=R}^{N} (n-R)\, P(n) = \sum_{n=4}^{5} (n-4) P(n) = P(5) = 0.0453 \tag{18}$$

$$E[I] = \sum_{n=0}^{R-1}(R-n)P(n) = \sum_{n=0}^{3}(4-n)P(n) = 4P(0) + 3P(1) + 2P(2) + P(3) = 2.085 \quad (19)$$

$$E[B] = R - E[I] = 4 - 2.085 = 1.915 \quad (20)$$

$$P_B = \sum_{n=R}^{N} P(n) = \sum_{n=4}^{5} P(n) = P(4) + P(5) = 0.136 \quad (21)$$

$$Ws = Ls/\lambda = 1.949/2 = 0.9745 \text{ and } Wq = Lq/\lambda = 0.0453/2 = 0.0223 \quad (22)$$

The distribution of steady-state probabilities is depicted in Figure 5. The relevant system performance measures, such as Ls, Lq, E[B] and Ws, are shown in the left-lower part of Figure 5. The average number of customers in the QS and the queue buffer are 1.949 and 0.0457, respectively. The average waiting times in the system and the queue buffer are 0.9745 and 0.0223, respectively.

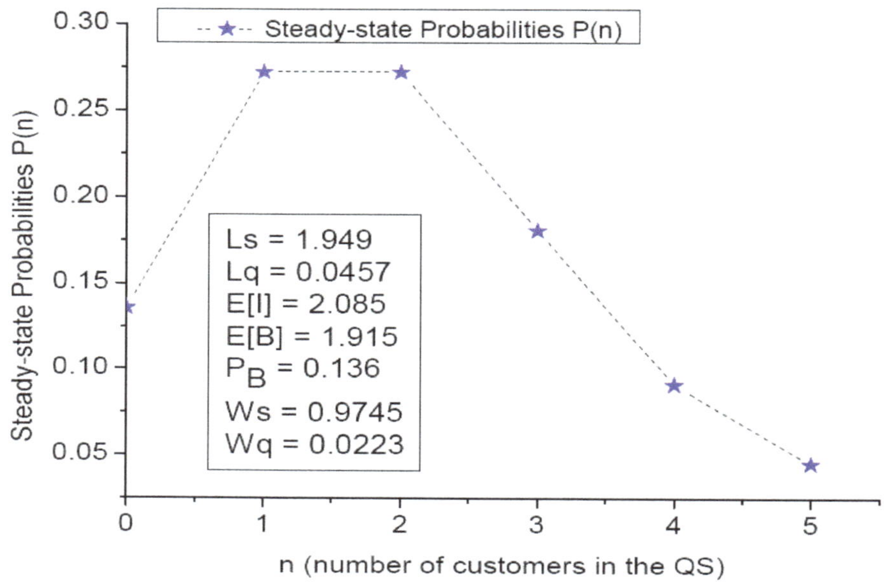

Figure 5. Steady-state probabilities with parameters (R, N, λ, μ) = (4, 5, 2, 1).

5. Issue on Decision Support for HED Management

5.1. Evaluation Formulation on Cost

The strategy to minimize the total cost of the operating horizon is referred to as the optimal policy. Like all medical institutions, the cost pattern is important for gaining long-term and stable hospital management. To optimize the cost, we developed a steady-state expected cost function per unit time for an M/M/R/N queuing system, in which the parameter vector of (R, N, λ, μ) and the average waiting times (Lq) are considered as decision variables. The cost element C_W is defined as the waiting cost per unit time (or cost rate) per customer (HED patient) present in the system. Our goal is to provide decision support for determining the optimal number of servers R, say R*, to optimize the cost function. To formulate the cost function, some cost parameters are defined in the following vector form as follows:

Cq = cost per unit time when one customer is waiting for service,
Cs = cost per unit time when one customer joins the system and is served,
(C_B, C_I) = cost per unit time when one server is (busy, idle).

Using the definitions of each cost element with its corresponding feature, the cost function F(R, N) can be developed in association with the system metrics Ls, P_B, Lq, E[I], and E[B], which are given in Equations (10)–(12), (7) and (8), respectively. It is noted that the steady-state probabilities for two segments are given in Equations (2) and (3). The probability that there is no customer in the system, P(0), is given by Equation (4).

$$\begin{aligned} F(R, N) &= Cq\,Lq + Cs\,(Ls - Lq) + C_B\,E[B] + C_I\,E[I] = (Cq - Cs)\,Lq + Cs\,Ls - C_B\,E[B] + C_I\,E[I] \\ &= (Cq - Cs)\,\frac{\rho^R P(0)}{R!}\sum_{j=0}^{N-R}[j\cdot(\rho_s)^j] + Cs\,\{\sum_{n=0}^{R-1} n\cdot\frac{\rho^n}{n!}P(0) + \frac{\rho^R P(0)}{R!}\sum_{j=0}^{N-R}[j\cdot(\rho_s)^j] + R\cdot \\ &\quad \frac{\rho^R}{R!}\frac{[1-(\rho_s)^{N-R+1}]}{(1-\rho_s)}\} + C_B\,(R - \sum_{n=0}^{R-1}(R-n)\,P(n)) + C_I\,[\sum_{n=0}^{R-1}(R-n)\,P(n)] \end{aligned} \tag{23}$$

The cost function F(R, N) in Equation (23) is expressed in terms of basic parameters, such as (R, N, λ, μ), and cost elements. It is noted that the utilization parameters of the unit server and system is given by $(\rho, \rho_S) = (\lambda/\mu, \lambda/(R\mu))$, respectively. The state probability functions P(n) for two segments are given in Equations (2) and (3), which are quite complex for the control parameter R. To find the optimal profile on the cost function, it is necessary to show the existence of convexity or unimodality of F(R, N). However, this mathematical task is difficult to implement. The cost function F(R, N) is unimodal; that is, it has a single relative minimum.

5.2. Evaluation of Cost Optimization

Equation (23) shows that the parameter R occurs not only at the location of in-line items, but also at the upper limit of the summation symbol Σ, which makes F(R, N) a highly nonlinear and complex function. Instead, practical numerical examples are presented and intensively studied by applying the proposed models. The optimization evaluation is firstly probed in terms of cost patterns in this subsection. For illustrative purposes, we first study the effect of varying R while keeping N constant, and then varying N while keeping R constant. All simulations are performed with the MATLAB platform with custom MATLAB scripts. The exemplified system parameters are listed as vector forms as follows:

(a) Average arrival rate of patients (λ) = 2.5, 3.0, and 3.5,
(b) Average service rate of a server (μ) = 1,
(c) Cost rate: $(Cq, Cs, C_B, C_I,) = (200, 150, 120, 100)$,
(d) N = 15 for emergency departments of small and medium size.

Contour plots may provide the best graphical representation of the optimization problem, and also possess a powerful visualization that permits the solutions of the optimization problem by inspection. To validate the analytical solution, the graphical results were obtained and are shown in Figure 6A, where three cost contours with the black box, red circle, and blue triangle icons are depicted along the Y-axis in terms of λ = 2.5, 3.0, and 3.5, respectively. Generally, a higher patient arrival rate implies that the medical service cost is higher, so the blue line marked with the triangle icon (λ = 3.5) is situated over the red line marked with a circle (λ = 3.0). To clearly show the crucial region surrounded by the dashed-line rectangle in Figure 6A, enlarged detail is depicted in Figure 6B. In Figure 6B, the critical region is between R = 3 and R = 9 on the X-axis. The optimal cost value with the corresponding optimal R* is shown for each contour.

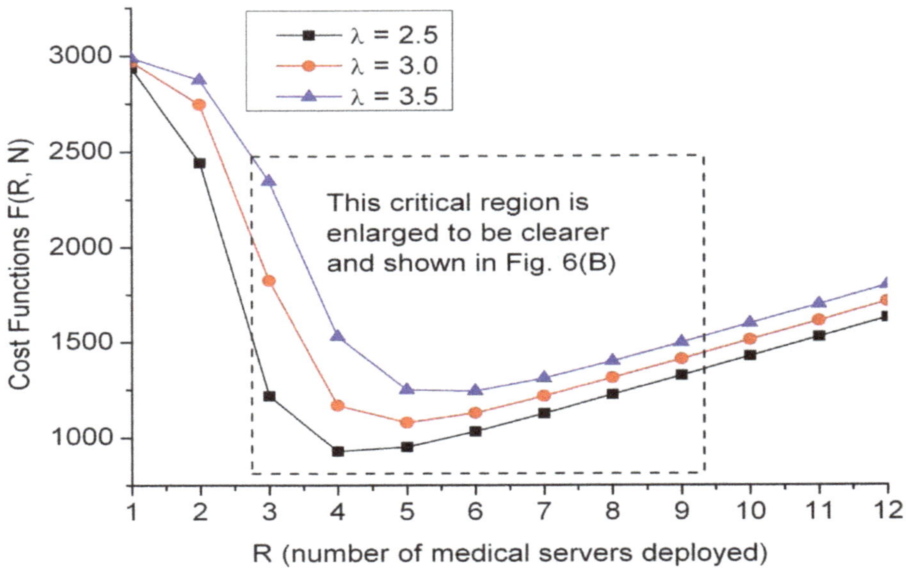

(A)

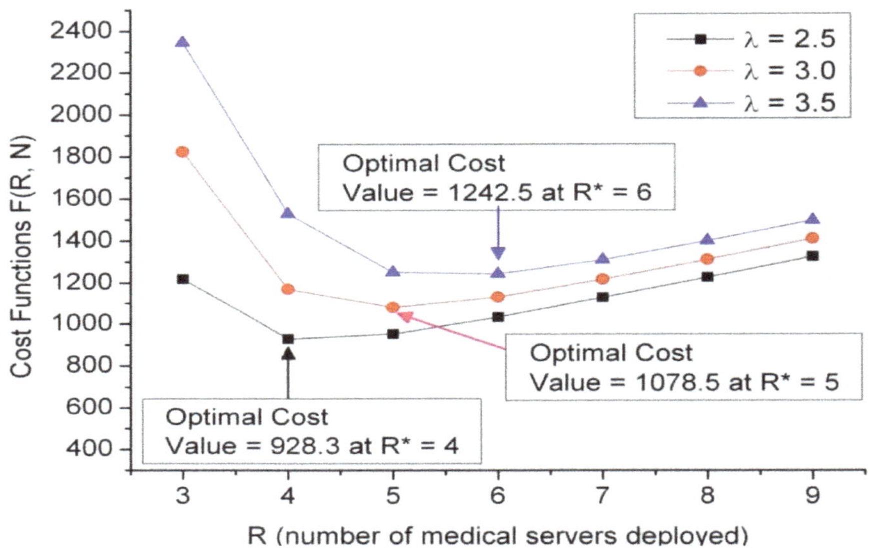

(B)

Figure 6. (**A**). Optimal cost patterns shown in terms of three average arrival rates. (**B**) An enlarged diagram showing the optimal cost data from Figure 6A.

5.3. Issues on Cost Profile under the Constraint of Average Waiting Time

In view of performance evaluation, the average waiting time (AWT) can also be regarded as a measure of performance committed to the HED patients, and of a yardstick for comparing the effectiveness of the deployment of the staffing providers in a quantitative manner. Practically, it is reasonable for management experts to guarantee an AWT target level when they want to alleviate the sense of worry for potential HED patients. Logically, the higher the number of staffing providers deployed, the higher the cost. Hence, the proposed approach explores the issue of decision support for optimal cost under the constraint of the AWT at some target level.

In Figure 7 with the double-Y axis, the left Y-axis and the right Y-axis are set to be the cost values and the average waiting time (AWT), respectively. Observing the solid-line contour marked with black rectangles (i.e., the left Y-axis), the optimal cost value F(R, N) = 1242.5, which occurs at R* = 6 based on the similar parameters in Figure 6A with the average arrival rate $\lambda = 3.5$. However, the corresponding

AWT approaches 6.84 units, which is a reference metric for decision-making. The proposed generic model could be used for general insights into the issues faced in deploying multiple staffing providers for a disease chain or a single department like the Department of Pediatrics shown in the middle right-handed location of the ground floor in Figure 1. On the right Y-axis, the dash-curve marked with a red star shows the variation profile of the performance metric for AWT.

During the busy time-window for a specific disease chain in HED, patients may spend hours in crowded waiting rooms before seeing a doctor. Those who choose to tolerate longer waiting times expose themselves to others who may have a contagious illness. To alleviate such an occasional impact, one straight approach for reducing the waiting time is to deploy more staffing providers for that specific disease chain. The simulation results in Figure 7 provide an exemplified decision reference on re-deploying the amount of staffing providers to alleviate the waiting time.

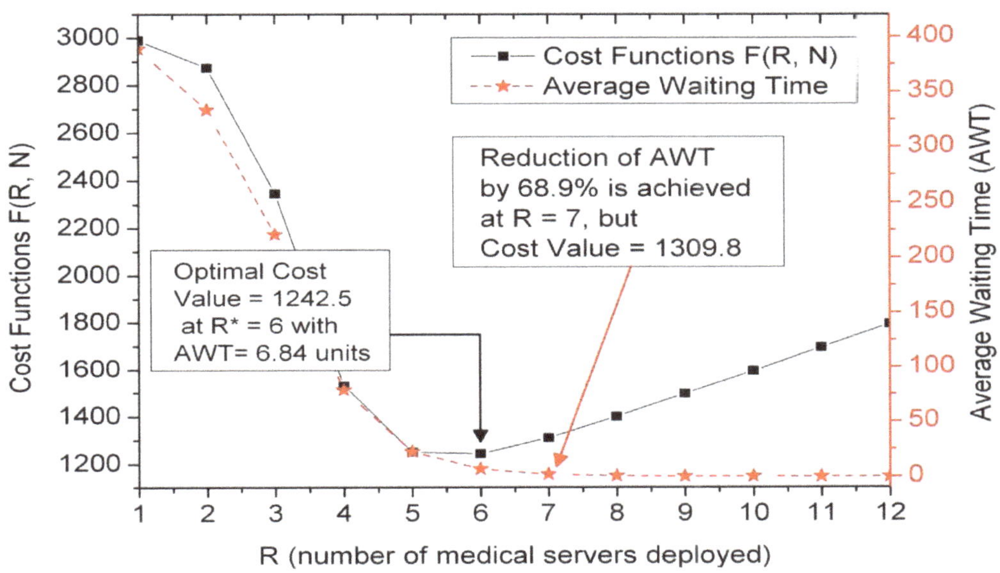

Figure 7. Decision support on optimal cost at R* = 7 under the constraint of reduction of AWT (average waiting time) by 68.9%, which is calculated from ((6.84–2.13)/6.84) × 100%.

Then an issue emerges from the judgment: how many extra staffing providers are needed to gain a reduction in the AWT by some level (for example, 50%) without over-provisioning? Observing the red-star contour with the right Y-axis in Figure 7, it is found that the AWT can be reduced by 68.9% at R* = 7 (shown by the red dash-line) at the expense of only adding one staffing provider and cost values F(R* = 7, N) = 1309.8, compared to the minimum cost F(R = 6, N) = 1242.5. The detailed numerical data are listed in Table 1 with a range of R from unity to 12. The value of AWT for R = 12 is less than 0.01 and then marked to be 0 for clarity. In other words, the proposed approach can provide a quantitative decision support on the trade-off study between the cost profile and the amount of staffing providers in HED deployment.

Table 1. Numerical data on AWT and the corresponding cost values for the range of R from unity to 12.

R	Cost Values	AWT	R	Cost Values	AWT
1	2990.0	388.57	7	1309.9	2.13
2	2873.9	333.42	8	1399.5	0.65
3	2345.8	220.77	9	1496.3	0.19
4	1530.2	78.57	10	1595.4	0.05
5	1250.7	22.51	11	1695.1	0.01
6	1242.5	6.84	12	1795.0	0

AWT, average waiting time.

5.4. Application Profile in a Window-by-Window Way

This work addressed the issue of the mathematical modelling to evaluate scenarios for deployment of medical resources to the HED, and also aimed to provide feasible applications iteratively to approaching an effective decision support in terms of deploying appropriate staffing providers to alleviate the impact on HED crowding. Patients who want to receive medical services always arrive randomly, and they require immediate services available at that time. If the service facility is operating at peak capacity when they arrive, they are obliged to wait in line (queue) with patience in the case of a shortage in staffing level. The surges and changes in HED activity may occur from time to time in terms of various time-widows with associated system parameters, as shown in Figure 8.

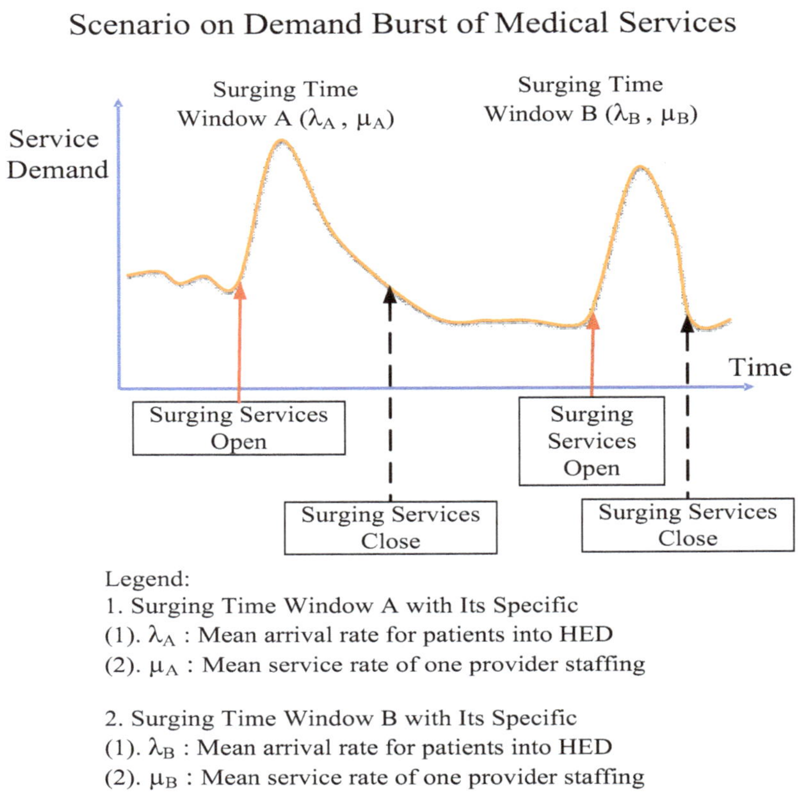

Figure 8. Iterative applications exemplified by various time-windows.

In Figure 8, each unique time-window may represent a specific surge time-period, wherein larger numbers of patients nearby the hospital are delivered to HED after some disaster or traffic event has occurred. In modeling language, the proposed modeling approaches can be applied in a window-by-window way that each specific time window can be approximated by its λ (average arrival rate) and μ (average service rate) in association with various practical historical data. For example, supposing that the surge in time window B of Figure 8 represents some middle-level traffic event, then the system parameters λ_B (average arrival rate) and μ_B (average service rate) may be approximated by some existing past and experienced parameters for the baseline, and then the cost function F(R, N) (23) may be applied iteratively to approach the cost optimization in a window-by-window way.

6. Conclusions

In terms of patient flow and available resources, an efficient generic methodology to optimize the performance of the HED platform has been addressed in this research. The proposed queue-based approach provides HED administrators with an efficient deployment of staffing providers to optimize the cost profile. Conceptually, the HED service platform was mapped into an M/M/R/N queuing system, and illustrated using appropriate figures and materials in the work. To gain insight into the queuing model, the mathematical derivation was detailed for the application need as well.

Based on the quantitative analysis, the M/M/R/N queue model was applied and derived, and then the relevant system metrics were established in a brand-new manner. The mathematical expression for cost function was established for evaluation requirements. In regards to verification, the relevant experimental results were obtained in terms of integration configurations on cost optimization and average waiting time. Instead of chaotic management, the proposed generic methodology may provide feasible applications for approaching an effective decision support in terms of deploying appropriate staffing providers to alleviate the impact on HED crowding.

Author Contributions: Conceptualization, F.-C.J.; Data curation, Y.-J.C. and C.-H.L.; Formal analysis, C.-M.S.; Investigation, C.-H.L.; Methodology, C.-M.S. and Y.-M.W.; Project administration, Y.-J.C.; Resources, C.-T.Y.; Software, C.-T.Y.; Supervision, F.-C.J.; Validation, C.-M.S.; Writing—original draft, F.-C.J. and Y.-M.W.; Writing—review & editing, F.-C.J. and C.-T.Y.

References

1. Zengin, S.; Guzel, R.; Al, B.; Kartal, S.; Sarcan, E.; Yildirim, C. Cost analysis of a university hospital's adult emergency service. *J. Acad. Emerg. Med.* **2013**, *12*, 71–75. [CrossRef]
2. Simonet, D. Cost reduction strategies for emergency services: Insurance role, practice changes and patients accountability. *Health Care Anal.* **2009**, *17*, 1–19. [CrossRef] [PubMed]
3. Cremonesi, P.; Di Bella, E.; Montefiori, M. Cost analysis of emergency department. *J. Prev. Med. Hyg.* **2010**, *51*, 157–163. [PubMed]
4. Cooper, R.B. *Introduction to Queuing Theory*, 2nd ed.; Elsevier Science Publishing Co., Inc.: New York, NY, USA, 1990.
5. Gross, D.; Shortle, J.F.; Thompson, J.M.; Harris, C. *Fundamentals of Queuing Theory*, 4th ed.; John Wiley &Sons, Inc.: New York, NY, USA, 2008.
6. Finamore, S.R.; Sheila, S.A. Shorting the wait: A strategy to reduce waiting times in the emergency department. *J. Emerg. Nurs.* **2009**, *35*, 509–514. [CrossRef] [PubMed]
7. Green, L.V.; Soares, J.; Giglio, J.F.; Green, R.A. Using queuing theory to increase the effectiveness of emergency department provider staffing. *Acad. Emerg. Med.* **2006**, *13*, 61–68. [CrossRef] [PubMed]
8. Derlet, R.W.; Richards, J.R.; Kravitz, R.L. Frequent overcrowding in U.S. emergency departments. *Acad. Emerg. Med.* **2001**, *8*, 151–155. [CrossRef] [PubMed]
9. Kennedy, J.; Rhodes, K.; Walls, C.A.; Asplin, B.R. Access to emergency care: Restricted by long waiting times and cost and coverage concerns. *Ann. Emerg. Med.* **2004**, *43*, 567–573. [CrossRef] [PubMed]
10. Hoot, N.R.; Aronsky, D. Systematic review of emergency department crowding: Causes, effects, and solutions. *Ann. Emerg. Med.* **2008**, *52*, 126–136. [CrossRef] [PubMed]
11. Ding, R.; Zeger, S.L.; McCarthy, M.L.; Pines, J.M. Comparison of methods for measuring crowding and its effects on length of stay in the emergency department. *Acad. Emerg. Med.* **2011**, *18*, 1269–1277.
12. Kaushal, A.; Zhao, Y.; Peng, Q.; Strome, T.; Weldon, E.; Zhang, M.; Chochinov, A. Evaluation of fast track strategies using agent-based simulation modeling to reduce waiting time in a hospital emergency department. *Socio Econ. Plan. Sci.* **2015**, *50*, 18–31. [CrossRef]
13. Vass, H.; Szabo, Z.K. Application of queuing model to patient flow in emergency department. Case study. *Procedia Econ. Financ.* **2015**, *32*, 479–487. [CrossRef]
14. Taichung Veterans General Hospital (TVGH): Departments of Medical Services. Available online: http://www.vghtc.org.tw/ (accessed on 5 December 2019).
15. Fletcher, A.; Worthington, D. What is a 'generic' hospital model?—A comparison of 'generic' and 'specific' hospital models of emergency patient flows. *Health Care Manag. Sci.* **2009**, *12*, 374–391. [CrossRef]
16. Hoot, N.R.; Leblanc, L.J.; Jones, I.; Levin, S.R.; Zhou, C.; Gadd, C.S.; Aronsky, D. Forecasting emergency department crowding: A discrete event simulation. *Ann. Emerg. Med.* **2008**, *52*, 116–125. [CrossRef]

17. Cochran, J.K.; Roche, K.T. A multi-class queuing network analysis methodology for improving hospital emergency department performance. *Comput. Oper. Res.* **2009**, *36*, 1497–1512. [CrossRef]
18. McManus, M.L.; Long, M.C.; Cooper, A.; Litvak, E. Queuing theory accurately models the need for critical care resources. *Anesthesiology* **2004**, *100*, 1271–1276. [CrossRef]
19. Marmor, Y.N.; Wasserkrug, S.; Zeltyn, S.; Mesika, Y.; Greenshpan, O.; Carmeli, B.; Shtub, A.; Mandelbaum, A. Toward simulation-based real-time decision-support systems for emergency departments. In Proceedings of the 2009 Winter Simulation Conference (WSC), Austin, TX, USA, 13–16 December 2009.
20. Oh, C.; Novotny, A.M.; Carter, P.L.; Ready, R.K.; Campbell, D.D.; Leckie, M.C. Use of a simulation-based decision support tool to improve emergency department throughput. *Oper. Res. Health Care* **2016**, *9*, 29–39. [CrossRef]

15

Cerebral White Matter Hyperintensity as a Healthcare Quotient

Kaechang Park [1,*,†], Kiyotaka Nemoto [2,†], Yoshinori Yamakawa [3], Fumio Yamashita [4], Keitaro Yoshida [2], Masashi Tamura [2], Atsushi Kawaguchi [5], Tetsuaki Arai [2] and Makoto Sasaki [4]

1 Research Organization for Regional Alliance, Kochi University of Technology, Kochi 782-0003, Japan
2 Department of Psychiatry, Faculty of Medicine, University of Tsukuba, Tsukuba 305-8575, Japan; kiyotaka@nemotos.net (K.N.); keicima0154@gmail.com (K.Y.); tamuramas@gmail.com (M.T.); 4632tetsu@md.tsukuba.ac.jp (T.A.)
3 ImPACT Program of Council for Science, Technology and Innovation (Cabinet Office, Government of Japan), Tokyo 100-8974, Japan; yamakawa@bi-lab.org
4 Division of Ultrahigh Field MRI, Institute for Biomedical Sciences, Iwate Medical University, Morioka 028-3694, Japan; fyamashi@iwate-med.ac.jp (F.Y.); masasaki@iwate-med.ac.jp (M.S.)
5 Center for Comprehensive Community Medicine, Faculty of Medicine, Saga University, Saga 849-8501, Japan; akawa@cc.saga-u.ac.jp
* Correspondence: park.kaechang@kochi-tech.ac.jp
† These authors contributed equally to this work.

Abstract: To better understand the risk factors and optimal therapeutic strategies of cerebral white matter hyperintensity (WMH), we examined a large population of adults with and without various vascular risk factors (VRFs) or vascular risk conditions (VRCs), such as hypertension (HT), diabetes mellitus (DM), and dyslipidemia (DLP), including the comorbidities. We assessed two participant groups having no medical history of stroke or dementia that underwent brain checkup using magnetic resonance imaging (MRI): 5541 participants (2760 men, 2781 women) without VRCs and 1969 participants (1169 men, 800 women) who had received drug treatments for VRCs and the combination of comorbidities. For data analysis, we constructed WMH-brain healthcare quotient (WMH-BHQ) based on the percentile rank of WMH volume. This metric has an inverse relation to WMH. Multiple linear regression analysis of 5541 participants without VRCs revealed that age, systolic blood pressure (SBP), Brinkman index (BI), and female sex were significant factors lowering WMH-BHQ, whereas body mass index (BMI), male sex, fasting blood sugar, and triglyceride levels were increasing factors. The Kruskal–Wallis test and Dunn tests showed that WMH-BHQs significantly increased or decreased with BMI or SBP and with BI classification, respectively. Regarding the impact of impaired fasting glucose and abnormal lipid metabolism, there were almost no significant relationships. For 1969 participants who had HT, DM, and DLP, as well as their comorbidities, we found that DLP played a substantial role in increasing WMH-BHQ for some comorbidities, whereas the presence of HT and DM alone tended to decrease it. Cerebral WMH can be used as a healthcare quotient for quantitatively evaluating VRFs and VRCs and their comorbidities.

Keywords: white matter hyperintensity; MRI; healthcare quotient; chronic

1. Introduction

Cerebral vessel diseases are classified as large vessels diseases (LVDs) or small vessels diseases (SVDs) based on whether the diameters of the vessels involved are larger than a few millimeters or smaller than several hundred micrometers, respectively [1,2]. Both categories can be noninvasively diagnosed using magnetic resonance imaging (MRI) [3]. With regard to risk factors, many longitudinal studies have reported that LVD can be responsible for stroke, cognitive decline, and dementia [1–4]. Hypertension (HT), diabetes mellitus (DM), and dyslipidemia (DLP), three primary vascular risk conditions (VRCs) in developed countries, are risk factors for LVD [5,6]. Although HT is an obvious risk factor for SVD, the roles of DM and DLP remain disputable [7,8]. Compared with LVD, SVD has not yet been sufficiently studied with regard to its onset and development. The pathological complexity of SVD, such as arteriosclerosis, hyalinosis, blood–brain barrier disruption, and venous collagenosis, have long complicated our ability to fully comprehend its many aspects [1,8]. For SVD studies using MRI, it is difficult to include large numbers of participants who have various conditions ranging from preclinical to chronic HT, DM, and DLP, partly because SVD is mostly asymptomatic and does not have hospital follow-up like LVD. To clarify the whole range of cerebral vessel damages, a large scale epidemiological study of SVD including preclinical or chronic HT, DM, and DLP is essential.

Brain MRIs show four major features of SVD: lacuna stroke, white matter hyperintensity (WMH), cerebral microbleeds, and visible perivascular spaces [9]. In our study, we focused on WMHs, also known as leukoaraiosis, which are commonly observed in the general population, particularly among individuals with preclinical or chronic HT, DM, and DLP. WMHs are recognized in >60% of people over 60 years old [10] and >30% of people with the age range from 40 to 50 years in Japan, where MRI examination is incorporated as part of health checkups in connection with a screening program called Brain Dock [11,12]. WMHs are regarded as disappearance of arterioles and capillary arteries caused by aging, HT, and reduced cerebral blood flow [9,13]. WMHs are also significantly associated with recurrent stroke, cognitive decline, and dementia [2,5].

Numerous efforts have been made to develop MRI-based measures of health status, such as the concept of "brain age", which reportedly reflects the mortality of an individual [14]. Our team earlier proposed brain healthcare quotients (BHQs) based on gray matter volume or fractional anisotropy and found significant associations between these proffered metrics and various physical factors, such as obesity, high blood pressure (BP), and daily personal schedules, as well as social factors, including subjective socioeconomic status, subjective well-being, and the adoption of a postmaterialism view of life [15]. In this cross-sectional study, we proposed another BHQ based on WMH, which begins to appear in early middle age and increases in frequency with age. Using an extensively large database obtained from 8921 participants who were examined through MRI as part of the Brain Dock component of a routine health checkups, we analyzed two groups of individuals with VRFs: those without VRCs and those with VRCs receiving drug treatment for high BP, impaired fasting glucose (IFG), or abnormal lipid metabolism (ALM), each of which chronically results in the onset of HT, DM, or ALM, respectively. In the drug treatment group, the BHQs of WMH were compared according to the comorbidity of HT, DM, or DLP because these VRCs commonly combine together. Nonetheless, the relationship between WMH and comorbidity remains remarkably unclear [9,10,13]. To help make progress in this area, we designed and executed a large scale, cross-sectional study covering healthy and non-healthy states ranging from preclinical to chronic HT, DM, and DLP to examine whether WMH can be used as a healthcare quotient to maintain a healthy state or prevent the onset and development of VRCs.

2. Materials and Methods

2.1. Participants

Data were collected between January 2013 and April 2017 from the brain dock center (BDC) affiliated with Kochi University of Technology. From BDC, we enrolled 8921 healthy participants without a history of cerebral stroke, who underwent the brain dock health checkups only once. Although we were interested in the WMH of individuals with various medical backgrounds, participants who had been clinically diagnosed with HT, DM, and DLP but had not been treated with drugs were excluded (n = 1411). Thus, 5541 participants (2760 males, 2781 females; age, 20–89 years; mean age ± SD, 51.38 ± 9.80 years; median age, 51 years) with no medical history for HT, DM, and DLP were selected for analysis (Table 1). Here, the term "medical history" refers to the drug treatment history before and at the time of enrollment in the study. In addition, the following participants were also enrolled for analysis based on the examination results at BDC that compared WMH-BHQ of the participants with no medical history with that of those with a medical history of HT, DM, and DLP or their comorbidities (n = 1969).

Table 1. Number and age distribution of participants without and with hypertension (HT), diabetes mellitus (DM), and/or dyslipidemia (DLP).

	Total	Male	Female	Mean Age ± SD (Years)	Median Age (Years)
No medical history	5541	2760	2781	51.4 ± 9.8	51
HT only	1074	622	422	59.5 ± 9.3	59
DM only	150	114	36	59.3 ± 9.8	59
DLP only	299	124	175	56.9 ± 8.7	57
HT + DLP	220	124	96	60.0 ± 9.0	59
HT + DM	124	97	27	60.8 ± 9.0	60
DM + DLP	35	19	16	57.0 ± 7.6	57
HT + DM + DLP	67	39	28	60.4 ± 7.6	59

All participants lived in Kochi Prefecture, visited BDC, and underwent brain MRI as part of their routine health checkups. They also answered a questionnaire on their past and present medical history and lifestyles, such as smoking. Health checkups included systolic blood pressure (SBP), body mass index (BMI), Brinkman index (BI; multiplying the average number of cigarettes smoked per day by the number of years the person has smoked), and various blood chemistry test items, including hemoglobin A1c (HbA1c), fasting blood sugar (FBS), triglycerides (TG), and high- density lipoprotein (HDL) and low-density lipoprotein (LDL) cholesterol. Based on these tests, BMI, BI, High BP, IFG, and ALM were classified according to the criteria shown in Table 2.

Table 2. Classification of body mass index (BMI), Brinkman index (BI), high blood pressure (BP), and criteria of impaired fasting glucose (IFG) and abnormal lipid metabolism (ALM).

	Classification and Criteria
BMI	Underweight, BMI < 18.5; normal, 18.5 ≤ BMI < 25, overweight, 25 ≤ BMI< 30; and obese, BMI ≥ 30
BI	BI = 0, 0 < BI < 400, and BI ≥ 400
High BP	Systolic blood pressure (SBP) < 139, 140 ≤ SBP < 160, SBP ≥ 150
IFG	A (fasting blood sugar (FBS) < 100 and HbA1c < 5.6%) B (100 ≤ FBS < 100 or 5.6% ≤ HbA1c < 6.0%) C (110 ≤ FBS < 126 or 6.0% ≤ HbA1c < 6.5%) D (FBS ≥ 126 or HbA1c ≥ 6.5%)
ALM	Triglycerides (TG); TG < 29, 30 ≤ TG< 140, 140 ≤ TG< 400, and TG ≥ 400 Ratios of LDL to HDL (LH ratio): LH ratio < 1, 1 ≤ LH ratio < 1.5, 1.5 ≤ LH ratio < 2, 2 ≤ LH ratio < 2.5, and LH ratio ≥ 2.5

2.2. *Automated Measurement of WMH Volume*

A 1.5 Tesla MRI system (ECHELON Vega; Hitachi Medical Corporation, Tokyo, Japan) was used to perform MRI examinations for WMH diagnosis. The imaging protocol included T2-weighted spin-echo (repetition time/echo time (TR/TE) = 5800/96 ms), T1-weighted spin-echo (TR/TE = 520/14 ms), and fluid-attenuated inversion recovery (FLAIR; TR/TE = 8500/96 ms; inversion time = 2100 ms) images as described previously [16]. Images were obtained as 27 transaxial slices per scan. The slice thickness was 5 mm, with no interslice gap, as described previously [11,16]. Measurement of WMH volume was needed to evaluate the severity, especially for levels more than the maximum of the Fazekas scale. In our study, WMHs were automatically segmented and quantified for their volume using the following procedure. First, the FLAIR images were segmented into gray and white matter and cerebrospinal fluid space using SPM12, which also yielded the intensity inhomogeneity corrected image (IICI) [17,18]. Then, IICI was anatomically normalized into the template space using advanced normalization tools. A region-of-interest delineating the middle cerebellar peduncle was applied to the anatomically normalized IICI to estimate the intensity distribution of normal white matter of each subject. IICI in native space was then normalized for its intensity in the brain region segmented by the gray and white matter. The intensity normalized IICI was thresholded using a 3.5 SD cutoff to segment WMH, with search regions limited to WMH mask. The WMH volume (WMHV) was calculated by multiplying the voxel size by slice thickness. Finally, the measured WMH was automatically colored red to be detected by the first author (K.P.) who were a neurosurgeon trained enough to confirm the presence and location of WMH.

2.3. *WMH-BHQ, a Novel Quotient Based on WMHV*

Based on the WMHV of each participant, we constructed a new metric, the WMH-BHQ in that higher values are better and the median value for a given set of subjects is 100. In other words, this new metric was devised to convert WMHV to the standardized scale so that one can easily understand whether the WMHV of a subject is more or less than the median. In the development of this metric, we realized that the distribution of WMHV is skewed, and therefore, we used the percentile rank to define WMH-BHQ, which is the percentage of scores in its frequency distribution that are equal to or lower than it. For example, a test score that is greater than 75% of the scores of people taking the test is said to be at the 75th percentile, where 75 is the percentile rank. From the raw WMHV we obtained the percentile ranking for each subject (WMHV percentile), where zero means the lowest WMHV and 100 percentile means that the participant has the highest WMHV in the group. From this ranking method, a cumulative probability curve was estimated so that the percentile rank with newer data could be calculated with this curve. This estimation was based on the nonparametric density estimation and implemented by using the polspline function in the "polspline" package with R 3.4.3. We then defined this new brain health metric, WMH-BHQ, to be:

$$\text{WMH-BHQ} = 100 + 15 \times (50 - \text{WMHV percentile})/24, \quad (1)$$

With this formula, the median value, which was equivalent to the 50th percentile, generates a WMH-BHQ equal to 100. Likewise, the 74th and 26th percentiles produce BHQ 85 and 115, respectively. Originally, we considered directly using interquartile range (i.e., 75th and 25th percentiles). However, if the newer data were beyond the range of original data, an error would be produced. To avoid this prospect, we used the value 24 instead of 25 in the denominator. As a result, the WM-BHQ of 95% of our subjects ranged from 70.31 to 130. A lower WMH-BHQ means a higher and more problematic level of WMHV. A histogram of the WMH-BHQ values of our subjects with upward sloping curve implies "well-being" of brain health and a downward slope shows "not well-being" in terms of WMH.

2.4. *Statistical Analysis*

WMHV and WMH-BHQ data were not normally distributed. Thus, Mann–Whitney *U* and Kruskal–Wallis tests were utilized to evaluate the associations between WMHs and VRCs or other possible risk factors by comparing the differences between group distributions. The groups were defined by the presence or absence of VRCs or by standard criteria and classifications of risk factors described in the upper paragraphs. When the null hypotheses were rejected in the Kruskal–Wallis tests, we used Dunn tests [18] for pairwise comparisons. The p values were then adjusted using the Benjamini–Hochberg procedure [19], which controls the false discovery rate for multiple comparisons. Multiple regression analyses were performed to examine complex associations among multiple variables while controlling for the effect of potential confounding factors [20]. All statistical analyses except for the Benjamini–Hochberg procedure were performed using the Statistical Package for the Social Sciences software version 22 (IBM Corp., Armonk, NY, USA) [20]. Adjusted p values based on the Benjamini–Hochberg procedure were calculated using a Microsoft Excel (Microsoft Inc, Redmond, WA, USA) spreadsheet [21].

2.5. *Standard Protocol Approvals, Registrations, and Participant Consents*

Written informed consent was received from all participants and this study was reviewed and approved by the institutional review board of Kochi University of Technology.

2.6. *Data Availability*

Anonymized data might be shared by request.

3. Results

3.1. *WMH-BHQ of Participants with no Medical History According to Age Decades*

As shown in Figure 1a, the contour of the histogram for our metric WMH-BHQ changed remarkably across the different ages of the participants in this study. For subjects in their 40s, it was up right, while for those in their 50s, it was symmetric like a rainbow curve, and those in their 60s, 70s, and 80s generated plots shifting up and to the left as the age decades increased. In terms of WMH-BHQ, brain health obviously declined with age, as shown by the box plot in Figure 1b. The Kruskal–Wallis test and Dunn tests showed that all pairwise comparisons were significant except for those between 70s and 80s (p = 0.076). The WMHV histogram was asymptotic with a peak volume of <5 mL; therefore, WMH-BHQ was clearly superior to WMHV with regard to visualization and understanding of changes occurring over the age decades.

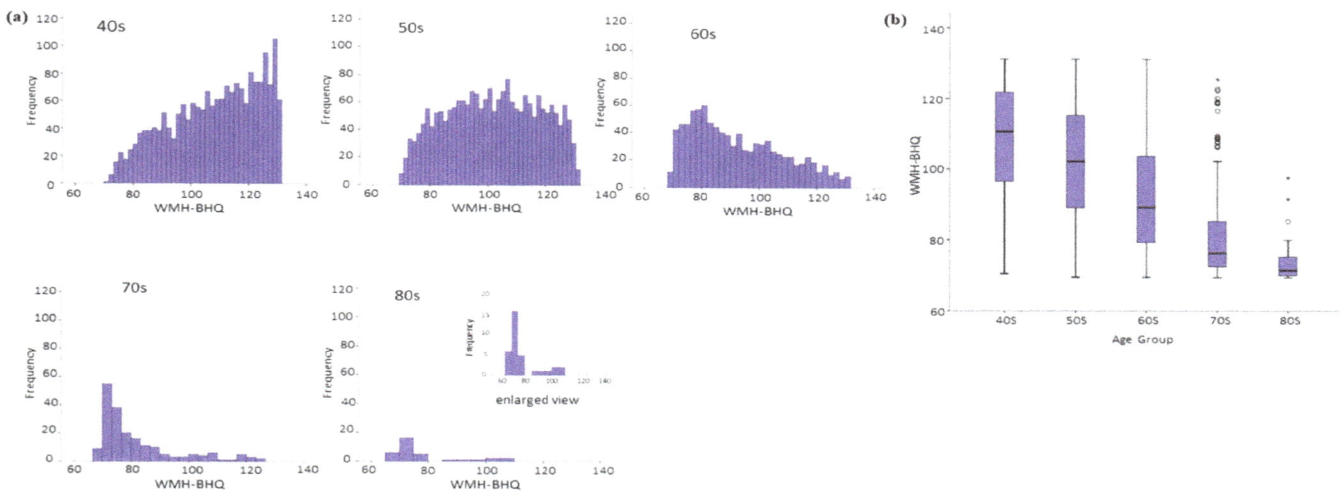

Figure 1. Histograms (**a**) and box plots (**b**) of WMH-BHQ with no medical history according to age decades of 40s, 50s, 60s, 70s, and 80s.

3.2. *WMH-BHQ Histograms of Sex*

There was a distinct difference in WMH-BHQ between males and females (Figure 2). The histogram of males was a trapezoid with an upward slope, while that of females showed a plateau, suggesting that females are more susceptive to WMH than males.

Compared with results across the various age decades, the Mann–Whitney U test showed a clear sex difference for participants younger than their 50s but not for participants in their 60s and beyond (Table 3).

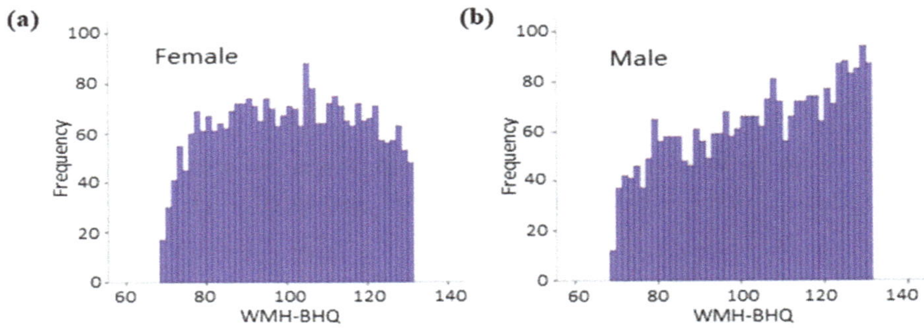

Figure 2. WMH-BHQ Histograms of females (**a**) and males (**b**).

Table 3. Mann-Whitney U test of white matter hyperintensity brain healthcare quotient (WMH-BHQ) without medical history according to genders and age decades.

Mann-Whitney U (M-W U) Test							
	Male		Female				
Age Decade	N	Mean Rank	N	Mean Rank	M-W U	Z	P
30s	351	276.7	239	323.1	35361	−3.24	0.001
40s	955	855.0	865	971.8	359991	−4.74	0.001
50s	920	971.9	1117	1057.8	470485.5	−3.28	0.001
60s	437	449.5	460	448.5	100299.5	−0.05	0.957
70s	89	88.0	82	83.9	3473	−0.54	0.586
80s	8	14.9	18	12.9	61	−0.61	0.541

3.3. *Analysis of WMH-BHQ Risk Factors: No VRCs*

Multiple linear regression analysis of participants without VRCs was performed using age, sex, BMI, BI, SBP, HbA1c, FBS, TG, HDL, and LDL as independent variables and WMH-BHQ as a dependent variable (Table 4). A stepwise model was adapted for variable selection procedure. Female or male sex was a significant risk factor lowering or raising WMH-BHQ, respectively. The increases in age, SBP, and BI were significantly associated with the decrease in WMH-BHQ, whereas the increases in BMI, FBS, and TG were significantly associated with the increase in WMH-BHQ. HbA1c, HDL, and LDL were excluded after the stepwise regressions.

Table 4. Multiple linear regression analysis for white matter hyperintensity brain healthcare quotients (WMH-BHQ) risk factors.

Model	Unstandardized Coefficients		Standardized Coefficients	t	*p*	95% Confidence Interval for B	
	B	Standard Error	Beta			Lower Bound	Upper Bound
(Constant)	125.170	2.256		55.49	<0.001	120.750	129.595
Age	−0.064	0.022	−0.377	−29.53	<0.001	−0.708	−0.620
Body mass index (BMI)	0.693	0.070	0.135	9.86	<0.001	0.556	0.831
Systolic blood pressure (SBP)	−0.079	0.015	−0.074	−5.41	<0.001	−0.108	−0.051
Brinkman index (BI)	−0.003	0.001	−0.049	−3.88	<0.001	−0.004	−0.001
Fasting blood glucose (FBG)	0.045	0.015	0.038	2.96	0.003	0.015	0.074
Triglycerides (TG)	0.008	0.003	0.036	2.75	0.006	0.002	0.013

3.4. *WMH-BHQ without VRCs: the Effect of Three Classifications and Two Criteria*

We explored in detail the impact of differing values for BMI, BI, high BP and the criteria of IFG and ALM. Regarding BMI, the box plots in Figure 3a showed that WMH-BHQ significantly increased as the classification of BMI became larger. The Kruskal–Wallis test and the following Dunn tests showed all pairwise comparisons to be significantly different. BMI was also positively associated with WMH-BHQ. The effect of cigarette smoking, as measured by the BI, was that lower levels were associated with higher WMH-BHQ values. In particular, a BI value of 0 (Dunn test; $p < 0.001$) and 0–400 ($p < 0.001$) revealed significantly better bran brain health than levels above 400 (Figure 3b).

Also, from Figure 4a, it is apparent that WMH-BHQ declined as SBP increased. Regarding high BP, WMH-BHQs of ≥400 ($p < 0.010$) and 0–400 ($p < 0.001$) revealed significant decreases compared with levels of ≥400 (Figure 4a). For IFG, a significant relationship existed only between (FBS < 100 and HbA1c < 5.6%) and (FBS ≥ 100 and <110 or HbA1c ≥ 5.6% and < 6.0%) ($p < 0.001$), although the other pair matches showed no significance (Figure 4b). TG showed a significant relationship only between 30 ≤ TG < 149 and 150 ≤ TG < 399 ($p = 0.001$), although the other pair matches showed no significance (Figure 4c). The LH ratio showed significant differences between 1 ≤ LH ratio < 1.5 and 2.5 ≤ LH ratio ($p = 0.010$) and between 1.5 ≤ LH ratio < 2.0 and 2.5 ≤ LH ratio ($p = 0.018$), although the other pair matches showed no significance (Figure 4d).

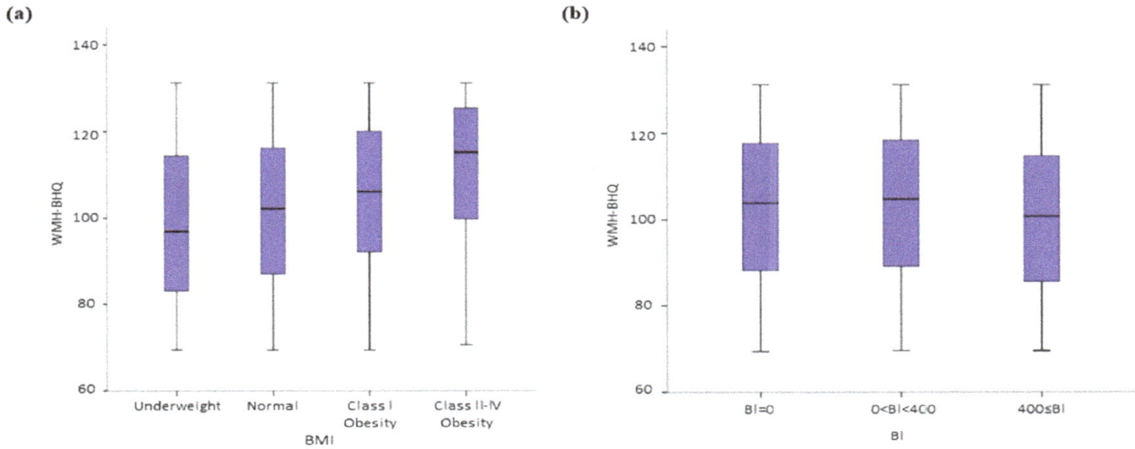

Figure 3. Box plots of WMH-BHQ with no medical history according to (**a**) Body Mass Index (BMI) and (**b**) Brinkman Index (BI).

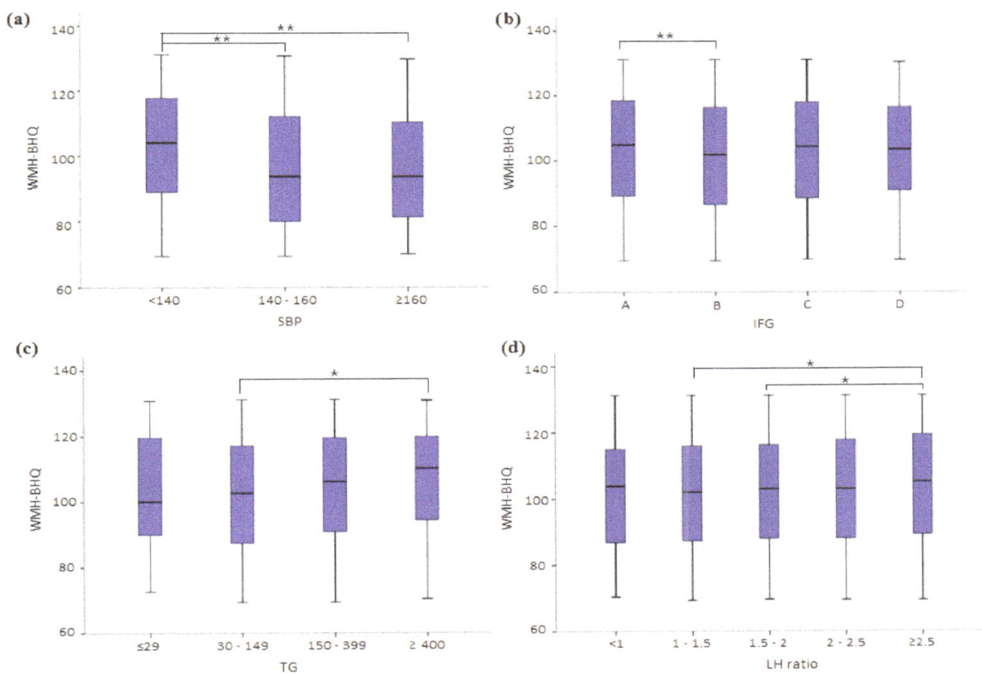

Figure 4. Box plots of WMH-BHQ with no medical history according to (**a**) systolic BP (SBP), (**b**) triglyceride (TG), (**c**) impaired fasting glucose (IFG) criteria, and d) the ratios of LDL to HDL (LH ratio). (**d**) A: fasting blood sugar (FBS) < 100 and HbA1c < 5.6; B: 100 ≤ FBS < 110 or 5.6 ≤ HbA1c < 6.0; C: 110 ≤ FBS < 126 or 6.0 ≤ HbA1c < 6.5; D: FBS ≥ 126 or HbA1c ≥ 6.5. * $p < 0.05$; ** $p < 0.001$

3.5. WMH-BHQ with VRCs and Their Comorbidities

WMH-BHQ histograms showed a downward slope for HT, while those of DM and DLP are almost plateaued compared with HT (Figure 5a). We also analyzed WMH-BHQ patterns regarding various multimorbidities, specifically, HT+DM, HT+DLP, DM+DLP, and HT+DM+DLP. Somewhat surprisingly, DM+DLP and HT+DM+DLP showed no downward slopes. Box plots showed that "no medical history" had the highest and HT+DM had the lowest median WMH-BHQs (Figure 5b). The Kruskal–Wallis test and the following Dunn test showed that all but DLP+DM had a significant difference in mean rank compared with no medical history (Table 5).

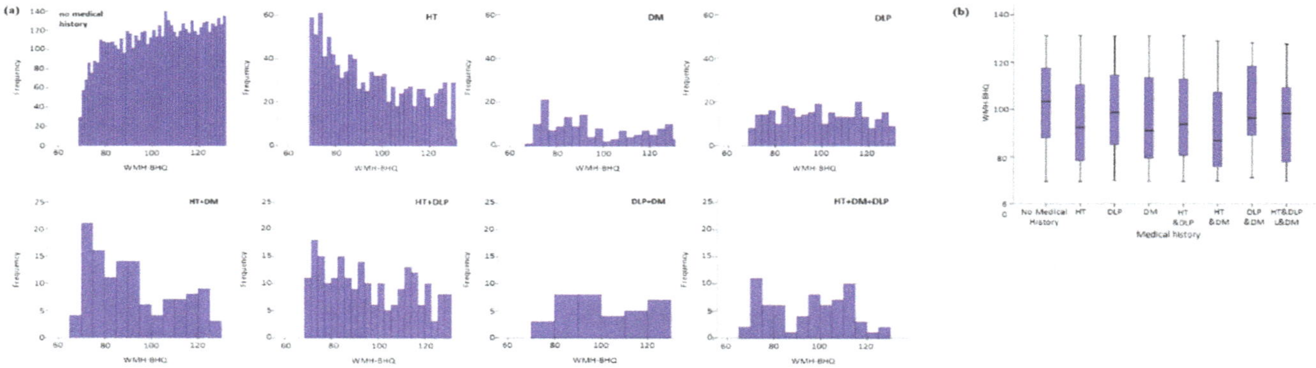

Figure 5. Histograms (**a**) and box plots (**b**) of WMH-BHQ according to no medical history, single morbidity, and multiple comorbidities. HT: Hypertension, DM: Diabetes mellitus, DLP: Dyslipidemia.

Table 5. Dunn test of WMH-BHQ among no medical history, hypertenstion (HT), diabetes mellitus (DM), dyslipidemia (DLP), and the comorbidities.

Pairwise Comparison by Dunn Test						
Comparison 1	**Comparison 2**	**Test Statistic**	**SD**	**Z**	**Unadjusted p-Value**	**Adjusted p-Value**
No medical history	HT	911.74	72.29	12.61	<0.001	<0.001
	DLP	368.32	128.72	2.86	0.004	0.015
	DM	793.29	179.40	4.42	<0.001	<0.001
	HT + DLP	765.91	149.05	5.14	<0.001	<0.001
	HT + DM	1307.35	196.87	6.64	<0.001	<0.001
	DLP + DM	188.32	367.63	0.51	0.608	0.710
	HT + DLP + DM	928.24	266.47	3.48	<0.001	0.002
HT	DLP	−543.42	141.77	−3.83	<0.001	0.001
	DM	−118.45	188.98	−0.63	0.531	0.676
	HT + DLP	−145.83	160.45	−0.91	0.363	0.485
	HT + DM	395.61	205.63	1.92	0.054	0.098
	DLP + DM	−723.42	372.40	−1.94	0.052	0.098
	HT + DLP + DM	16.49	273.01	0.06	0.952	0.952
DLP	DM	424.97	216.93	1.96	0.050	0.098
	HT + DLP	397.59	192.58	2.07	0.039	0.098
	HT + DM	939.03	231.58	4.06	<0.001	<0.001
	DLP + DM	−180.00	387.33	−0.47	0.642	0.719
	HT + DLP + DM	559.91	293.05	1.91	0056	0.098
DM	HT + DLP	−27.38	229.57	−0.12	0.905	0.939
	HT + DM	514.06	263.15	1.95	0.051	0.098
	DLP + DM	−604.97	406.99	−1.49	0.137	0.211
	HT + DLP + DM	134.94	318.59	0.42	0.672	0.724
HT + DLP	HT + DM	541.44	243.46	2.22	0.026	0.073
	DLP + DM	−577.59	394.55	−1.46	0.143	0.211
	HT + DLP + DM	162.32	302.53	0.54	0.592	0.710
HT+DM	DLP + DM	−1119.08	414.99	−2.70	0.007	0.022
	HT + DLP + DM	−379.12	328.74	−1.15	0.249	0.348
DLP+DM	HT + DLP + DM	739.91	452.18	1.64	0.102	0.168

In addition, there was a statistically significant difference in the mean rank of WMH-BHQ between DLP and HT ($p = 0.001$), and a marginally significant difference between DLP and DM ($p = 0.098$). Furthermore, there were significant differences in the mean rank of WMH-BHQ between DLP and HT+DM ($p < 0.001$) and between HT+DM and DM+DLP ($p = 0.022$). These results show that DLP may positively affect WMH-BHQ, or at least, DLP appears unlikely to be a negative factor in this regard.

4. Discussion

Age was the strongest risk factor positively related to WMH on multiple regression analysis. In addition to age, SBP and BI were positive factors for WMH, which is consistent with prior reports [4,5]. Conversely, female sex, FBS, TG, and BMI were negative factors for WMH. The reason for sex differences in WMH remains unclear although the risk factors for LVD include male sex [22,23]. Recently, a population-based cognitively unimpaired cohort study with participants aged >70 years demonstrated that females had significantly greater WMHV than males [24]. Although our study examined the percentile of WMHV, the female susceptibility to WMH was significantly observed in participants aged <60 years but not in those aged >60 years (Table 3). The average menopausal age in Japan is around 50 years, but the differences across individuals are also regarded as substantial. Further study of the exact menopausal age is needed to elucidate the influence of sex hormones. If anything, sex differences according to age may contribute to the development of sex-specific preventive strategies against WMH progression linking to stroke and dementia.

Regarding fasting blood glucose and triglycerides, both β values were relatively low and the Kruskal–Wallis test showed no significant relationships according to IGF and ALM criteria. Fasting blood glucose and triglycerides may not be so heavily involved in WMH onset and development. Conversely, BMI was a powerful negative factor that increased the strength according to BMI criteria. BMI is an obesity index, whereas the others indicate waist circumstance (WC) and hip-waist ratio (HWR) [25]. Obesity directly depends on the amount of adipose tissue that can increase without weight gain. Obesity can be evaluated more accurately by WC or HWR than BMI, especially in the elderly [25]. Instead of BMI, WC was used for multiple regression analysis and yielded similar result as that with BMI, a negative factor of WMH. That obesity appears to suppress WMH may be because some growth factors for vessels are reportedly secreted from adipose tissue [26]. For example, angiopoietin-like protein 4 (ANGPTL4) is a member of the angiopoietin family, which encodes a secretory glycoprotein highly expressed in adipose tissue and liver and placenta [27]. ANGPTL4 and/or other vascular trophic factors are delivered from adipose tissue to the brain small vessels and may prevent WMH onset and progression. Further study will be needed to validate the hypothesis.

The existence and progression of WMH in the brain can be visually recognized through WMH-BHQ before or after VRCs such as HT, DM, and DLP emerge, that is, at any progression of morbidity from preclinical to chronic stages. The visible changes of WMH in the brain readily force patients to make efforts to control VRCs, linking to the prevention of stroke or dementia, and can determine when to start drug treatments or how to promote nondrug therapies, such as low calorie and salt diets and/or physical exercise. For example, HT diagnosis based on BP values remains unreflective of organ damages caused by a high BP. If WMH was accurately grasped by means of the new metric WMH-BHQ and efficiently treated according to the change in this measure, the damages due to HT in the brain and entire body could be minimized. Thus, WMH-BHQ may be regarded as an effective indicator that can help us to visualize brain damages and estimate the health of the whole body in terms of cerebral small vessel damages. Another advantage of WMH-BHQ is that it is based on percentile and ranking order, which enables minimization of measurement bias compared with WMHV, which heavily depends on scanning conditions and the abilities of MRI equipment.

Regarding comorbidity, HT+DM yielded lower WMH-BHQs than the other double morbidities (HT+DLP and DM+DLP) as well as triple morbidities (HT+DM+DLP), although this may be due to the possible ceiling effect of the WMH volume associated with the VRF. Multimorbidity is becoming a global challenge to prevent stroke and extend lifespan [28,29]. A nationally representative cross-sectional study of more than 1.4 million persons in Scotland showed that a diagnosis of stroke significantly became more common as the number of morbidities increased [30]. Additional comorbidities are widely considered to decrease health with a destructive metabolic domino effect [29]. In our study, however, DLP may have a suppressive or preventive effect on WMH in comorbidity, although the Scotland study did not describe DLP at all. According to the ALM criteria, there were no significant differences in WMH-BHQ. This evidence might imply some effect of statins, usual drugs for DLP, rather than DLP pathology. Several meta-analyses of placebo-controlled randomized trials suggest that statins may be beneficial in reducing the overall incidence of stroke [31,32]. It remains to be determined whether statins prevent onset and development of stroke through suppression of WMH. In our study, the numbers of DLP and DM patients were extremely smaller than those with HT. Further validation needs a larger number of participants with DLP and DM for the next follow-up study. In the near future, MRI parameters could be assessed through artificial intelligence pivoting on data mining [33,34]. Such approach together with the identification of biomarkers based on novel nanotechnology or biomedical engineering platforms would allow to propose new biosignatures for risk stratification in neurovascular patients [35].

Limitations

The Brain Dock program utilizes an MRI-based approach to preventive medicine that was uniquely developed in Japan, aiming at early detection of unruptured cerebral aneurysms. At Brain Dock, health checks are conducted for a vast number of participants, and therefore, a large database could be built for brain research. Our study covered approximately 9000 participants living in Kochi Prefecture, Japan, and a single MRI machine was used throughout the study. Thus, the selection and information bias in this study could be minimized. However, our study included a bias of socioeconomic state involved, whereas one-fourth of the participants belonged to the white-collar class, such as public officials with moderate yearly incomes. The socioeconomic impact of this proportion is likely considered significant on WMH and the onset as well as the progression of VRCs to no small extent. The usage of 1.5 T MRI yields lower measurement of WMH volume as compared with 3 T MRI [36]. Nevertheless, the difference in magnetic power may be minimized in case of WMH-BHQ using the percentile of WMH volume. Our study was designed as a cross-sectional approach and only referred to the associations with WMHs at preclinical and chronic stages of VRCs. The next step will involve a prospective cohort study to certify the causal validation of WMH-BHQ using participants undergoing Brain Dock examinations more than twice.

5. Conclusions

In this study, we showed that cerebral white matter hyperintensities can be used as a healthcare quotient for quantitatively evaluating vascular risk factors or vascular risk conditions. Because of easiness of interpretation (Higher WMH-BHQ is better for brain in terms of cerebral vascular risk), WMH-BHQ might be useful for both clinicians and patients/inidividuals to pay their attentions to reduce cerebral vascular risks.

Author Contributions: Conceptualization, K.P. and K.N.; methodology, K.N. and K.Y.; software, F.Y.; validation, M.T., T.A. and M.S.; formal analysis, K.Y.; investigation, M.S.; resources, K.P.; data curation, K.P.; writing—original draft preparation, K.P.; writing—review and editing, K.N.; visualization, A.K.; supervision, M.S.; project administration, K.P.; funding acquisition, Y.Y.

Acknowledgments: We thank Miho Kawai for assistance with questionnaires in our Brain Dock.

References

1. Pantoni, L. Cerebral small vessel disease: From pathogenesis and clinical characteristics to therapeutic challenges. *Lancet Neurol.* **2010**, *9*, 689–701. [CrossRef]
2. Debette, S.; Markus, H.S. The clinical importance of white matter hyperintensities on brain magnetic resonance imaging: Systematic review and meta-analysis. *BMJ* **2010**, *341*, c3666. [CrossRef] [PubMed]
3. Salat, D.H. Imaging small vessel-associated white matter changes in aging. *Neuroscience* **2014**, *276*, 174–186. [CrossRef] [PubMed]
4. Zeestraten, E.A.; Lawrence, A.J.; Lambert, C.; Benjamin, P.; Brookes, R.L.; Mackinnon, A.D.; Morris, R.G.; Barrick, T.R.; Markus, H.S. Change in multimodal MRI markers predicts dementia risk in cerebral small vessel disease. *Neurology* **2017**, *89*, 1869–1876. [CrossRef]
5. Ding, J.; Sigurðsson, S.; Jonson, P.V.; Eiriksdottir, G.; Charidimou, A.; Lopez, O.L.; van Buchem, M.A.; Guðnason, V.; Launer, L.J. Large perivascular spaces visible on magnetic resonance imaging, cerebral small vessel disease progression, and risk of dementia: The age, gene/environment susceptibility-reykjavik study. *JAMA Neurol.* **2017**, *74*, 1105–1112. [CrossRef]
6. Baradaran, H.; Al-Dasuqi, K.; Knight-Greenfield, A.; Giambrone, A.; Delgado, D.; Ebani, E.J.; Kamel, H.; Gupta, A. Association between Carotid plaque features on CTA and cerebrovascular ischemia: A systematic review and meta-analysis. *AJNR Am. J. Neuroradiol* **2017**, *38*, 2321–2326. [CrossRef]
7. Staals, J.; Makin, S.D.; Doubal, F.N.; Dennis, M.S.; Wardlaw, J.M. Stroke subtype, vascular risk factors, and total MRI brain small-vessel disease burden. *Neurology* **2014**, *83*, 1228–1234. [CrossRef]
8. Pantoni, L.; Garcia, J.H. Pathogenesis of leukoaraiosis: A review. *Stroke* **1997**, *28*, 652–659. [CrossRef]
9. Lin, J.; Wang, D.; Lan, L.; Fan, Y. Multiple factors involved in the pathogenesis of white matter lesions. *Biomed. Res. Int.* **2017**, *2017*, 1–9. [CrossRef]
10. Habes, M.; Erus, G.; Toledo, J.B.; Zhang, T.; Bryan, N.; Launer, L.J.; Rosseel, Y.; Janowitz, D.; Doshi, J.; Van der Auwera, S.; et al. White matter hyperintensities and imaging patterns of brain ageing in the general population. *Brain* **2016**, *139*, 1164–1179. [CrossRef]
11. Park, K.; Yasuda, N.; Toyonaga, S.; Yamada, S.M.; Nakabayashi, H.; Nakasato, M.; Nakagomi, T.; Tsubosaki, E.; Shimizu, K. Significant association between leukoaraiosis and metabolic syndrome in healthy subjects. *Neurology* **2007**, *69*, 974–978. [CrossRef] [PubMed]
12. Bokura, H.; Yamaguchi, S.; Iijima, K.; Nagai, A.; Oguro, H. Metabolic syndrome is associated with silent ischemic brain lesions. *Stroke* **2008**, *39*, 1607–1609. [CrossRef] [PubMed]
13. Assayag, E.B.; Eldor, R.; Korczyn, A.D.; Kliper, E.; Shenhar-Tsarfaty, S.; Tene, O.; Molad, J.; Shapira, I.; Berliner, S.; Volfson, V.; et al. Type 2 diabetes mellitus and impaired renal function are associated with brain alterations and poststroke cognitive decline. *Stroke* **2017**, *48*, 2368–2374. [CrossRef] [PubMed]
14. Cole, J.H.; Ritchie, S.J.; Bastin, M.E.; Valdés Hernández, M.C.; Muñoz Maniega, S.; Royle, N.; Corley, J.; Pattie, A.; Harris, S.E.; Zhang, Q.; et al. Brain age predicts mortality. *Mol. Psychiatry* **2018**, *23*, 1385–1392. [CrossRef] [PubMed]
15. Nemoto, K.; Oka, H.; Fukuda, H.; Yamakawa, Y. MRI-based brain healthcare quotients: A bridge between neural and behavioral analyses for keeping the brain healthy. *PLoS ONE* **2017**, *12*, e0187137. [CrossRef] [PubMed]
16. Park, K.; Nakagawa, Y.; Kumagai, Y.; Nagahara, M. Leukoaraiosis, a common brain magnetic resonance imaging finding, as a predictor of traffic crashes. *PLoS ONE* **2013**, *8*, e57255. [CrossRef] [PubMed]
17. Ashburner, J. SPM: A history. *Neuroimage* **2012**, *62*, 791–800. [CrossRef]
18. Dunn, O.J. Multiple comparisons among means. *J. Am. Stat. Assoc.* **1961**, *56*, 52–64. [CrossRef]
19. Benjamini, Y.; Hochberg, Y. Controlling the false discovery rate: A practical and powerful approach to multiple testing. *J. R. Stat. Soc. Ser. B. Stat. Methodol.* **1995**, *57*, 289–300. [CrossRef]
20. Darlington, R. Multiple regression in psychological research and practice. *Psychol. Bull.* **1968**, *69*, 161–182. [CrossRef]
21. IBM Corp. *IBM SPSS Statistics for Windows*; Version 22.0; IBM Corp: Armonk, NY, USA, 2013.
22. Schulz, U.G.; Rothwell, P.M. Differences in vascular risk factors between etiology subtypes of ischemic stroke: Importance of population-based studies. *Stroke* **2003**, *34*, 2050–2059. [CrossRef] [PubMed]

23. Verhaaren, B.F.; Vernooij, M.W.; de Boer, R.; Hofman, A.; Niessen, W.J.; van der Lugt, A.; Ikram, M.A. High blood pressure and cerebral white matter lesion progression in the general population. *Hypertension* **2013**, *61*, 1354–1359. [CrossRef] [PubMed]
24. Fatemi, F.; Kantarci, K.; Graff-Radford, J.; Preboske, G.M.; Weigand, S.D.; Przybelski, S.A.; Knopman, D.S.; Machulda, M.M.; Roberts, R.O.; Mielke, M.M. Sex differences in cerebrovascular pathologies on FLAIR in cognitively unimpaired elderly. *Neurology* **2018**, *90*, e466–e473. [CrossRef] [PubMed]
25. World Health Organization. *Obesity and Overweight [Fact Sheet]*; World Health Organization: Geneva, Switzerland, 2011.
26. Corvera, S.; Gealekman, O. Adipose tissue angiogenesis: Impact on obesity and type-2 diabetes. *Biochim. Biophys. Acta* **2014**, *1842*, 463–472. [CrossRef] [PubMed]
27. La Paglia, L.; Listì, A.; Caruso, S.; Amodeo, V.; Passiglia, F.; Bazan, V.; Fanale, D. Potential role of ANGPTL4 in the cross talk between metabolism and cancer through PPAR signaling pathway. *PPAR Res.* **2017**, *17*, 8187–8235. [CrossRef] [PubMed]
28. Kabboord, A.D.; van Eijk, M.; Fiocco, M.; van Balen, R.; Achterberg, W.P. Assessment of comorbidity burden and its association with functional rehabilitation outcome after stroke or hip fracture: A systematic review and meta-analysis. *J. Am. Med. Dir. Assoc.* **2016**, *17*, 1066.e13–1066.e21. [CrossRef]
29. Hole, B.; Salem, J. How long do patients with chronic disease expect to live? A systematic review of the literature. *BMJ Open* **2016**, *6*, e012248. [CrossRef]
30. Gallacher, K.I.; Batty, G.D.; McLean, G.; Mercer, S.W.; Guthrie, B.; May, C.R.; Langhorne, P.; Mair, F.S. Stroke, multimorbidity and polypharmacy in a nationally representative sample of 1,424,378 patients in Scotland: Implications for treatment burden. *BMC Med.* **2014**, *12*, 151. [CrossRef]
31. Chróinín, D.N.; Asplund, K.; Åsberg, S.; Callaly, E.; Cuadrado-Godia, E.; Díez-Tejedor, E.; Di Napoli, M.; Engelter, S.T.; Furie, K.L.; Giannopoulos, S.; et al. Statin therapy and outcome after ischemic stroke: Systematic review and meta-analysis of observational studies and randomized trials. *Stroke* **2013**, *44*, 448–456. [CrossRef]
32. Choi, J.Y.; Seo, W.K.; Kang, S.H.; Jung, J.M.; Cho, K.H.; Yu, S.; Oh, K. Statins improve survival in patients with cardioembolic stroke. *Stroke* **2014**, *45*, 1849–1852. [CrossRef]
33. Garg, R.; Oh, E.; Naidech, A.; Kording, K.; Prabhakaran, S. Automating ischemic stroke subtype classification using machine learning and natural language processing. *J. Stroke Cerebrovasc. Dis.* **2019**, *28*, 2045–2051. [CrossRef] [PubMed]
34. Schirmer, M.D.; Dalca, A.V.; Sridharan, R.; Giese, A.K.; Donahue, K.L.; Nardin, M.J.; Mocking, S.J.T.; McIntosh, E.C.; Frid, P.; Wasselius, J.; et al. White matter hyperintensity quantification in large scale clinical acute ischemic stroke cohort. The MRI-GENIE study. *Neuroimage Clin.* **2019**, *23*, 101884. [CrossRef] [PubMed]
35. Ganau, L.; Prisco, L.; Ligarotti, G.K.I.; Ambu, R.; Ganau, M. Understanding the pathological basis of neurological diseases through diagnostic platforms based on innovations in biomedical engineering: New concepts and theranostic perspectives. *Medicines (Basel)* **2018**, *5*, 22. [CrossRef] [PubMed]
36. Perri1, C.D.; Dwyer, M.G.; Wack, D.S.; Cox, J.L.; Hashmi, K.; Saluste, E.; Hussein, S.; Dalaker, T.O.; Schirda, C.; Bastianello, S. White Matter Hyperintensities on 1.5 and 3 Tesla Brain MRI in Healthy Individuals. *J. Biomed. Gr. Comput.* **2013**. [CrossRef]

16

Characteristics of Mild Cognitive Impairment in Northern Japanese Community-Dwellers from the ORANGE Registry

Yu Kume [1], Tomoko Takahashi [2], Yuki Itakura [3], Sangyoon Lee [4], Hyuma Makizako [5], Tsuyosi Ono [6], Hiroyuki Shimada [4] and Hidetaka Ota [3,*]

1. Department of Occupational Therapy, Graduate School of Medicine, Akita University, Akita 010-8543, Japan; kume.yuu@hs.akita-u.ac.jp
2. Integrated Community Support Center, Public Health and Welfare Department, City Hall of Yokote, Akita 013-0525, Japan; takahashi-tomoko-d@city.yokote.lg.jp
3. Advanced Research Center for Geriatric and Gerontology, Akita University, Akita 010-8543, Japan; itacie15@gmail.com
4. Center for Gerontology and Social Science, National Center for Geriatrics and Gerontology, Obu, Aichi 474-8511, Japan; sylee@ncgg.go.jp (S.L.); shimada@ncgg.go.jp (H.S.)
5. Department of Physical Therapy, School of Health Sciences, Faculty of Medicine, Kagoshima University, Kagoshima 890-8544, Japan; makizako@health.nop.kagoshima-u.ac.jp
6. Omori Municipal Hospital, Akita 013-0525, Japan; onot@oomorihp.jp

* Correspondence: hidetaka-ota@med.akita-u.ac.jp

Abstract: A gradually increasing prevalence of mild cognitive impairment (MCI) is recognized in the super-aging society that Japan faces, and early detection and intervention in community-dwellers with MCI are critical issues to prevent dementia. Although many previous studies have revealed MCI/non-MCI differences in older individuals, information on the prevalence and characteristics of MCI in rural older adults is limited. The aim of this study was to investigate differential characteristics between older adults with and without MCI. The investigation was conducted over one year from 2018 to 2019. Participants were recruited from Akita in northern Japan. Neuropsychological assessments were applied to classify MCI, including the National Center for Geriatrics and Gerontology Functional Assessment Tool (NCGG-FAT) and the Touch panel-type Dementia Assessment Scale (TDAS) based on the Alzheimer's disease assessment scale. Our samples consisted of 103 older adults divided into 54 non-MCI and 49 MCI. The MCI group had lower scores of all cognitive items. Our results showed that individuals with MCI had significantly slower walking speed (WS) and worse geriatric depression scale (GDS) compared to non-MCI. In addition, WS was significantly associated with some cognitive items in non-MCI, but not in MCI. Finally, we showed that predictive variables of MCI were WS and GDS. Our study provides important information about MCI in rural community-dwellers. We suggest that older adults living in a super-aging society should receive lower limb training, and avoiding depression in older adults through interaction of community-dwellers may contribute to preventing the onset of MCI.

Keywords: older adults living in super-aging society; mild cognitive impairment; walking speed; depression

---

1. Introduction

Mild cognitive impairment (MCI) is a transitional state of cognition between normal ageing and dementia that may progress to dementia. MCI is defined by subjective or objective evidence of cognitive decline greater than expected for the individual's age and education level but that does not interfere notably with activities of daily life, and the early detection and prevention of MCI are a challenge to prevent dementia in older adults [1]. Within established processes for making a diagnosis of MCI [2], some factors in its early detection remain unclear, as well as predictors of reversion from MCI to normal cognition. Differences between individuals without MCI and those with MCI have been studied and reported, which shows that many factors such as a lack of exercise [3], cerebrovascular factors [4], and anxiety [5] affect cognitive function. Especially, it is appreciated that cognitive and physical impairments in older adults are related through shared pathophysiological mechanisms [6]. Some studies show that older adults with MCI compared to individuals without MCI perform more poorly not just on neurocognitive performance, but also on complex motor and psychomotor domains [7–9], and exhibit greater gait impairment [10–14]. Recently, it has become clear that MCI and physical frailty are related. The physical phenotype of frailty is represented by low levels of lean body mass, muscle strength, gait performance, physical activity, and exhaustion [15]. Gait performance of the frailty is associated with cognitive decline and MCI conversion to AD as reported by [9,16]. Therefore, investigating close associations between MCI and physical function has important implications for improving diagnostic acuity of MCI and targeting interventions to prevent dementia and disability among older adults.

To clarify the dementia risk associated with MCI or early stage dementia, a nationwide clinical registry called the Organized Registration for the Assessment of dementia on Nationwide General consortium toward Effective treatment (ORANGE) is ongoing in Japan [17]. The recruitment of many registrants has been in progress in several regions of Japan from 2017, and we performed an extending preclinical trial in a cohort in northern Japan up to 2019. As is well known, gradual growth of the older population has been experienced in Japan. Especially, northern rural areas in Japan (Akita prefecture) are the most super-aging society in the world (e.g., the number of individuals over aged 75 in Akita is estimated to reach 205,000 people by 2025 [18]). Although there are few epidemiological data regarding MCI in rural areas of Japan, several studies have reported MCI profiles in older adults [19,20]. Most of them are focused on the prevalence of MCI or the conversion rate to dementia, and the detailed cognitive profile (e.g., attention, executive function, information coding skill, etc.) of MCI is not covered, as well as scarce epidemiological data regarding health-related variables such as physical performance and mental status. Therefore, we analyzed the data of a prospective cohort in northern Japan. In this study, we investigated which factors were related to MCI status according to the National Center for Geriatrics and Gerontology Functional Assessment Tool (NCGG-FAT) [21,22] and the Touch panel-type Dementia Assessment Scale (TDAS) [23,24] based on the Alzheimer's disease assessment scale (ADAS) [25]. To clarify the characteristics of rural older adults with MCI, we focused on three points as follows. First, we mainly compared cognitive function, physical performance, and depressive symptoms in MCI individuals with those in non-MCI individuals. Second, we examined correlations between physical performance and cognitive and mental function in each group (i.e., non-MCI group and MCI group). Finally, a binomial logistic regression model was estimated to determine predictive factors for MCI in rural older adults in Japan.

2. Experimental Section

2.1. Participants and Study Design

The participants were recruited in a rural area in Akita with a small population (total 32,440) with a super-aged rate of 38.7% according to public information, from 2018 to 2019. The inclusion criteria were age 65 years and over, having walking ability without personal assistance, and living at home. The exclusion criteria were dementia, major depression, severe hearing or visual impairment, stroke, Parkinson's disease, other neurological disease, intellectual disability, need for support or care as certified by the Japanese public long-term care insurance system due to disability, and inability to complete cognitive tests at the baseline assessment. The study was approved by the ethics committee of the Faculty of Medicine, Akita University (approval No. 1649) and was performed in accordance with the Declaration of Helsinki II. Informed consent was obtained from all participants. According to sample size calculations using G*Power for unpaired t test [26], we estimated a sample size of 64 participants per group to detect a clinically significant effect with $\alpha = 0.05$, power = 80%, and effect size = 0.50.

2.2. *Assessment and Outcome*

After obtaining informed consent from each participant, demographics (age, gender, and education) and health variables (body mass index (BMI), medical history of hypertension and diabetes, frail phenotype, medication and Geriatric Depression Scale-15 (GDS)) were collected according to the ORANGE protocol. A questionnaire sent in advance by mail was self-described by each participant, including age, gender, educational duration, presence of hypertension and diabetes (e.g., yes or no), amount of medications, and GDS (e.g., score range from 0 to 15, as indexed more depressive symptoms in higher scores). Height and weight to calculate BMI were measured by public health nurses. Five components of the National Center for Geriatrics and Gerontology-Study of Geriatric Syndromes (NCGG-SGS) [27] based on the Fried frailty index [15] were applied to assess frailty: (i) self-reported unintentional weight loss (i.e., a decrease of 2–3 kg over six months [28]), (ii) self-reported exhaustion (i.e., presence of fatigue for two weeks [28]), (iii) self-reported low physical activity (i.e., no exercise habit for a week [29]), (iv) weakness (i.e., grip strength (GS) less than 26/18 kg for male/female [30]): GS was measured using a Smedley-type handheld dynamometer (GRIP-D; Takei Ltd., Niigata, Japan), and (v) slow walking speed (WS) (i.e., less than 1.0 m/s in 5 m walking test [29]): walking time was measured over a 2.4-m distance in seconds using infrared sensors and participants' WS (m/s) was calculated. They were used to define robust (score of zero), pre-frail (score of 1 to 2), and frail (score of 3 to 5). The frail index of NCGG-SGS is almost equal to the original index of Fried's study [15] except the modified cut-off values for slowness and weakness are appropriate criteria for physical frailty assessments in the Japanese older population [31,32]. The present study also applied NCGG-FAT and TDAS based on ADAS to assess cognitive function in the participants and to divide the participants into non-MCI and MCI groups. All the variables of five frail components, the NCGG-FAT and TDAS were evaluated by trained public health nurses throughout a comprehensive health checkup in a local spot.

2.3. *Components of NCGG-FAT*

The computerized multidimensional neurocognitive test was performed on an iPad (Apple, Cupertino, CA, USA) with a 9.7-inch touch display. The task instructions were presented with a letter size of at least 1.0×1.0 cm^2 on the display. For this study, a trained operator supported each participant by setting up the tablet PC and running each test. Participants completed the NCGG-FAT subtests as follows.

2.3.1. Tablet Version of Word Recognition (WR)

This test is comprised of two computerized tasks of immediate recognition and delayed recall. In the first task of immediate recognition, participants were instructed to memorize 10 words, each of which was displayed for 2 s on the tablet PC. After that, a total of 30 words including 10 target and 20 distracter words were shown to participants, and they were required to select the 10 target words immediately. This task was repeated for three trials. The average number of correct answers was recorded as a score ranging from 0 to 10. In another task, participants were asked to correctly recall the 10 target words after 20 min. The number of correctly recalled target words was scored ranging from 0 to 10. Finally, we calculated the sum score of the two tasks of immediate recognition and delayed recall.

2.3.2. Tablet Version of Trail Making Test Version A (TMT-A) and Version B (TMT-B)

In the Trail Making Test Version A (TMT-A) task, participants were instructed to touch the target numbers in a sequence as rapidly as possible. Target numbers from 1 to 15 were randomly displayed on the tablet panel. In addition, the Trail Making Test Version B (TMT-B) instructions required participants to touch target numbers (e.g., 1–15) and letters in turn. The required time (seconds) to complete each task was recorded, within a maximum time of 90 s.

2.3.3. Tablet Version of Symbol Digit Substitution Task (SDST)

In the Symbol Digit Substitution Task (SDST), nine pairs of numbers and symbols were shown in the upper part of the tablet display. A target symbol was shown in the center of the tablet panel, and selectable numbers were displayed at the bottom. Participants were asked to touch the number corresponding to the target symbol shown in the central part of the tablet display as rapidly as possible. The number of correct numbers within 90 s was recorded.

2.4. Components of TDAS

The TDAS test was presented on a 14-inch touch panel display. The TDAS subtests consisted of seven of the ADAS-cog test items (11 test items) and two other tasks. Participants were instructed verbally or visually by the computer to complete the TDAS subtests as follows.

2.4.1. WR

The WR test was a computerized test based on the WR task of ADAS-cog. At the start of instructions for this task, 12 target words were individually presented on the display for 3 s each at 2 s intervals. After demonstrating the target words, the computer randomly displayed 24 words consisting of 12 target words and 12 non-target words. Participants were then instructed to respond by touching the displayed button of 'yes', 'no', or 'unknown' in response to the question regarding whether the word had been shown previously. Participants completed the trial three times. The total number of incorrect responses for three trials was recorded, with a maximum score of 72.

2.4.2. Following a Command

This task was modified from the command task of ADAS-cog. The computer presented 10 selectable icons labelled from 0 to 9 and then required participants to touch the number specified. The number of incorrect responses in two trials was scored with a maximum score of 2.

2.4.3. Orientation

This task was based on the orientation task of ADAS-cog. The computer displayed four screens in sequence. On each screen, participants were asked to touch selectable icons and answer what year, month, day, and weekday it is. The number of incorrect responses was scored with a maximum score of 4.

2.4.4. Visual-Spatial Perception

This task was modified from the constructional praxis task of ADAS-cog to evaluate visual-spatial perception. ADAS-cog requires subjects to copy the geometric forms presented. The computer first presented four screens displaying a target geometric form (i.e., a square, rhombus, cube, or triangular prism) for 5 s each. Participants were then required to correctly select the target form in response to a question task including the target form and four non-target forms. The number of incorrect responses was scored with a maximum score of 4.

2.4.5. Naming Fingers

This test assessed whether participants can name the fingers correctly, using the protocol of ADAS-cog. Participants were asked to correctly respond to a picture question of a hand marked with a red circle, by touching an icon labelled with the five finger names. An incorrect response was scored as one point, with a maximum score of 5.

2.4.6. Object Recognition

This task was based on the naming objects task of ADAS-cog. Participants were instructed to touch the correct usage icon (e.g., a pair of scissors, comb or broom) of five selectable icons labelled with the purpose of usage. Three trials were completed, and an incorrect response was scored as one point (maximum score = 3).

2.4.7. Accuracy of Order of a Process

This task was modified from the ideational praxis of ADAS-cog. The computer displayed seven icons labelled randomly with seven actions. Participants were asked to correctly touch the icons in order. The number of incorrect responses was recorded, with a maximum score of 5.

2.4.8. Money Calculation

This task assessed the money calculation ability of each participant. Participants needed to combine coins equal to an amount of money from various denominations of coins displayed on the screen. Three trials were completed, and an incorrect response was scored as one point (maximum score = 3).

2.4.9. Clock Time Recognition

This task included three kinds of question regarding clock time recognition. Participants were instructed to correctly state the time shown on a clock displayed on the screen. The number of incorrect responses was recorded, with a maximum score of 3.

2.5. MCI Classification by NCGG-FAT and TDAS

According to Petersen's report [2] in which individuals who showed cognitive impairment but were independent in activities of daily living were defined as having MCI, we applied MCI classification according to the cutoff point of NCGG-FAT or TDAS. For all cognitive subtests of NCGG-FAT, the standardized threshold in each corresponding domain for defining impairment in Japanese population-based cohorts consisting of older community-dwellers is a score more than 1.5 standard deviations (SD) below the age- and education-specific mean [21]. In TDAS, decreasing scores indicate cognitive improvement (range of scores from 0 to 101), and total scores ranging from 7 to 13 were classified as MCI [23].

3. Analyses

According to results of the normalization test (Kolmogorov–Smirnov test), Age, Height, Weight, and BMI were used by the unpaired t test. Gender (% female), Hypertension (% Yes), Diabetes (% Yes), Weight loss (% Yes), Poor energy (% Yes), and Low physical activity level (% Yes) were analyzed by chi-squared test for 2 × 2 contingency, except for Pearson's chi-square test for Frail phenotype (%, robust/pre-frail/frail) for 2 × 3 contingency. Mann–Whitney test was applied for GS (kg), WS (m/s), Amount of medications (n), Education (years), GDS-15 (score), and cognitive measurements of NCGG-FAT and TDAS (Table 1).

Table 1. Characteristics of participants with and without mild cognitive impairment (MCI).

Variables	Non-MCI Group $n = 54$		MCI Group $n = 49$		p Value	
	Mean	SD	Mean	SD		
Age (years)	74.1	6.1	74.4	5.7	0.84	
Gender (% female)	53.7%		55.1%		0.89	
Height (cm)	155.0	8.2	156.0	8.5	0.53	
Weight (kg)	57.9	11.4	60.0	10.1	0.34	
Body Mass Index (kg/m^2)	24.0	3.7	24.6	3.5	0.41	
	%		%		**p Value**	
Hypertension (% Yes)	63.0%		61.2%		0.86	
Diabetes (% Yes)	20.4%		26.5%		0.46	
Frail five components						
Frail phenotype (%, robust/pre-frail/frail)	50%/50%/0%		43%/47%/10%		0.054	
(i) Weight loss (% Yes)	11.1%		14.3%		0.63	
(ii) Poor energy (% Yes)	16.7%		26.5%		0.22	
(iii) Low physical activity level (% Yes)	13.0%		18.4%		0.45	
	Median	**IQR**	**Median**	**IQR**	**p Value**	
(iv) Grip strength (kg)	25.2	12.0	22.9	9.0	0.25	
(v) Walking speed (m/s)	1.3	0.4	1.2	0.3	0.03	*
Amount of medications (n)	3.0	3.0	4.0	4.0	0.17	
Education (years)	12.0	3.0	12.0	3.0	0.18	
GDS-15 total score (score)	2.0	2.0	3.0	4.0	0.046	*
NCGG-FAT						
Word recognition (score)	11.7	3.8	8.0	4.2	0.000	***
Tablet version of TMT-A (s)	19.0	6.0	27.0	11.0	0.000	***
Tablet version of TMT-B (s)	33.5	18.0	46.0	44.5	0.000	***
Tablet version of SDST (score)	42.0	12.0	33.0	12.5	0.000	***
TDAS						
TDAS total score (score)	2.0	3.0	7.0	9.0	0.000	***

* $p < 0.05$, ** $p < 0.01$, *** $p < 0.001$, Mann–Whitney test was applied for Education (years), Amount of medications (n), GDS-15 total score (score), Grip strength (kg), Walking speed (m/s), and cognitive measurements of NCGG-FAT and TDAS. Age, height, weight, and BMI were analyzed by unpaired t test, and gender (% female), hypertension (% Yes), diabetes (% Yes), weight loss (% Yes), poor energy (% Yes), and low physical activity level (% Yes) were analyzed by chi-squared test, except for Pearson's chi-square test for frail phenotype (%, robust/pre-frail/frail). SD, standard deviation; IQR, interquartile range; Loss weight, Loss weight more than 3 kg in six months; TMT-A, Trail Making Test A version; TMT-B, Trail Making Test B version; SDST, Symbol Digit Substitution Task; TDAS, Touch Panel-type Dementia Assessment Scale; GDS-15, Geriatric Depression Scale.

As the variables of WS, GS, subtests of NCGG-FAT, TDAS, and GDS-15 total score were not statistically normalized from the Kolmogorov–Smirnov test, Spearman correlation analysis for interval scales was applied to analyze the relationship among Age, GS, WS, subtests of NCGG-FAT, TDAS, and GDS total score for each group (Table 2).

The values of $p_{\mathrm{in}} = 0.2$ and $p_{\mathrm{out}} = 0.25$ were set up to select independent variables from Tables 1 and 2 for input into a binominal logistic regression model. The regression model was performed by a method of likelihood ratio, and set up the MCI classification as the dependent variable and predictors (i.e., independent variables) according to the following regression models; (i) 11 predictors of Model I include Age, GS, WS, Amount of medications, Education, WR, TMT-A, B, and SDST of NCGG-FAT, TDAS, and GDS-15 total score. (ii) Ten predictors of Model II except for TDAS score include Age, GS, WS, Amount of medications, Education, WR, TMT-A, B, and SDST of NCGG-FAT, and GDS-15 total score. Finally, (iii) six predictors of Model III except for all cognitive variables included Age, GS, WS, Amount of medications, Education, and GDS-15 total score. The model adaptation was examined by Hosmer–Lemeshow test (Table 3). SPSS Version 26.0 for Windows (SPSS Inc., Chicago. IL, USA) was used for analysis, and the level of significance was set at $p = 0.05$.

Table 2. Correlations for each group (non-MCI and MCI).

Variables	Non-MCI Group (n = 54)							MCI Group (n = 49)						
	WS	GS	WR	TMT-A	TMT-B	SDST	TDAS	WS	GS	WR	TMT-A	TMT-B	SDST	TDAS
Age (years)	−0.37 **	−0.21	−0.51 **	0.55 **	0.66 **	−0.66 **	0.05	−0.37 *	−0.04	−0.33 *	0.43 **	0.49 **	−0.47 **	0.25
BMI (kg/m^2)	0.08	0.24	0.18	0.05	0.05	0.02	0.00	−0.19	0.08	0.19	0.01	−0.01	0.03	−0.04
Education (years)	0.19	−0.01	0.03	−0.36 **	−0.35 **	0.15	−0.13	−0.02	0.28	0.09	−0.13	−0.10	0.29	−0.45 **
Medications (n)	0.06	−0.22	−0.11	−0.02	0.22	0.01	−0.16	−0.24	0.25	0.04	−0.03	0.07	−0.07	0.06
WS (m/s)	1.00	0.26	0.42 **	−0.31 **	−0.35 **	0.44 **	−0.05	1.00	−0.08	−0.08	−0.18	−0.07	0.12	−0.06
GS (kg)	0.26	1.00	0.18	−0.09	−0.02	0.22	0.31 *	−0.08	1.00	0.06	0.16	−0.12	0.16	−0.11
GDS-15 (score)	0.16	0.01	0.03	0.00	−0.01	−0.04	0.00	0.03	−0.16	0.12	−0.13	−0.28	0.12	−0.14

* $p < 0.05$, ** $p < 0.01$, Statistics represent Spearman r correlations for each parameter. BMI, body mass index; WS, walking speed; GS, grip strength; WR, word recognition; TMT-A, Trail Making Test A version; TMT-B, Trail Making Test B version; SDST, Symbol Digit Substitution Task; TDAS, Touch Panel-type Dementia Assessment Scale; GDS-15, Geriatric Depression Scale-15.

Table 3. Multiple comparison among binomial logistic regression models depending on MCI classification with odds ratio.

Model	Coefficient (β)	Odds Ratio	95% CI	*p* Value
Model I				
Age (years)	−0.27	0.77	0.66, 0.89	0.000
TMT-B (s)	0.08	1.09	1.04, 1.14	0.001
SDST (score)	−0.12	0.88	0.80, 0.97	0.012
TDAS total score (score)	0.65	1.91	1.37, 2.68	0.000
Model II				
Age (years)	−0.26	0.77	0.67, 0.88	0.000
WR (score)	−0.55	0.58	0.44, 0.76	0.000
TMT-A (s)	0.17	1.19	1.07, 1.33	0.001
TMT-B (s)	0.05	1.05	1.01, 1.10	0.025
GDS-15 total score (score)	0.32	1.37	1.07, 1.77	0.014
Model III				
Walking speed (m/s)	−2.29	0.10	0.02, 0.69	0.020
GDS-15 total score (score)	0.20	1.22	1.04, 1.43	0.015

Reference group for analysis was non-MCI group. Model I: Model χ^2 test, $p < 0.0001$; The Hosmer–Lemeshow test, $p = 0.12$; Percentage of correct classifications = 87.4%. Model II: Model χ^2 test, $p < 0.0001$; The Hosmer–Lemeshow test, $p = 0.84$; Percentage of correct classifications = 84.5%. Model III: Model χ^2 test, $p = 0.002$; The Hosmer–Lemeshow test, $p = 0.02$; Percentage of correct classifications = 59.2%. CI, confidence interval; WR, word recognition; TMT-A, Trail Making Test A version; TMT-B, Trail Making Test B version; SDST, Symbol Digit Substitution Task; TDAS, Touch Panel-type Dementia Assessment Scale; GDS, Geriatric Depression Scale-15.

4. Results

Our samples consisted of 103 older participants divided into 54 non-MCI people and 49 MCI people. We confirmed that the MCI group had significantly lower scores or longer required times of all cognitive items including WR test, TMT-A, B, SDST and TDAS scores than the non-MCI group ($p < 0.0001$) (Table 1). Demographic and health data including Age, Gender, BMI, presence of Hypertension or Diabetes, Frail phenotype, presence of Weight loss, Poor energy, Low physical activity level, Amount of medications, and Education showed no significant difference between the non-MCI group and MCI group. Of physical assessments, WS was significantly different between the groups ($p = 0.03$), whereas GS was not different ($p = 0.25$). Moreover, the MCI group showed a worse score of GDS ($p = 0.046 < 0.05$). Next, we examined correlations between physical performance, cognitive and mental function in each group (Table 2). According to the results of Spearman correlation analysis, WS was associated with some items of cognitive subtests including WR, TMT-A, B, and SDST in the non-MCI group ($|r| > 0.30$, $p < 0.01$), but these were not significant in the MCI group except for correlations between cognitive items and Age or Education. Finally, we performed an analysis to determine explanatory variables for MCI with reference to non-MCI by binomial logistic regression analysis (Table 3). According to a result of Phi coefficient of association, all the nominal scales including Gender (Phi coefficient = 0.01, $p = 0.89$), presence of Hypertension (Phi coefficient = 0.02, $p = 0.86$) and Diabetes (Phi coefficient = 0.07, $p = 0.46$), Weight loss (Phi coefficient = 0.05, $p = 0.63$), Poor energy (Phi coefficient = 0.12, $p = 0.22$), Low physical activity level (Phi coefficient = 0.08, $p = 0.45$) were not significantly associated with MCI classification, and they were not included into predictors for the regression model. Three regression models were estimated according to the predictors of Age, GS, WS, Amount of medications, Education, WR, TMT-A, B, SDST, TDAS, and GDS-15 total score. Model I that included them demonstrated that the classification of MCI had a significant association with Age, TMT-B, SDST, and TDAS. Next, Model II except for T-DAS score from Model I was applied to estimate a specific cognitive profile in MCI. Model II demonstrated that the classification of MCI had a significant association with Age, WR, TMT A, B, and GDS-15 total score. Finally, considering the self-explanatory effect of cognitive items, Model III except for all cognitive variables from Model II was applied to clarify the classification of MCI.

As shown in Model III, WS and GDS-15 total score were extracted as explanatory variables of MCI (Table S1). In the three estimated models, the results of Hosmer–Lameshow test showed adaptability of 87.4% ($p = 0.12$) in Model I, 84.5% ($p = 0.84$) in Model II, and 59.2% ($p = 0.02$) in Model III.

5. Discussion

In this study, we found characteristics of MCI in northern Japanese community-dwellers of super-aging society had slower WS and tendency to depression. Aging continues in the subjects of our survey area, and the population ratio 65 years or older reached 38.7% (July, 2019). Actually, the prevalence of MCI in this study was higher (47.6%) compared with other rural areas which were previously reported to be about 10%–30% [29,33]. Additionally, some wealthy urban areas different from our rural area showed that characteristics of MCI were greater with older age and less education than non-MCI [34,35]. Although this high prevalence and multifactorial approach may be due to different methods, it could also be because our community-dwellers living in an area of heavy snowfall in northern Japan experience a more negative impact on gait performance [36] and a potentially high incidence of depressive symptoms [37] because of fewer opportunities to go out and participate in social activities. In fact, we showed an association between cognitive function and demographic and health data including age, gender, BMI, medical history, medication, frailty phenotype, education, physical performance, and GDS in older adults living in a super-aging society (Table 1). We found that recognized risk factors for MCI including age, gender, BMI, presence of hypertension or diabetes, frailty phenotype, education, and amount of medications were not different, but WS and GDS were significantly different between the groups. We also found that WS was significantly associated with some cognitive items including SDST and TMT in the non-MCI group, but not in the MCI group (Table 2). The regression models demonstrated that MCI had a significant association with age, executive function, information coping speed, and composite cognitive performance, indicating that these are predictive variables for the presence of MCI. However, because of the effect of variables on these cognitive scores (Model I), we applied Models II and III (Table 3). Model II excluding composite cognitive performance, as indexed in the TDAS score, demonstrated that MCI had a significant association with age, WR, attention, executive function, and GDS. Compatible with the results of Reinvang et al. [38], attention and executive dysfunction in neuropsychological tests could be early symptoms of MCI. Especially, the variables of SDST and TMT are recognized to reflect psychomotor processing and executive function [39], and several studies have reported that they are rapidly altered in MCI subjects [40,41]. Although they justify its use for the detection of cognitive impairment in older adults, most of these tests have numerous limitations (the problem of novelty, lack of sensitivity and specificity, patient cognitive reserve, etc.) [42,43]. This recent observation underscores the need to find new detection indicators for cognitive impairment. With this in perspective, a new approach associates WS of older adults with the presence of cognitive impairment.

Interestingly, in Model III excluding all cognitive domains, WS and GDS were selected as explanatory variables although the percentage of correct classifications was not so good in the Hosmer–Lameshow test. These findings indicate that the variables WS and GDS can potentially distinguish the presence or absence of MCI; therefore, they provide suggestive information on the presence of MCI. Recently, some studies have focused on both cognition and locomotor performance as predictors of adverse outcomes in community-dwellers with MCI [44,45]. In particular, slow gait speed at usual pace has been implicated in the onset of adverse outcomes, such as disability [46], cognitive impairment [47], institutionalization, falls [48,49], and mortality [50]. As previously reported, the association between slowing of walking and MCI is supported by shared neurological findings that include a smaller right hippocampus [51]. This finding underscores walking–brain behavior relationships and the value of WS as an early indicator of dementia risk. However, thus far, there is insufficient information to state that WS can potentially predict adverse outcomes in older community-dwellers, and more specific investigations need to be performed. Moreover, we showed that GS was no different between the groups ($p = 0.25$), suggesting that reinforcement of lower, but not upper, limb muscular strength may be a critical target in rehabilitation. Likewise, recent studies have indicated that lower extremity motor dysfunction may be a feature of MCI [52], but little is known about the nature and biological mechanism such as myokines of lower extremity motor dysfunction associated with MCI. Regarding WS and a cognitive function, the concept of frailty has become a geriatric topic recently. Although we could not include frailty as global score in the correlation analysis or binomial regression analysis because the distribution of a frail group according to the frailty phenotype was greatly biased (e.g., % of robust/pre-frail/frail, 50%/50%/0% in the non-MCI group, 43%/47%/10% in the MCI group) (Table 1), some studies have reported that a physical frailty is associated with MCI and a reduction of WS in five items of the Fried index mostly reflect the occurrence of MCI and disability [31,53]. MCI with concomitant physical frailty may be considered to fulfil the criteria for cognitive frailty [54]. In this regard, we believe that the cognitive frailty concept has potential advantages in better stratifying the risk profiles of older adults with MCI. In a comparison between the groups, MCI also showed significantly higher depressive scores as indexed in the GDS. Concerning geriatric depression in MCI, cross-sectional research has shown that the association between depressive symptoms, as indexed in the Korean version of GDS, and memory or executive function was significantly greater in individuals with MCI than in those with AD [55]. Additionally, survival analysis followed for 6.28 years on average, indicating that the presence of MCI is a poor predictive factor in individuals with depressive symptoms as indexed in the GDS [56]. Thus, geriatric depressive symptoms in individuals with MCI need to be carefully screened in rural community-dwellers.

The limitations of our research need to be considered in developing our future research. First, the NCGG-FAT and TDAS used to classify individuals with MCI in this study were a tablet PC version of cognitive measurement tools based on the MCI criteria reported by Petersen [2], and evaluation of the accuracy of MCI's classification is essential for worldwide research. Second, our cohort was comprised of a localized group of individuals in one rural area of northern Japan, whose actual sample size (n = 103) did not reach the calculated required sample size (n = 128) due to difficulty sampling and recruiting in a depopulated, small rural area. Third, considering younger age was associated with MCI, we could not take the association into consideration. Fourth, although focusing this study on frailty concept was important, we guessed it was difficult to analyze frail status in detail due to bias of frail samples between the groups (e.g., 0% of the non-MCI group, 10% of the MCI group). Further examination concerning frailty is warranted in future research. Finally, we hypothesize that cognitive domains, gait performance, and tendency to depression might be associated with MCI status. For the three regression models in this study, WS and GDS were selected as explanatory variables in Model III. However, further research with sufficient adaptability should be carried out with a large sample size in multiple rural districts. These limitations need to be considered when interpreting this study's findings.

6. Conclusions

In conclusion, WS and GDS were shown to be potential predictive variables of MCI in our study, and we consider they provide important information about characteristics of MCI in rural community-dwellers. It is suggested that older individuals living in a super-aging society should work on training lower limb muscular strength, and avoiding depression in older adults by interaction of community-dwellers may contribute to prevention of the onset of MCI.

Author Contributions: Conceived the trial and participated in the study design: H.S., H.M., S.L., and H.O. Recruited and collected data: T.T., Y.I., T.O., and H.O. Analyzed data: Y.K. and H.O. All authors participated in interpretation of the results. Y.K. and H.O. drafted the manuscript, and all authors contributed to critical review and revision of the manuscript. H.O. takes responsibility for the manuscript as a whole.

Acknowledgments: The authors would like to thank all of participants for their enthusiasm in contributing to this project and making this study possible. We would also like to thank Soichi Kagaya (Akita University) for his management, and all staff at Yokote Hall and Omori Hospital who provided assistance in performing the assessments, and AMED for financial support.

References

1. Petersen, R.C.; Stevens, J.C.; Ganguli, M.; Tangalos, E.G.; Cummings, J.L.; DeKosky, S.T. Practice parameter: Early detection of dementia: Mild cognitive impairment (an evidence-based review). Report of the Quality Standards Subcommittee of the American Academy of Neurology. *Neurology* **2001**, *56*, 1133–1142. [CrossRef] [PubMed]
2. Petersen, R.C. Mild cognitive impairment as a diagnostic entity. *J. Intern. Med.* **2004**, *256*, 183–194. [CrossRef] [PubMed]
3. Öhman, H.; Savikko, N.; Strandberg, T.E.; Pitkälä, K.H. Effect of physical exercise on cognitive performance in older adults with mild cognitive impairment or dementia: A systematic review. *Dement. Geriatr. Cogn. Disord.* **2014**, *38*, 347–365. [CrossRef] [PubMed]
4. McKetton, L.; Cohn, M.; Tang-Wai, D.F.; Sobczyk, O.; Duffin, J.; Holmes, K.R.; Poublanc, J.; Sam, K.; Crawley, A.P.; Venkatraghavan, L.; et al. Cerebrovascular resistance in healthy aging and mild cognitive impairment. *Front. Aging Neurosci.* **2019**, *11*, 79. [CrossRef]
5. Mirza, S.S.; Ikram, M.A.; Bos, D.; Mihaescu, R.; Hofman, A.; Tiemeier, H. Mild cognitive impairment and risk of depression and anxiety: A population-based study. *Alzheimers Dement.* **2017**, *13*, 130–139. [CrossRef]
6. Panza, F.; Seripa, D.; Solfrizzi, V.; Tortelli, R.; Greco, A.; Pilotto, A.; Logroscino, G Targeting cognitive frailty: Clinical and neurobiological roadmap for a single complex phenotype. *J. Alzheimers Dis.* **2015**, *47*, 793–813. [CrossRef]
7. Kluger, A.; Gianutsos, J.G.; Golomb, J.; Ferris, S.H.; George, A.E.; Franssen, E.; Reisberg, B. Patterns of motor impairment in normal aging, mild cognitive decline, and early Alzheimer's disease. *J. Gerontol. B Psychol. Sci. Soc. Sci.* **1997**, *52*, 28–39. [CrossRef]
8. McGough, E.L.; Kelly, V.E.; Logsdon, R.G.; McCurry, S.M.; Cochrane, B.B.; Engel, J.M.; Teri, L. Associations between physical performance and executive function in older adults with mild cognitive impairment: Gait speed and the timed "up & go" test. *Phys. Ther.* **2011**, *91*, 1198–1207.
9. Aggarwal, N.T.; Wilson, R.S.; Beck, T.L.; Bienias, J.L.; Bennett, D.A. Motor dysfunction in mild cognitive impairment and the risk of incident Alzheimer disease. *Arch. Neurol.* **2006**, *63*, 1763–1769. [CrossRef]
10. McGough, E.L.; Cochrane, B.B.; Pike, K.C.; Logsdon, R.G.; McCurry, S.M.; Teri, L. Dimensions of physical frailty and cognitive function in older adults with amnestic mild cognitive impairment. *Ann. Phys. Rehabil. Med.* **2013**, *56*, 329–341. [CrossRef]
11. Fitzpatrick, A.L.; Buchanan, C.K.; Nahin, R.L.; DeKosky, S.T.; Atkinson, H.H.; Carlson, M.C.; Williamson, J.D. Associations of gait speed and other measures of physical function with cognition in a healthy cohort of elderly persons. *J. Gerontol. A Biol. Sci. Med. Sci.* **2007**, *62*, 1244–1251. [CrossRef]
12. Montero-Odasso, M.; Muir, S.W.; Speechley, M. Dual-task complexity affects gait in people with mild cognitive impairment: The interplay between gait variability, dual tasking, and risk of falls. *Arch. Phys. Med. Rehabil.* **2012**, *93*, 293–299. [CrossRef] [PubMed]
13. Doi, T.; Makizako, H.; Shimada, H.; Yoshida, D.; Ito, K.; Kato, T.; Ando, H.; Suzuki, T. Brain atrophy and trunk stability during dual-task walking among older adults. *J. Gerontol. A Biol. Sci. Med. Sci.* **2012**, *67*, 790–795. [CrossRef] [PubMed]
14. Hooghiemstra, A.M.; Ramakers, I.H.G.B.; Sistermans, N.; Pijnenburg, Y.A.L.; Aalten, P.; Hamel, R.E.G.; Melis, R.J.; Verhey, F.R.; Olde Rikkert, M.G.; Scheltens, P.; et al. Gait speed and grip strength reflect cognitive impairment and are modestly related to incident cognitive decline in memory clinic patients with subjective cognitive decline and mild cognitive impairment: Findings from the 4C Study. *J. Gerontol. A Biol. Sci. Med. Sci.* **2017**, *72*, 846–854. [CrossRef] [PubMed]

15. Fried, L.P.; Tangen, C.M.; Walston, J.; Newman, A.B.; Hirsch, C.; Gottdiener, J.; Seeman, T.; Tracy, R.; Kop, W.J.; Burke, G.; et al. Cardiovascular Health Study Collaborative Research G. Frailty in older adults: Evidence for a phenotype. *J. Gerontol. A Biol. Sci. Med. Sci.* **2001**, *56*, M146–M156. [CrossRef] [PubMed]
16. Buchman, A.S.; Boyle, P.A.; Wilson, R.S.; Tang, Y.; Bennett, D.A. Frailty is associated with incident Alzheimer's disease and cognitive decline in the elderly. *Psychosom. Med.* **2007**, *69*, 483–489. [CrossRef] [PubMed]
17. Saji, N.; Sakurai, T.; Suzuki, K.; Mizusawa, H.; Toba, K. ORANGE investigators. ORANGE's challenge: Developing wide-ranging dementia research in Japan. *Lancet Neurol.* **2016**, *15*, 661–662. [CrossRef]
18. Japanese Ministry of Health; Labour and Welfare. Health and Welfare Bureau for the Elderly. Long-Term Care Insurance System of Japan. 2016. Available online: https://www.mhlw.go.jp/english/policy/care-welfare/care-welfare-elderly/dl/ltcisj_e.pdf (accessed on 17 June 2019).
19. Wada-Isoe, K.; Uemura, Y.; Nakashita, S.; Yamawaki, M.; Tanaka, K.; Yamamoto, M.; Shimokata, H.; Nakashima, K. Prevalence of dementia and mild cognitive impairment in the rural island Town of Ama-cho, Japan. *Dement. Geriatr. Cogn. Dis. Extra* **2012**, *2*, 190–199. [CrossRef]
20. Ishikawa, T.; Ikeda, M.; Matsumoto, N.; Shigenobu, K.; Brayne, C.; Tanabe, H. A longitudinal study regarding conversion from mild memory impairment to dementia in a Japanese community. *Int. J. Geriatr. Psychiatry* **2006**, *21*, 134–139. [CrossRef]
21. Makizako, H.; Shimada, H.; Park, H.; Doi, T.; Yoshida, D.; Uemura, K.; Tsutsumimoto, K.; Suzuki, T. Evaluation of multidimensional neurocognitive function using a tablet personal computer: Test-retest reliability and validity in community-dwelling older adults. *Geriatr. Gerontol. Int.* **2013**, *13*, 860–866. [CrossRef]
22. Shimada, H.; Makizako, H.; Doi, T.; Lee, S.; Lee, S. Conversion and reversion rates in Japanese older people with mild cognitive impairment. *J. Am. Med. Dir. Assoc.* **2017**, *18*, e801–e808. [CrossRef] [PubMed]
23. Inoue, M.; Jinbo, D.; Nakamura, Y.; Taniguchi, M.; Urakami, K. Development and evaluation of a computerized test battery for Alzheimer's disease screening in community-based settings. *Am. J. Alzheimers Dis. Other Dement.* **2009**, *24*, 129–135. [CrossRef] [PubMed]
24. Inoue, M.; Jimbo, D.; Taniguchi, M.; Urakami, K. Touch Panel-type Dementia Assessment Scale: A new computer-based rating scale for Alzheimer's disease. *Psychogeriatrics* **2011**, *11*, 28–33. [CrossRef] [PubMed]
25. Mohs, R.C.; Cohen, L. Alzheimer's Disease Assessment Scale (ADAS). *Psychopharmacol. Bull.* **1988**, *24*, 627–628.
26. Faul, F.; Erdfelder, E.; Buchner, A.; Lang, A.G. Statistical power analyses using G*Power 3.1: Tests for correlation and regression analyses. *Behav. Res. Methods* **2009**, *41*, 1149–1160. [CrossRef]
27. Shimada, H.; Makizako, H.; Lee, S.; Doi, T.; Lee, S.; Tsutsumimoto, K.; Harada, K.; Hotta, R.; Bae, S.; Nakakubo, S.; et al. Impact of cognitive frailty on daily activities in older persons. *J. Nutr. Health Aging* **2016**, *20*, 729–735. [CrossRef]
28. Fukutomi, E.; Okumiya, K.; Wada, T.; Sakamoto, R.; Ishimoto, Y.; Kimura, Y.; Chen, W.L.; Imai, H.; Kasahara, Y.; Fujisawa, M.; et al. Relationships between each category of 25-item frailty risk assessment (Kihon Checklist) and newly certified older adults under Long-Term Care Insurance: A 24-month follow-up study in a rural community in Japan. *Geriatr. Gerontol. Int.* **2015**, *15*, 864–871. [CrossRef]
29. Shimada, H.; Makizako, H.; Doi, T.; Yoshida, D.; Tsutsumimoto, K.; Anan, Y.; Uemura, K.; Ito, T.; Lee, S.; Park, H.; et al. Combined Prevalence of Frailty and Mild Cognitive Impairment in a Population of Elderly Japanese People. *J. Am. Med. Dir. Assoc.* **2013**, *147*, 518–524. [CrossRef]
30. Chen, L.K.; Liu, L.K.; Woo, J.; Assantachai, P.; Auyeung, T.W.; Bahyah, K.S.; Chou, M.Y.; Chen, L.Y.; Hsu, P.S.; Krairit, O.; et al. Sarcopenia in Asia: Consensus Report of the Asian Working Group for Sarcopenia. *J. Am. Med. Dir. Assoc.* **2014**, *15*, 95–101. [CrossRef]
31. Makizako, H.; Shimada, H.; Doi, T.; Tsutsumimoto, K.; Suzuki, T. Impact of physical frailty on disability in community-dwelling older adults: A prospective cohort study. *BMJ Open* **2015**, *5*, e008462. [CrossRef]
32. Tsutsumimoto, K.; Doi, T.; Makizako, H.; Hotta, R.; Nakakubo, S.; Makino, K.; Suzuki, T.; Shimada, H. The association between anorexia of aging and physical frailty: Results from the national center for geriatrics and gerontology's study of geriatric syndromes. *Maturitas* **2017**, *97*, 32–37. [CrossRef] [PubMed]
33. Shimada, H.; Makizako, H.; Doi, T.; Tsutsumimoto, K.; Lee, S.; Suzuki, T. Cognitive impairment and disability in older Japanese adults. *PLoS ONE* **2016**, *11*, e0158720. [CrossRef] [PubMed]
34. Kluger, A.; Gianutsos, J.G.; Golomb, J.; Wagner, A., Jr.; Wagner, D.; Scheurich, S. Clinical features of MCI: Motor changes. *Int. Psychogeriatr.* **2008**, *20*, 32–39. [CrossRef] [PubMed]

35. Ravaglia, G.; Forti, P.; Montesi, F.; Lucicesare, A.; Pisacane, N.; Rietti, E.; Dalmonte, E.; Bianchin, M.; Mecocci, P. Mild cognitive impairment: Epidemiology and dementia risk in an elderly Italian population. *J. Am. Geriatr. Soc.* **2008**, *56*, 51–58. [CrossRef]
36. Mizumoto, A.; Ihira, H.; Makino, K.; Saitoh, S.; Ohnishi, H.; Furuna, T. Physical activity changes in the winter in older persons living in northern Japan: A prospective study. *BMC Geriatr.* **2015**, *15*, 43. [CrossRef]
37. Lewy, A.J.; Emens, J.S.; Songer, J.B.; Sims, N.; Laurie, A.L.; Fiala, S.C.; Buti, A.L. Winter depression: Integrating mood, circadian rhythms, and the sleep/wake and light/dark cycles into a bio-psycho-social-environmental model. *Sleep Med. Clin.* **2009**, *4*, 285–299. [CrossRef]
38. Reinvang, I.; Grambaite, R.; Espeseth, T. Executive dysfunction in MCI: Subtype or early symptom. *Int. J. Alzheimers Dis.* **2012**, *2012*, 936272. [CrossRef]
39. Lowry, K.A.; Brach, J.S.; Nebes, R.D.; Studenski, S.A.; VanSwearingen, J.M. Contributions of cognitive function to straight- and curved-path walking in older adults. *Arch. Phys. Med. Rehabil.* **2012**, *93*, 802–807. [CrossRef]
40. Chapman, R.M.; Mapstone, M.; McCrary, J.W.; Gardner, M.N.; Porsteinsson, A.; Sandoval, T.C.; Guillily, M.D.; DeGrush, E.; Reilly, L.A. Predicting conversion from mild cognitive impairment to Alzheimer's disease using neuropsychological tests and multivariate methods. *J. Clin. Exp. Neuropsychol.* **2011**, *33*, 187–199. [CrossRef]
41. Clark, L.R.; Schiehser, D.M.; Weissberger, G.H.; Salmon, D.P.; Delis, D.C.; Bondi, M.W. Specific measures of executive function predict cognitive decline in older adults. *J. Int. Neuropsychol. Soc.* **2012**, *18*, 118–127. [CrossRef]
42. Brooks, B.L.; Strauss, E.; Sherman, E.M.S.; Iverson, G.L.; Slick, D.J. Developments in neuropsychological assessment: Refining psychometric and clinical interpretive methods. *Can. Psychol.* **2009**, *50*, 196–209. [CrossRef]
43. Weston, A.L.; Weinstein, A.M.; Barton, C.; Yaffe, K. Potentially inappropriate medication use in older adults with mild cognitive impairment. *J. Gerontol. A Biol. Sci. Med. Sci.* **2010**, *65*, 318–321. [CrossRef] [PubMed]
44. Perrochon, A.; Kemoun, G. The Walking Trail-Making Test is an early detection tool for mild cognitive impairment. *Clin. Interv. Aging* **2014**, *9*, 111–119. [CrossRef] [PubMed]
45. Mielke, M.M.; Roberts, R.O.; Savica, R.; Cha, R.; Drubach, D.I.; Christianson, T.; Pankratz, V.S.; Geda, Y.E.; Machulda, M.M.; Ivnik, R.J.; et al. Assessing the temporal relationship between cognition and gait: Slow gait predicts cognitive decline in the Mayo Clinic Study of Aging. *J. Gerontol. A Biol. Sci. Med. Sci.* **2013**, *68*, 929–937. [CrossRef] [PubMed]
46. Abe, T.; Kitamura, A.; Taniguchi, Y.; Amano, H.; Seino, S.; Yokoyama, Y.; Nishi, M.; Narita, M.; Ikeuchi, T.; Fujiwara, Y.; et al. Pathway from gait speed to incidence of disability and mortality in older adults: A mediating role of physical activity. *Maturitas* **2019**, *123*, 32–36. [CrossRef] [PubMed]
47. Abellan van Kan, G.; Rolland, Y.; Andrieu, S.; Bauer, J.; Beauchet, O.; Bonnefoy, M.; Cesari, M.; Donini, L.M.; Gillette Guyonnet, S.; Inzitari, M.; et al. Gait speed at usual pace as a predictor of adverse outcomes in community-dwelling older people an International Academy on Nutrition and Aging (IANA) Task Force. *J. Nutr. Health Aging* **2009**, *13*, 881–889. [CrossRef]
48. Kyrdalen, I.L.; Thingstad, P.; Sandvik, L.; Ormstad, H. Associations between gait speed and well-known fall risk factors among community-dwelling older adults. *Physiother. Res. Int.* **2019**, *24*, e1743. [CrossRef]
49. Nakakubo, S.; Doi, T.; Makizako, H.; Tsutsumimoto, K.; Hotta, R.; Kurita, S.; Kim, M.; Suzuki, T.; Shimada, H. Association of walk ratio during normal gait speed and fall in community-dwelling elderly people. *Gait Posture* **2018**, *66*, 151–154. [CrossRef]
50. Veronese, N.; Stubbs, B.; Volpato, S.; Zuliani, G.; Maggi, S.; Cesari, M.; Lipnicki, D.M.; Smith, L.; Schofield, P.; Firth, J.; et al. Association between gait speed with mortality, cardiovascular disease and cancer: A systematic review and meta-analysis of prospective cohort studies. *J. Am. Med. Dir. Assoc.* **2018**, *19*, 981–988. [CrossRef]
51. Rosso, A.L.; Verghese, J.; Metti, A.L.; Boudreau, R.M.; Aizenstein, H.J.; Kritchevsky, S.; Harris, T.; Yaffe, K.; Satterfield, S.; Studenski, S.; et al. Slowing gait and risk for cognitive impairment: The hippocampus as a shared neural substrate. *Neurology* **2017**, *89*, 336–342. [CrossRef]
52. Boyle, P.A.; Wilson, R.S.; Buchman, A.S.; Aggarwal, N.T.; Tang, Y.; Arvanitakis, Z.; Kelly, J.; Bennett, D.A. Lower extremity motor function and disability in mild cognitive impairment. *Exp. Aging Res.* **2007**, *33*, 355–371. [CrossRef] [PubMed]

53. Park, E.Y.; Park, S.M.; Kim, J.H. Psychometric properties of the geriatric quality of life-dementia in older adults with dementia or mild cognitive impairment living in nursing homes. *BMC Geriatr.* **2019**, *19*, 281. [CrossRef] [PubMed]
54. Kelaiditi, E.; Cesari, M.; Canevelli, M.; Van Kan, G.A.; Ousset, P.J.; Gillette-Guyonnet, S.; Ritz, P.; Duveau, F.; Soto, M.E.; Provencher, V.; et al. Cognitive frailty: Rational and definition from an (IANA/IAGG) international consensus group. *J. Nutr. Health Aging* **2013**, *17*, 726–734. [CrossRef] [PubMed]
55. Lee, C.H.; Kim, D.H.; Moon, Y.S. Differential associations between depression and cognitive function in MCI and AD: A cross-sectional study. *Int. Psychogeriatr.* **2019**, *31*, 1151–1158. [CrossRef] [PubMed]
56. Steffens, D.C.; McQuoid, D.R.; Potter, G.G. Amnestic mild cognitive impairment and incident dementia and Alzheimer's disease in geriatric depression. *Int. Psychogeriatr.* **2014**, *26*, 2029–2036. [CrossRef]

17

Relationships between Multimorbidity and Suicidal Thoughts and Plans among Korean Adults

Youn Huh [1], Ga Eun Nam [2,*], Yang-Hyun Kim [2] and Jun Hyung Lee [1,*]

1 Department of Family Medicine, Inje University Ilsan Paik Hospital, College of Medicine, Inje University, 170, Juhwa-ro, Ilsanseo-gu, Goyang-si, Gyeonggi-do, Seoul 10380, Korea
2 Department of Family Medicine, Korea University Anam Hospital, Korea University College of Medicine, 73, Goryeodae-ro, Seongbuk-gu, Seoul 02841, Korea
* Correspondence: namgaaa@daum.net (G.E.N.); leeddoll@naver.com (J.H.L.)

Abstract: Multimorbidity and suicide rates are rising simultaneously among Korean adults. To address this issue, we assessed the association between multimorbidity and suicidal behavior among adults aged ≥19 years in Korea. We analyzed the data from the 2017 Korea National Health and Nutrition Examination Survey. Multimorbidity was defined as experiencing two or more chronic diseases. We compared the presence of suicidal thoughts and plans according to multimorbidity using chi-square test, and examined the associations between multimorbidity and suicidal thoughts and plans using multiple binary logistic regression analyses. Multimorbidity was found in 30.8% of total participants. As the number of chronic diseases increased, the percentage of thoughts and plans tended to increase ($p < 0.001$ and $p = 0.002$). Among participants with multimorbidities, 8.5% had suicidal thoughts, whereas only 3.4% without multimorbidity had such thoughts ($p < 0.001$). Participants with multimorbidity had significantly higher odds of suicidal thoughts (OR = 2.14; 95% CI = 1.54–2.97) and suicidal plans (OR = 2.01; 95% CI = 1.08–3.73) compared to those without multimorbidity after adjusting confounding variables. **Conclusion:** People with multimorbidity had a higher prevalence of suicidal thoughts and plans. Early detection of and intervention for suicidal thoughts and plans are critical for suicide prevention among people with multimorbidity.

Keywords: chronic disease; multimorbidity; suicidal thoughts; suicidal plans

---

1. Introduction

The National Commission on Chronic Illness in the United States defines chronic illness as permanent illnesses accompanied by disability due to complication or injury, and those requiring special training for rehabilitation, long-term protection, monitoring, and treatment [1]. These individuals require continuous and comprehensive medical intervention, and communication and self-care is necessary [2]. Multimorbidity refers to the state of having multiple chronic illnesses simultaneously, potentially mixed with acute illnesses as well [3]. Unlike the concept of co-morbidity, which refers to how the impact of indicator diseases are influenced by co-morbid illnesses, the concept of multimorbidity is firmly centered on individuals with multimorbidity [4].

There has been an increase of chronic illnesses following the extension of longevity in society. As expected, in South Korea the prevalence of chronic illnesses and multimorbidity has been shown to increase with age. An analysis of older adults with one or more chronic illnesses revealed that 70.9% of older adults with chronic illnesses have multimorbidity, reaching an average of 4.1 chronic illnesses [5]. Another study found that older patients with multimorbidity had an average of 5.1 chronic illnesses, whereas patients without multimorbidity tended to have an average of 1.6 [5]. There have been several studies on the definition of multimorbidity [3,6]. Because people with two or more chronic medical conditions are more common than those with three or more chronic medical conditions, former status is more frequently accepted as the definition of multimorbidity [6]. Studies adopting this definition reported that multimorbidity better reflected poor quality of life, impaired functioning, and increased use of medical facilities such as emergency admissions, particularly with higher numbers of coexisting conditions [7–11].

Suicide is one of the leading causes of death worldwide [12]. Among the countries in the Organization for Economic Co-operation and Development (OECD) as of 2012, the suicide rate (per the OECD standard population of 100,000 people) in South Korea was 29.1, which is the highest out of all OECD countries (average is 12.5). The specific risk factors associated with suicide among adults include depression and other mental disorders, illnesses, loss of function, the death of a partner, and other traumatic incidents [13]. By comparison, according to a 2006 report by the World Health Organization (WHO), the general risk factors of suicide include low socioeconomic status, education level, loss of a job, social stress, mental disorders, illnesses, and chronic pain [14,15]. One study found that 34% of people with suicidal thoughts have plans for suicide, 72% of people who plan for suicide actually attempt suicide, and 26% of people who have suicidal thoughts attempt suicide impulsively without having elaborated a prior plan to do so [16]. Therefore, suicidal thoughts and suicidal plans are important when discussing suicide.

Multimorbidity is associated with suicide-related risk, and primary care and mental health clinics need to evaluate for suicide ideation for patients with multimorbidity [17]. To address the impact of these issues, we aimed to investigate the increase in suicide-related variables in multimorbidity among Korean adults. Specifically, we examined the prevalence of suicidal thoughts and plans among adults who participated in the Korea National Health and Nutrition Examination Survey (KNHANES) in 2017, depending on whether they had multimorbidity.

2. Methods

2.1. Participants and Data

Drawing on raw data from the second year of the 7th KNHANES of 2017, we initially selected a total of 8127 individuals. Among them, we excluded people aged ≤18 years (n = 1938) and those who had any missing variables (n = 395), because people under the age of 18 did not perform suicide-related questionnaire in the 7th KNHANES of 2017. Finally, 5794 adults were considered in our analyses.

The KNHANES is a cross-sectional health surveillance system that assesses the status of and trends in national health and nutrition of South Korea to identify vulnerable groups to be prioritized in health policies, as well as evaluate whether existing health policies and projects are effective. It provides data on smoking habits, drinking habits, physical activities, and obesity, as well as various other statistics required by the WHO and OECD. The KNHANES comprises a health interview survey, a nutrition survey, a health examination survey, and data on demographic characteristics, diet, and health collected through personal interviews. Physical examinations along with blood and urine sampling were carried out at a mobile examination center. A stratified, multistage probability sampling design was used to select the household units that participated in the survey [18].

Our study adhered to the principles of the Declaration of Helsinki and was approved by the Institutional Review Board of Ilsan Paik Hospital (No. ISPAIK IRB 12 February 2017). Requirement of informed consent was waived because anonymous and de-identified information was used.

2.2. Research Variables

The chronic illnesses surveyed in the 7th KNHANES included hypertension, dyslipidemia, cerebral infarction (stroke), myocardial infarction, angina, osteoarthritis, rheumatoid arthritis, osteoporosis, tuberculosis, asthma, allergic rhinitis, depression, renal failure, atopic dermatitis, diabetes mellitus, thyroid disease, stomach cancer, liver cancer, colon cancer, breast cancer, cervical cancer, lung cancer, thyroid cancer, other cancers, hepatitis B, hepatitis C, and cirrhosis. Participants who self-reported not currently having a disease or a doctor's diagnosis of a disease were regarded as not having it; by contrast, participants who self-reported having a disease or a doctor's diagnosis of one were defined as having a chronic illness. Of these, stomach cancer, liver cancer, colon cancer, breast cancer, cervical cancer, lung cancer, thyroid cancer, and other cancers were combined into an overarching "cancer" category.

In the mental health section of surveys, participants were asked to answer the following questions (employing answer options of yes, no, or I do not know/no answer): "Have you seriously considered suicide in the last year?" and "Have you seriously planed suicide in the last year?"

People who had smoked at least 100 cigarettes in their lifetime and continued smoking at the time of survey were defined as current smokers. People who consumed at least one alcoholic beverage per month in a year prior to the survey were considered alcohol drinkers and those who did not were considered non-drinkers. Education level was categorized into two groups depending on whether participants had achieved a higher qualification than middle school graduation or not. Monthly personal income level was divided into two groups: the lowest quartile group and the second-lowest to highest quartile group.

2.3. Analysis Method

We combined the raw data from the 2017 KNHANES according to the KNHANES raw data analysis guidelines. Based also on a complex sample design, we conducted all analyses by assigning a dispersed stratification estimation, stratification variables, and weighted sample values. We divided participants who had 2 or more of the above-stated chronic illnesses as multimorbidity based on the definition used in the previous study [6]. Subsequently, a chi-square test was performed to evaluate proportions of suicidal thoughts and plan according to the number of chronic illness or the presence of multimorbidity. Then, to determine the association of suicidal thoughts and plans with multimorbidity, we conducted a multiple binary logistic regression analysis and calculated the odd ratio (OR) and 95% confidence intervals (CIs). Model 1 did not adjust. Model 2 adjusted for sex and age. Model 3 adjusted for sex, age, education, personal income, smoking status, and alcohol consumption. Since there are studies showing that income and education level are related the risk of suicide, we adjusted these variables [14,15]. Stratified analyses according to sex and age were also performed. All analyses were performed using SPSS Statistics 21.0 (IBM Corp., Armonk, NY, USA).

3. Results

3.1. Participants' General Characteristics

Participants' demographics are shown in Table 1. A total of 5794 adults were included. Of the entire sample, 30.8% had multimorbidity. The proportion of patients with multimorbidity increased with age. The proportion of women with multimorbidity was higher than that of men. In addition, the ratio of people with multimorbidity was higher when education level or income was low. Regarding smoking, the percentage of patients with multimorbidity was the highest among ex-smokers. The proportion of patients with multimorbidity was higher in non-drinkers than in drinkers.

Table 1. General characteristics of participants. Data are presented as % (standard error (SE)).

		Without Multimorbidity (n = 4007)		Multimorbidity (n = 1787)		p-Value
		n	% (SE)	n	% (SE)	
Age (years)	19–40	1531	91.7 (0.9)	135	8.3 (0.9)	<0.001
	41–64	1890	73.4 (1.0)	746	26.6 (1.0)	
	≥65	586	39.6 (1.5)	906	60.4 (1.5)	

Table 1. *Cont.*

		Without Multimorbidity (n = 4007)		Multimorbidity (n = 1787)		p-Value
		n	% (SE)	n	% (SE)	
Sex	Male	1836	77.2 (1.0)	723	22.8 (1.0)	<0.001
	Female	2171	72.4 (1.1)	1064	27.6 (1.1)	
Personal income	≤1st quartile	536	52.9 (1.7)	597	47.1 (1.7)	<0.001
	≥2nd quartile	3471	78.8 (0.8)	1190	21.2 (0.8)	
Education (years)	≤9	843	49.7 (1.4)	973	50.3 (1.4)	<0.001
	≥10	3164	82.4 (0.8)	814	17.6 (0.8)	
Smoking status	Never smoker	2491	74.0 (1.1)	1151	26.0 (1.1)	<0.001
	Former smoker	737	70.5 (1.6)	391	29.5 (1.6)	
	Current smoker	779	81.1 (1.4)	245	18.9 (1.4)	
Alcohol consumption	Non-drinker	1605	67.4 (1.2)	1019	32.6 (1.2)	<0.001
	Alcohol drinker	2402	79.9 (0.9)	768	20.1 (0.9)	

3.2. Suicidal Thoughts and Plans According to the Number of Chronic Diseases

Regarding suicidal ideation, 5.0% of participants had suicidal thoughts and 1.3% had suicidal plans. In the absence of chronic diseases, suicidal thoughts were present in 2.7% of the cases, and suicidal plans were present in 0.6%. If the patients had one chronic disease, suicidal thoughts were present in 4.5% of the cases, and suicidal plans were present in 1.6%. Suicidal thoughts and plans were present in 9.7%, and 2.2% of participants who had more than 3 chronic diseases, respectively. As the number of chronic diseases increased, the proportions of suicide thoughts and plans tended to increase ($p < 0.001$ and $p = 0.002$) (Table 2).

Table 2. Suicidal thoughts and plans according to the number of chronic diseases. Data are presented as % (standard error (SE)). * Obtained by using chi-square test.

		Number of Chronic Diseases				
		0 (n = 2348)	1 (n = 1659)	2 (n = 943)	≥3 (n = 844)	p-Value *
Suicidal thoughts (−)	n	2279	1589	877	761	<0.001
	% (SE)	97.3 (0.4)	95.5 (0.7)	92.5 (1.3)	90.3 (1.3)	
Suicidal thoughts (+)	n	69	70	66	83	
	% (SE)	2.7 (0.4)	4.5 (0.7)	7.5 (1.3)	9.7 (1.3)	
Suicidal plans (−)	n	2332	1637	925	824	0.002
	% (SE)	99.4 (0.2)	98.4 (0.4)	98.0 (0.5)	97.8 (0.5)	
Suicidal plans (+)	n	16	22	18	20	
	% (SE)	0.6 (0.2)	1.6 (0.4)	2.0 (0.5)	2.2 (0.5)	

3.3. Suicidal Thoughts and Plans According to the Presence of Multimorbidity

Table 3 shows the relationship between multimorbidity and suicidal thoughts and plans. While 3.4% of adults without multimorbidity were found to have suicidal thoughts, 8.5% of adults with multimorbidity had such thoughts ($p < 0.001$). As for suicide plans, 2.1% of adults with multimorbidity and 1.0% without multimorbidity were found to have them, respectively ($p = 0.003$).

Table 3. Suicidal thoughts and plans among participants with and without multimorbidities. Values are presented as weighted % (standard error (SE)). * Obtained by using chi-square test.

	Without Multimorbidity (n = 4007)		Multimorbidity (n = 1787)		p-Value *
	n	% (SE)	n	% (SE)	
Suicidal thoughts (−)	3868	96.6 (0.4)	1638	91.5 (1.0)	<0.001
Suicidal thoughts (+)	139	3.4 (0.4)	149	8.5 (1.0)	
Suicidal plans (−)	3969	99.0 (0.2)	1749	97.9 (0.4)	0.003
Suicidal plans (+)	38	1.0 (0.2)	38	2.1 (0.4)	

3.4. Multivariable Logistic Regression Analysis Between Multimorbidity and Suicidal Thoughts and Plans

Table 4 presents multivariable logistic regression analysis results regarding the association of multimorbidity with suicidal thoughts and plans. Compared to participants without multimorbidity, participants with multimorbidity had significantly higher odds of suicidal thoughts in all adjusted models (OR, 95% CI: 2.65, 1.95–3.60 in model 1; 2.49, 1.82–3.40 in model 2; 2.14, 1.54–2.97 in model 3). Stratified analysis with sex and age showed similar findings. In men, the odds of suicide thoughts increased by 3.1 times among people with multimorbidity compared to those without multimorbidity after adjusting for all potential variables (OR, 95% CI: 3.09, 1.84–5.20 in model 3). The odds of suicide thoughts increased by 3.2 times in younger people (19–40 years) with multimorbidity compared with those without it (OR, 95% CI: 3.15, 1.43–6.97 in model 3). For suicidal plans, compared to participants without multimorbidity, participants with it had higher chances of suicidal plans (OR, 95% CI: 2.14, 1.30–3.54 in model 1; 2.26, 1.22–4.20 in model 2; 2.01, 1.08–3.73 in model 3). Suicidal plans were 2.3 times more prevalent in women with multimorbidity than in those without multimorbidity (OR, 95% CI: 2.30, 1.07–4.97 in model 2); however, this association was attenuated after further adjustment in model 3. Suicidal plans were 2.5 times more prevalent in middle aged people (41–64 years) with multimorbidity than in those without multimorbidity (OR, 95% CI: 2.54, 1.12–5.77 in model 3). On the other hand, there was no statistically significant association between multimorbidity and suicidal plans among younger or older men.

Table 4. Associations of multimorbidity and suicidal thoughts and plans. OR, odds ratio; CI, confidence interval. Model 1 was not adjusted. Model 2 was adjusted for sex and age. Model 3 was adjusted for sex, age, education, personal income, smoking status, and alcohol consumption. Values were calculated by multivariable logistic regression analysis.

	Suicidal Thoughts OR (95% CI)	p	Suicidal Plans OR (95% CI)	p
Total				
Model 1	2.65 (1.95–3.60)	<0.001	2.14 (1.30–3.54)	0.003
Model 2	2.49 (1.82–3.40)	<0.001	2.26 (1.22–4.20)	0.010
Model 3	2.14 (1.54–2.97)	<0.001	2.01 (1.08–3.73)	0.028
Sex				
Men				
Model 1	3.30 (2.06–5.28)	<0.001	2.33 (1.02–5.30)	0.044
Model 2	3.40 (2.05–5.65)	<0.001	2.29 (0.85–6.20)	0.101
Model 3	3.09 (1.84–5.20)	<0.001	2.00 (0.74–5.45)	0.172
Women				
Model 1	2.18 (1.57–3.04)	<0.001	1.97 (1.06–3.67)	0.032
Model 2	1.92 (1.33–2.76)	0.001	2.30 (1.07–4.97)	0.034
Model 3	1.63 (1.12–2.36)	0.011	2.01 (0.94–4.33)	0.073

Table 4. *Cont.*

	Suicidal Thoughts		Suicidal Plans	
	OR (95% CI)	*p*	OR (95% CI)	*p*
Age (years)				
19–40				
Model 1	3.15 (1.50–6.60)	0.003	2.30 (0.61–8.68)	0.220
Model 2	3.14 (1.50–6.58)	0.003	2.34 (0.62–8.77)	0.207
Model 3	3.15 (1.43–6.97)	0.005	2.04 (0.45–9.18)	0.350
41–64				
Model 1	2.58 (1.65–4.04)	<0.001	3.37 (1.48–7.68)	0.004
Model 2	2.55 (1.63–4.00)	<0.001	3.34 (1.48–7.55)	0.004
Model 3	1.83 (1.17–2.85)	0.008	2.54 (1.12–5.77)	0.026
≥65				
Model 1	1.87 (1.21–2.90)	0.005	1.16 (0.47–2.84)	0.750
Model 2	1.89 (1.21–2.96)	0.005	1.20 (0.48–2.97)	0.697
Model 3	1.89 (1.20–2.98)	0.006	1.20 (0.47–3.10)	0.700

4. Discussion

In this study, it was shown that 30.8% of the total population of the 7th KNHANES has multimorbidity with more than two chronic diseases. As other studies have shown, the prevalence of multimorbidity increases with age, [19] with 60.4% of people aged 65 and older having multimorbidity. The proportion of women found with multimorbidity is overwhelmingly higher than that of men, which is the same as in previous studies [20]. Further, this study found evidence that level of education and smoking and drinking habits are related to multimorbidity.

We verified differences in suicidal thoughts and plans according to whether participants had multimorbidity. A comparative analysis was performed on these two groups drawing on data from the 2017 waves of the 7th KNHANES. Participants who had multimorbidity had a significantly greater prevalence of suicidal thoughts compared to those without such group of diseases. It was also found that the higher the number of chronic diseases, the higher the percentage of suicidal thoughts and suicidal plans.

As life extension continues to increase in South Korea, it has become necessary to change the perception of diseases among adults. This new understanding is essential for properly managing patients with multimorbidity [3]. Multimorbidity is highly likely to occur from polypharmacy, adverse drug side effects, or competing medical recommendations [21–23]. Moreover, if a person has multimorbidity, their risk of suicide appears to increase. The concurrence of chronic illnesses can lead to a decline in functional state and increase in mortality; therefore, more emphasis must be placed on the comprehensive impact of multimorbidity on patients' overall health and quality of life [24].

When a stratified analysis was conducted by age, younger people with multimorbidity were more at risk of suicide than those without multimorbidity. In this study, the associations of multimorbidity with suicidal thoughts in older adults aged over 65 were lower than in other age groups and did not affect suicidal plans. However, the suicide rate among older adults is increasing as the population of this group increases. According to South Korea's statistics for 2014, the suicide rate is approximately 37.5 per 100,000 people aged in their 60s, 57.6 per 100,000 people aged in their 70s, and 78.6 per 100,000 people aged in their 80s, which are all much higher than the rates of 17.8 and 27.9 of people in their 20s and 30s, respectively. These rates indicate that older adults have a higher risk of suicide compared to other age groups [25]. It is also relevant to mention that suicide attempts among older adults are more likely to lead to death compared to other age groups [25,26]. However, unlike suicide in other age groups, suicide among older adults is generally not impulsive, and diverse realistic factors tend to contribute to its occurrence [26,27].

When a stratified analysis was conducted by sex, there was a significant difference of suicidal thoughts according to multimorbidity in men and women. In this study, the associations of multimorbidity with suicidal thoughts in men are higher than in women. This shows that there is a difference in suicide between women and men, corroborating other studies [28–30]. However, suicidal plans according to multimorbidity in men and women did not significantly differ.

Although this study provides reliable basic data on multimorbidity and suicidal thoughts and plans in a representative sample of Koreans, it does not go without limitations. First, because of their nature, cross-sectional studies cannot explain causal relationships between disease status and the various suicide-related relevant variables among adults. Furthermore, we evaluated only the presence of suicidal thoughts in the last year, without considering the frequency of these thoughts. Second, because participants' disease status was recorded based on self-reports, it is possible that biases affected the data. Third, we could not perform a detailed survey of assessed suicidal thoughts and plans, as we relied on previously written questions. In addition, while we might have considered some of the factors that influence suicidal thoughts, we could not account for all confounding variables. Finally, because older adults only accounted for a small proportion of all participants in the KNHANES, there was a major difference in the number of participants between disease groups. Therefore, there is the chance of false negatives and underestimation for some age-related results.

Previous studies have analyzed suicidal thoughts in relation to chronic illnesses; however, this study is unique in verifying whether participants had suicidal thoughts and plans according to whether they had multimorbidity. The presence of suicidal thoughts is a key risk factor for death by suicide. Suicidal behavior often recur in people who have previously attempted suicide, and suicide attempts often occur in people who frequently think about suicide [31,32]. Therefore, to prevent suicide, people with suicidal thoughts must be categorized as a high-risk group for suicide attempts and be cared for accordingly. By extension, it is necessary to consider multimorbidity in suicide prevention measures, as these individuals appear at risk of suicide. Interventions by medical professionals should, therefore, consider these thoughts as reflective of a person's mental health status [33]. Four weeks before suicide death, about 50% visited medical instructions such as outpatients, inpatients, and emergency room visits, and 83% of them visited within one year [34]. Therefore, it is necessary to screen suicidal risk for high-risk patients.

In conclusion, early detection and intervention regarding suicidal thoughts is essential in suicide prevention strategies for older adults with multimorbidity. Further research is needed to determine the suicide-related risk by chronic diseases and any clusters of chronic diseases.

Author Contributions: G.E.N., and Y.H. were the principal investigators. They contributed substantially to the study design, literature search, collection and assembly of data, data analyses and data interpretation. G.E.N., Y.H., and J.H.L. wrote all drafts and the final version of the report. Y.H., and J.H.L. analysed data and created all the tables. G.E.N., Y.H., Y.-H.K., and J.H.L. contributed to the conception and design of the study, the collection and assembly of data, data analyses and data interpretation. All authors contributed to preparation of the report and approved the final version. G.E.N., and J.H.L. had full access to all the data in the study and take responsibility for the integrity of the data and the accuracy of the data analysis and all authors had final responsibility for the decision to submit for publication.

References

1. Choi, Y.S. *Development of a Private Demonstration Model for Those with Frequent Chronic Diseases*, Kungmin Kŏn'gang Pohŏm Kongdan Kŏn'gang Pohŏm Chŏngchaek Yon'guwŏn. 2009.
2. Chung, Y.H.; Ko, S.J.; Kim, E.J. *Research on An Effective Method of Caring for Chronic Diseases*; Korea Institute for Health and Social Affairs: Sejong, Korea, 2013.
3. Van den Akker, M.; Buntinx, F.; Roos, S.; Knottnerus, J.A. Problems in determining occurrence rates of multimorbidity. *J. Clin. Epidemiol.* **2001**, *54*, 675–679. [PubMed]
4. Marengoni, A.; Winblad, B.; Karp, A.; Fratiglioni, L. Prevalence of chronic diseases and multimorbidity among the elderly population in Sweden. *Am. J. Public Health* **2008**, *98*, 1198–1200. [PubMed]
5. Chung, Y.H. Analysis of multiple chronic diseases among the elderly. *Health Welf. Issue Focus* **2013**, *196*, 1–8.

6. Fortin, M.; Bravo, G.; Hudon, C.; Vanasse, A.; Lapointe, L. Prevalence of multimorbidity among adults seen in family practice. *Ann. Fam. Med.* **2005**, *3*, 223–228. [PubMed]
7. Fortin, M.; Bravo, G.; Hudon, C.; Lapointe, L.; Dubois, M.F.; Almirall, J. Psychological distress and multimorbidity in primary care. *Ann. Fam. Med.* **2006**, *4*, 417–422.
8. Fortin, M.; Laponite, L.; Hudon, C.; VAnasse, A.; Ntetu, A.L.; Maltais, D. Multimorbidity and quality of life in primary care: A systematic review. *Health Qual. Life Outcomes* **2004**, *2*, 51. [PubMed]
9. Condelius, A.; Edberg, A.K.; Jakobsson, U.; Hallberg, I.R. Hospital admissions among people 65+ related to multimorbidity, municipal and outpatient care. *Arch. Gerontol. Geriatr.* **2008**, *46*, 41–55.
10. Bayliss, E.A.; Bayliss, M.S.; Ware, J.E.; Steiner, J.F. Predicting declines in physical function in persons with multiple chronic medical conditions: What we can learn from the medical problem list. *Health Qual. Life Outcomes* **2004**, *2*, 47.
11. Marengoni, A.; Angleman, S.; Melis, R.; Mangialasche, F.; Karp, A.; Garmen, A.; Meinow, B.; Fratiglioni, L. Aging with multimorbidity: A systematic review of the literature. *Ageing Res. Rev.* **2011**, *10*, 430–439.
12. World Health Organization. *Prevention of Suicide: Guidelines for the Formulation and Implementation of National Strategies*; World Health Organization: Geneva, Switzerland, 1996.
13. Lapierre, S.; Erlangsen, A.; Waern, M.; De Leo, D.; Oyama, H.; Scocco, P.; Gallo, J.; Szanto, K.; Conwell, Y.; Draper, B.; et al. A systematic review of elderly suicide prevention programs. *Crisis* **2011**, *32*, 88–98. [PubMed]
14. World Health Organization. *Preventing Suicide: A Resource at Work*; World Health Organization: Geneva, Switzerland, 2006.
15. Nock, M.K.; Borges, G.; Bromet, E.J.; Alonso, J.; Angermeyer, M.; Beautrais, A. Cross-national prevalence and risk factors for suicidal ideation, plans and attempts. *Br. J. Psychiatry* **2008**, *192*, 98–105. [PubMed]
16. Kessler, R.C.; Borges, G.; Walters, E.E. Prevalence of and risk factors for lifetime suicide attempts in the National Comorbidity Survey. *Arch. Gen. Psychiatry* **1999**, *56*, 617–626. [PubMed]
17. Kavalidou, K.; Smith, D.J.; O'Connor, R.C. The role of physical and mental health multimorbidity in suicidal ideation. *J. Affect. Disord.* **2016**, *209*, 80–85. [PubMed]
18. Kweon, S.; Kim, Y.; Jang, M.-J.; Kim, Y.; Kim, K.; Choi, S.; Chun, C.; Khang, Y.; Oh, K. Data resource profile: The Korea national health and nutrition examination survey (KNHANES). *Int J. Epidemiol.* **2014**, *43*, 69–77. [PubMed]
19. Fortin, M.; Stewart, M.; Poitras, M.E.; Almirall, J.; Maddocks, H. A systematic review of prevalence studies on multimorbidity: Toward a more uniform methodology. *Ann. Fam. Med.* **2012**, *10*, 142–151. [PubMed]
20. Van den Akker, M.; Buntinx, F.; Metsemakers, J.F.; Roos, S.; Knottnerus, J.A. Multimorbidity in general practice: Prevalence, incidence, and determinants of co-occurring chronic and recurrent diseases. *J. Clin. Epidemiol.* **1998**, *51*, 367–375. [PubMed]
21. Van Weel, C.; Schellevis, F.G. Comorbidity and guidelines: Conflicting interests. *Lancet* **2006**, *367*, 550–551.
22. Smith, S.M.; O'Kelly, S.; O'Dowd, T. GPs' and pharmacists' experiences of managing multimorbidity: A 'Pandora's box'. *Br. J. Gen. Pract.* **2010**, *60*, e285–e294.
23. Guthrie, B.; Payne, K.; Alderson, P.; McMurdo, M.E.; Mercer, S. Adapting clinical guidelines to take account of multimorbidity. *Br. Med. J. BMJ* **2012**, *345*, e6341.
24. Vogeli, C.; Shields, A.E.; Lee, T.A.; Gibson, T.B.; Marder, W.D.; Weiss, K.B.; Blumenthal, D. Multiple chronic conditions: Prevalence, health consequences, and implications for quality, care management, and costs. *J. Gen. Intern. Med.* **2007**, *22*, 391–395.
25. Korea, S. *Cause of Death Statistics 2014*; Statics Korea: Daejeon, Korea, 2014.
26. McIntosh, J.L. Suicide prevention in the elderly (age 65–99). *Suicide Life Threat. Behav.* **1995**, *25*, 180–192.
27. Mościcki, E.K. Epidemiology of suicide. *Int. Psychogeriatr.* **1995**, *7*, 137–148. [PubMed]
28. Lee, S.U.; Oh, I.H.; Jeon, H.J.; Roh, S. Suicide rates across income levels:retrospective cohort data on 1 million participatnts collected between 2003 and 2013 in South Korea. *J. Epidemiol.* **2017**, *27*, 258–264. [PubMed]
29. Chang, S.S.; Gunnell, D.; Sterne, J.A.; Lu, T.H.; Cheng, A.T. Was the economic crisis 1997–1998 responsible for rising suicide rates in East/Southeast Asia? A time-trend analysis for Japan, Hong Kong, South Korea, Taiwan, Singapore and Thailand. *Soc. Sci. Med.* **2009**, *68*, 1322–1331.
30. Hawton, K.; Arensman, E.; Wasserman, D.; Hultén, A.; Bille-Brahe, U.; Bjerke, T.; Crepet, P.; Deisenhammer, E.; Kerkhof, A.; De Leo, D.; et al. Relation between attempted suicide and suicide rates among young people in Europe. *J. Epidemiol. Community Health* **1998**, *52*, 191–194. [PubMed]

31. Bonner, R.L.; Rich, A.R. Toward a predictive model of suicidal ideation and behavior: Some preliminary data in college students. *Suicide Life Threat. Behav.* **1987**, *17*, 50–63.
32. Lester, D. A depression paradox theory of suicide. *Perssonal. Individ. Differ.* **1989**, *10*, 1103–1104.
33. Kim, H.S. A study on epistemology of Korean elder's suicidal thought. *J. Korean Gerontol. Soc.* **2002**, *22*, 159–172.
34. Ahmedani, B.K.; Simon, G.E.; Stewart, C.; Beck, A.; Waitzfelder, B.E.; Rossom, R.; Lynch, F.; Owen-Smith, A.; Hunkeler, E.M.; Whiteside, U.; et al. Health care contacts in the year before suicide death. *J. Gen. Intern. Med.* **2014**, *29*, 870–877.

18

Clinical Validation of Innovative Optical-Sensor-Based, Low-Cost, Rapid Diagnostic Test to Reduce Antimicrobial Resistance

Suman Kapur [1,*,†], Manish Gehani [1,†], Nagamani Kammili [2], Pankaj Bhardwaj [3], Vijayalakshmi Nag [3], Sudha M. Devara [2] and Shashwat Sharad [4,*]

1 Department of Biological Sciences, Birla Institute of Technology and Science, Pilani, Hyderabad Campus, Hyderabad, Telangana 500078, India; dr.manishgehani@gmail.com

2 Department of Microbiology, Gandhi Medical College and Hospital, Hyderabad, Telangana 500003, India; nagamaniy2k03@rediffmail.com (N.K.); sudha_devara@yahoo.com (S.M.D.)

3 All India Institute of Medical Sciences, Jodhpur, Rajasthan 342005, India; pankajbhardwajdr@gmail.com (P.B.); vijayalakshmi005@gmail.com (V.N.)

4 Center for Prostate Disease Research, Department of Surgery, Uniformed Services University of the Health Sciences and the Walter Reed National Military Medical Center, Bethesda, MD 20817, USA

* Correspondence: skapur@hyderabad.bits-pilani.ac.in (S.K.); ssharad@cpdr.org (S.S.);

† Suman Kapur and Manish Gehani contributed equally to this work.

Abstract: The antibiotic susceptibility test determines the most effective antibiotic treatment for bacterial infection. Antimicrobial stewardship is advocated for the rational use of antibiotics to preserve their efficacy in the long term and provide empirical therapy for disease management. Therefore, rapid diagnostic tests can play a pivotal role in efficient and timely treatment. Here, we developed a novel, rapid, affordable, and portable platform for detecting uropathogens and reporting antibiogram to clinicians in just 4 h. This technology replicates the basic tenets of clinical microbiology including bacterial growth in indigenously formulated medium, and measurement of inhibition of bacterial growth in presence of antibiotic/s. Detection is based on chromogenic endpoints using optical sensors and is analyzed by a lab-developed algorithm, which reports sensitivity to the antibiotic's panel tested. To assess its diagnostic accuracy, a prospective clinical validation study was conducted in two tertiary-care Indian hospitals. Urine samples from 1986 participants were processed by both novel/index test and conventional Kirby Bauer Disc Diffusion method. The sensitivity and specificity of this assay was 92.5% and 82%, respectively ($p < 0.0005$). This novel technology will promote evidence-based prescription of antibiotics and reduce the burden of increasing resistance by providing rapid and precise diagnosis in shortest possible time.

Keywords: urinary tract infection; rapid culture; antibiotic susceptibility testing (AST), evidence-based prescription; antibiotics; antimicrobial resistance (AMR), rapid diagnostics

1. Introduction

Healthcare challenges faced by developing countries are vastly different from those in developed nations. With very limited budget for healthcare, developing countries have not been able to put up any significant infrastructure to address their huge disease burden. In vitro diagnostic (IVD) tests provide the basis for most medical decision-making and play crucial role in limiting healthcare costs, since appropriate diagnostic tests performed in a timely manner i) improve patient care, ii) contribute to protecting consumers' health, iii) help to limit healthcare spending, iv) reduce the risk of trial-and-error treatment and over-prescription, v) shorten the time before treatment begins, and vi) decrease the length of hospital stays. Appropriate diagnosis can improve the effectiveness of treatments and avoid long-term complications for the infected patient. India harbors the world's largest burden of drug-resistant pathogens. Easy access, availability, and higher consumption of medicines have led to a disproportionately higher incidence of inappropriate use of antibiotics and greater levels of antimicrobial resistance (AMR) compared to developed countries [1]. It has been shown that the health sector in India suffers from gross inadequacy of funds, which will further result in conditions favorable for the development of drug resistance [2]. The high resistance of pathogens in the country, even to newer antibiotics, has led to the emergence of superbugs like New Delhi Metallo-beta-lactamase (NDM-1) [3]. By 2050, 2 million Indians are projected to die as a result of AMR [3]. Indians are the largest consumers of antibiotics worldwide, despite a decline in communicable diseases [3], due to a liberal policy for over-the-counter sale of antibiotics and irrational prescription of antibiotics. A study by Ganguly et al. highlighted the importance of rationalizing antibiotic use to limit AMR in India [4]. Irrational prescription happens due to a lack of fast point-of-use tests for evidence-based prescription, lack of infrastructure for bacterial culture and antibiotic susceptibility test (AST), and lack of awareness worldwide. Selective pressure from inappropriate use of antibiotics can lead to resistance via the emergence of mutant strains [5]. Unavailability of rapid point-of-use diagnostics to distinguish bacterial infections and suggest appropriate therapy is a major reason for irrational prescriptions of antibiotic/s.

Urinary tract infections (UTIs) lead to 23% of all antibiotic prescriptions in primary healthcare. Even in India, UTIs account for about 8.1 million prescriptions each year. Diagnosis of UTI is a multistep process including determination of pathogen load, identification, and AST requiring culture of sample, which takes around 48–72 h. Even if high-throughput automated systems like Vitek 2, Microscan Walkaway, or Phoenix are used, the results are not available faster than 28 h [6,7]. Conventional urine culture and AST method is not accessible to most clinicians practicing in low-resource settings. Even with access to lab testing facilities, but in the absence of any rapid test, clinicians are forced to prescribe antibiotics empirically. The empirical antibiotics used in the first 48–72 h prove to be ineffective against infection in approximately 33% cases [8–10]. Unresolved, relapsed UTIs tend to be resistant to previously used antibiotics [11]. Nearly 23% to 33% of the prescriptions for UTIs have been found to have no clinical justification [8–10]. Moreover, UTIs are also caused by non-bacterial organisms such as Candida (3% cases) [12], Trichomonas (17% cases) [13], Chlamydia (~16% cases) [14], and rarely Mycobacterium, Schistosoma haematobium, Adenovirus, BK polyomavirus, and mycoplasma [15], and cannot be treated by antibiotics that are empirically prescribed. Such unnecessary drug use is often harmful, and results in multidrug-resistant infections and reduced options for antimicrobial therapy [16]. An urgent need is perceived for developing suitable field operable test for prescribing targeted antibiotics [17]. Addressing the menace of antimicrobial resistance needs a scalable rapid diagnostic test, which gives detection, identification, quantification, and phenotypic antimicrobial susceptibility of bacteria within a minimum turn-around time and has an integrated technology platform for clinical adoption. This test should show high sensitivity and specificity, should be low cost for adoption in low-resource settings, and should be easy to use with minimal training [18,19].

Assays used for upstream screening to improve diagnostic yield of positive samples, like gram staining, dipstick with leukocyte esterase and nitrite, pus cell count [20], urine analysis and microscopy [21], chlorhexidine [22], interleukin-8 [23], Griess test [24], microstix [25], serum procalcitonin level [26], and urine catalase-based uriscreen test [27] have shown poor sensitivity and specificity. Novel antibody-based lateral flow immunoassay (RapidBac) [28], chromogenic limulus amoebocyte lysate assay [29], and flow cytometry-based systems (Accuri-6, UF 100, UF-1000i) [18,30,31] have shown high sensitivity and specificity but they do not provide identification of bacteria and its antimicrobial susceptibility. Forward light scattering systems like Uro-Quick (Alifax) and BacterioScan model 216 (BacterioScan Inc., St. Louis, MO, USA) provide detection of bacteria with antimicrobial susceptibility but do not identify the causative bacteria [32,33].

Molecular and proteomic technologies require overnight incubation on culture plates, and do not provide antimicrobial susceptibility [18]. Matrix Assisted Laser Desorption Ionization-Time Of Flight

(MALDI-TOF) is expensive to install [34], Fluorescence In Situ Hybridization (FISH) requires multiple probes for all uropathogens [18], while multiplex Polymerase Chain Reaction (PCR) platforms like GeneXpert Omni and Cepheid [18] do not provide quantification of significant bacteriuria and need multiple probes for all uropathogens. Application of these test to direct urine testing needs extensive sample preparation.

Genetic signature identification Confirming Active Pathogens Through Unamplified RNA Expression (CAPTURE) assay [35] identifies bacteria but does not give antimicrobial susceptibility. Time-lapse microscopy-based systems like oCelloScope (Phillips BioCell) [36] and Accelerate ID/AST (Accelerate Diagnostics) [37] provide both identification and antimicrobial susceptibility, but phenotypic measures for identification in direct urine are not precise and they are not easy to use in a clinical lab setting. Integrated microfluidic-Biosensor assays based on ion mobility spectrometry or colorimetric sensor arrays are cost effective and sensitive but their results get confounded by urine variability and in presence of low bacterial count [18]. Most of the newer technologies mentioned above are neither easy to use nor affordable in a resource-poor setting like public hospitals of India. In this study, we evaluated a rapid, portable, easy-to-use, less resource-intensive, and affordable technology, which provides bacterial identification and AST results within 4 h. This new technology integrates the basic tenets of clinical microbiology including bacterial growth in a medium optimized for uropathogens and measurement of inhibition of bacterial growth in presence of specific antibiotic, with detection of bacteria based on chromogenic endpoint by enzymatic hydrolysis of specific media cocktails by UTI causing bacteria. The optical sensor-based measurement of endpoint output is analyzed using indigenous software, based on a lab-developed statistical algorithm, which reports both the sensitivity of the pathogen to a customizable panel of antibiotics and bacterial load in the sample. This integrated technology platform can be used for diagnosing UTIs caused by bacteria and for suggesting effective antibiotics in all types of clinical settings as a preliminary triage test [38] to promote evidence-based prescription and minimize irrational use of antibiotics. The low cost of the test obliviates the need for upstream screening with poor sensitivity screening tests and promotes scalability for use in mass population. The objective of the present study was to evaluate the diagnostic accuracy of the novel test in UTI cases as compared to the gold standard urine culture method.

2. Materials and Methods

2.1. Study Design, Setting, and Population

The study was conducted over a 2-year period from January 2017 to December 2018, simultaneously in Gandhi Medical College and Hospital, Secunderabad located in Southern India, and All India Institute of Medical Sciences (AIIMS), Jodhpur located in Northern India. To ensure sufficient case load for achieving required sample size and to ensure that good lab practices are followed, Laboratory of Gandhi Hospital, which is the referral laboratory of State of Telangana, and AIIMS, which is a premiere tertiary care hospital, were chosen for this study.

2.2. Ethical Approval

The study was reviewed and approved by Institutional Ethics Review Committee of both institutions. Objectives of the study were explained to all participants in their native language and they were enrolled after obtaining a written informed consent. The study was conducted according to the principles expressed in the Declaration of Helsinki.

2.3. Study Oversight

This prospective clinical validation study was designed to evaluate diagnostic accuracy of the novel/index test with the reference gold standard urine culture and AST method. Eligible participants were referred by clinicians for urine culture and sensitivity test, based on a provisional diagnosis of UTI. Patients who received antibiotics in the preceding two weeks or had indwelling or suprapubic catheter were excluded. Consenting participants were evaluated in microbiology laboratory by history taking and review of medical records.

2.4. Test Methods for Bacterial Culture and Identification

Clean-catch mid-stream urine samples were collected from each enrolled participant in a sterile container and divided into two parts under sterile conditions. One part was used for routine urine culture and AST and the second for conducting the index test in the hospital premises itself. All samples were processed within 2 h of collection to avoid contamination/bacterial growth.

The index test was the novel test designed for direct quantitative detection and antibiotic sensitivity of bacteria found in human urine [39,40]. The test identifies common UTI-causing bacteria, namely *Escherichia coli*, *Klebsiella*, *Pseudomonas*, *Enterococcus*, *Proteus*, and *Staphylococcus* sp. This rapid method replicates the basic tenets of clinical microbiology, namely (1) growth of bacteria in a specialized medium, and (2) measuring the inhibition of growth of bacteria in the presence of an antibiotic. Detection is based on chromogenic endpoints. The output was analyzed using lab-developed algorithm-based software, which reports the sensitivity of the pathogen to the panel of antibiotics tested. The urine sample was collected in a sterile container. To harvest the bacteria, 10 mL urine was filtered through a sterile syringe with the help of a micro-filter attached to it and filtrate was discarded. After that, BITGEN, specially designed media for accelerated growth of uropathogens, was pushed through the filter in the vial to recover bacteria from the filter, shaken well, and then closed with the dropper cap. The bacteria were harvested in 3 mL of proprietary BITGEN medium. This was then set side at room temperature for about 5 min. Subsequently, four drops (~110–120 μL) of proprietary BITGEN medium containing harvested bacterial suspension was added into all the three strips—one pre-functionalized strip for identification of bacteria and two different 8-well strips, pre-loaded with antibiotics. All the strips were resealed and incubated at 37 °C for 4 h. A 4-h incubation period was found to be sufficient for all commonly found uropathogens accounting for 98% cases of UTIs. The media was optimized for nutrients and supports growth up to 8 h with a start bacterial number of 10^5 cells/mL [39]. BITGEN is a proprietary media that has chromogens sensitive to bacterial growth even at low numbers of bacteria and for rapid culture. The enzymatic hydrolysis of specific media cocktails used in this proprietary media metabolizes the chromogens. For identification of bacteria, the 8 wells in the identification strip had a cocktail of specific substrates, which were metabolized by specific bacterial types. Growth of bacteria in the well led to end product formation during the 4-h incubation. The use of optical sensor enables measuring of all color combinations and the lab-developed analytical software interprets the identification of the bacteria based on specific chromogenic endpoints produced as a consequence of specific metabolic activity of each bacterial type. For both identification and AST, the sample was loaded at the same time and incubated for the same length of time.

To identify susceptibility of pathogen, the above-mentioned two pre-functionalized antibiotic strips were used. Each of the antibiotic strips had 8 compartments and, except the first compartment (or reference well) of each of the two antibiotic strips, all the remaining 14 compartments were subjected to preloading by the chosen antibiotics. The preloaded antibiotics used were Amoxicillin, Gentamicin, Amikacin, Cefepime, Ofloxacin, Ciprofloxacin, Ceftriaxone, Piperacillin-Tazobactum, Cefotaxime, Cefuroxime, Tobramycin, Levofloxacin, Cefazolin, and Imipenem. The concentration and composition of the antibiotics were chosen as per Clinical and Laboratory Standards Institute (CLSI) guidelines [41].

In the case that the urine sample had pathogens, it was reflected in the first well of the antibiotic strips, referred to as the reference well of both the antibiotic strips as there is no inhibition of bacterial growth in this well. As per phenotypic AST of bacteria present, the remaining 14 compartments showed varied levels of bacterial growth depending on the bacterial susceptibility to the chosen antibiotics. The bacterial growth within the preloaded antibiotic compartment was represented by a change in color of the BITGEN, measured by chromogenic and nephelometric endpoints using an array of 64 photodiodes in an electronic optical sensor. The intensity of the color is a measure of the number of growing cells in the presence and absence of a particular antibiotic. The sensor output was analyzed using a proprietary lab-developed statistical algorithm, pre-installed on the reader, which provides ready-to-use results for sensitivity of the pathogen to the antibiotics tested, both as a display on liquid crystal display (LCD) screen and a printout for permanent records. The reader was also enabled to transfer results to other storage devices using a wireless module and/or a universal serial bus (USB) interface. In case of insufficient growth, the analytical software prompts for incubating for one additional hour and then if no growth is detected, the software reports the sample to be negative for presence of bacteria.

Further, for reference, standard universally accepted, conventional gold standard urine culture and Kirby Bauer method for AST was chosen. First, 10 μL of each urine sample was streaked on a chromogenic culture medium, chromID® CPS Elite Translucent using a calibrated ni-chrome wire loop of 4 mm by semi-quantitative method using surface streaking. The inoculated plates were incubated for 18–24 h at 37 °C. After incubation, in case growth of colonies was up to the tertiary streaking, it was considered as significant bacteriuria with 10^5 Colony Forming Units (CFU)/mL. Positive cultures were further processed for determining the AST by Kirby Bauer Disc Diffusion Method as per Clinical and Laboratory Standards Institute guidelines [41]. A suspension of each isolate was prepared to a McFarland standard and spread over Muller Hilton Agar using lawn culture method. Himedia discs with defined concentrations of antibiotics were placed over the culture. After incubation for 18 to 24 h at 37 °C, zones of growth inhibition around each antibiotic disc were measured to the nearest millimeter and a reference table was used to determine susceptibility. The American Type Culture Collection (ATCC) bacterial strains, namely *Enterococcus faecalis*, *Escherichia coli*, *Klebsiella pneumoniae*, *Pseudomonas aeruginosa*, and *Staphylococcus aureus*, were used for quality control in the entire process.

The cut-off for labelling both index as well as reference test as positive was pre-specified as 10^5 CFU/mL based on Infectious Diseases Society of America guidelines [42]. Neither the team performing the index test nor the one conducting urine culture and sensitivity was provided any clinical information about the participant/s. Both teams were also not informed about the results of the other test and, hence, the index test was conducted in a completely blinded manner.

2.5. Data Analysis

Collected data and results from both tests for each participant were compiled and analyzed by Statistical Package for the Social Sciences (SPSS) software (version 24). A contingency table was used for determining diagnostic accuracy and kappa statistics was used for agreement analysis. Further, 95% confidence interval (CI) was used to describe diagnostic accuracy, with p values of <0.05 considered as significant. Sample size was calculated to be 600 for estimating the sensitivity of the index test, based on a precision of 4% and confidence level of 95%, when the sensitivity of the new test was expected to be at least 50%. "Best-case scenario method" was used for indeterminate results and mixed growth. Samples with rare species, budding yeast cells, and contaminated samples were removed from final analysis for a "complete case analysis". No analysis of variability in diagnostic accuracy was performed with respect to age group or department, as it was not pre-specified in the study. The raw data generated from the study which was used to analyze these results has been made publicly available as a safe harbor file in online repository "Harvard Dataverse" [43].

2.6. Reagents

Analytical-grade chemicals required for preparation of BITGEN, identification strips, and antibiotic strips were procured from Sigma Chemicals, St Louis, MO, USA. Chromogenic culture media, Muller Hilton media, and antibiotic discs were procured from Himedia, India; chromID® CPS Elite Translucent from BioMérieux, France; 8-well strips and syringe filters from NUNC, Denmark; sterile syringes from Dispovan, India. The scanner/reader machine for novel test was obtained from Micro Lab Instruments,

Ahmedabad, India. The bacterial strains *Enterococcus faecalis* (ATCC29212), *Escherichia coli* (ATCC25922), *Klebsiella pneumoniae* (ATCC13883), *Pseudomonas aeruginosa* (ATCC27853), and *Staphylococcus aureus* (ATCC25923) were purchased from Himedia, India.

3. Results

3.1. Study Characteristics

Overall, 2001 eligible participants (1030 in AIIMS and 971 in Gandhi Hospital) were identified and 1986 participants (1022 in AIIMS and 964 in Gandhi Hospital) were enrolled in the study. Data of 1835 participants (982 in AIIMS and 853 in Gandhi Hospital) were included in the final analysis. A total of 55 samples (20 from AIIMS and 35 from Gandhi Hospital) with low sample volume could not be processed by the index test.

There were no indeterminate results reported by the index test in both the hospitals. One hundred and eleven participants (97 in AIIMS and 14 in Gandhi Hospital) with indeterminate reference standard urine culture results were reported as having no bacterial growth and were reclassified as true negatives using best-case scenario. Samples with mixed growth in both index and reference standard tests were considered positive for UTI. Fifty-five samples (5 from AIIMS and 50 from Gandhi Hospital) were reported as contaminated and not considered for final analysis. Since the index test is designed for identifying the most common bacteria only, 19 samples (6 from AIIMS and 13 from Gandhi Hospital) with budding yeast cells and 22 samples (9 from AIIMS and 13 from Gandhi Hospital) with rare bacteria (*Citrobacter*, *Acinetobacter*, *Morganella*, and *Providencia*) were also excluded from the final analysis. Thus, a total of 96 cases were excluded from final analysis after performing both tests (Figure 1). Table 1 summarizes the mean age, gender distribution, and referring departments. The majority of participants had cystitis, and more male patients were referred at AIIMS than Gandhi Hospital. Ninety-seven cases (10%) cases in AIIMS cohort and nine cases (1%) in Gandhi Hospital cohort had progressed to frank pyelonephritis.

Table 1. Characteristics of participants.

Characteristics	AIIMS [1] (n = 982)	Gandhi (n = 853)
Demographic characteristics		
Age (in years)		
Mean age	43.4	35.7
Minimum age	<1	1
Maximum age	95	90
Gender		
Male	631 (64.3%)	399 (46.8%)
Female	351 (35.7%)	454 (53.2%)
Referring Department		
Medical Specialties	193	481
Surgical Specialties	632	94
Pediatrics	67	138
Obstetrics and Gynecology	87	140
Radio-diagnosis	3	0
Clinical Syndrome		
Pyelonephritis	10%	1%
Cystitis	90%	99%

[1] AIIMS = All India Institute of Medical Sciences.

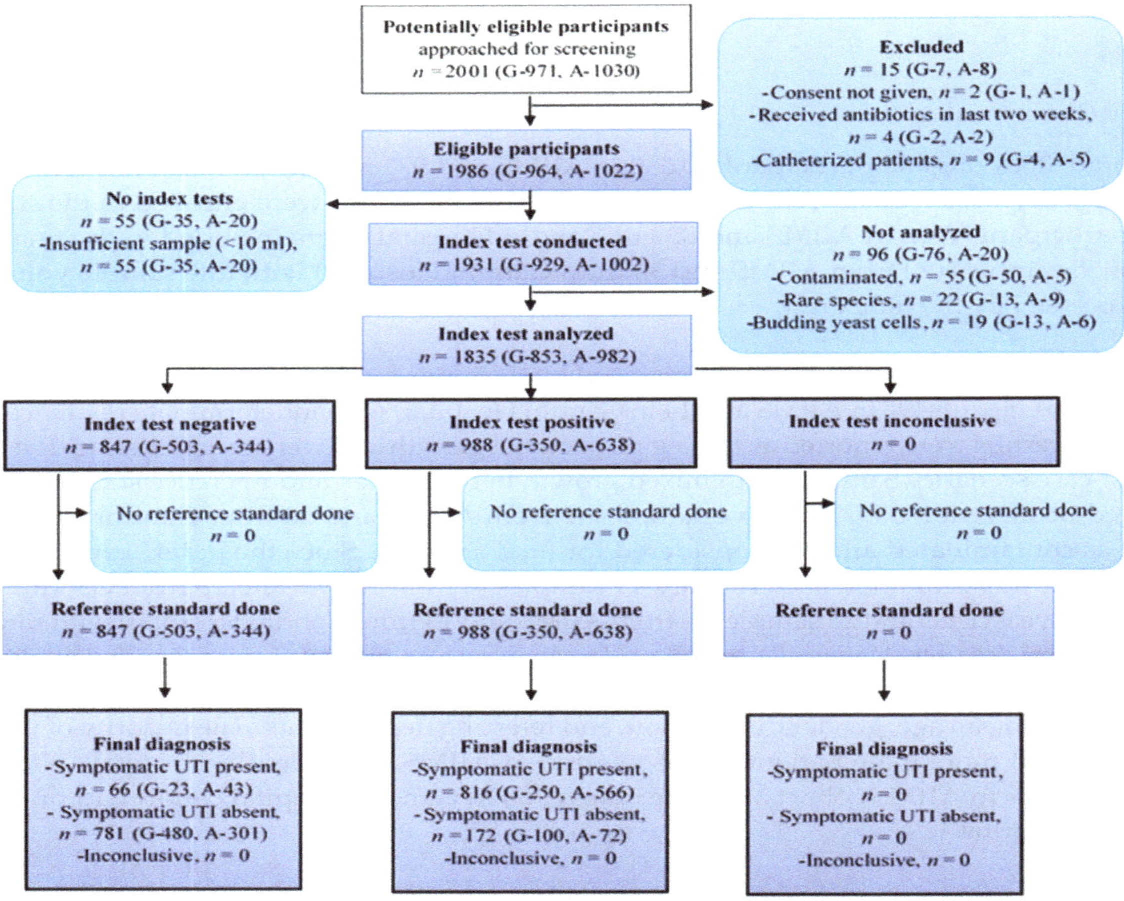

Figure 1. Flow of participants through the study—Standards for Reporting Diagnostic Accuracy (STARD) diagram (G = Gandhi Hospital, A = AIIMS).

3.2. *Test Performance*

There was no time gap between processing of samples by both tests. No adverse event occurred while performing index test or reference standard test since only urine sample collection was involved. In AIIMS, 609 cases, while in Gandhi Hospital, 273 cases, were diagnosed with symptomatic UTI based on positive culture results by conventional method. Furthermore, 953 participants (373 in AIIMS and 580 in Gandhi Hospital) with symptoms of UTI, showed low colony count on culture plates. Out of these, the index test reported 172 cases (72 in AIIMS and 100 in Gandhi Hospital) as positive, which were otherwise reported as negative by conventional method, 48 h post incubation.

3.2.1. Diagnostic Accuracy

AIIMS cohort showed a higher sensitivity (92.9%) while Gandhi Hospital cohort showed a marginally higher specificity (82.8%). The sensitivity and specificity in both the validation sites were within 95% confidence interval of the other hospital (Table 2). The sensitivity and specificity obtained by use of the novel test was well within the stipulated limits laid down in the recommendations issued by the European Urinalysis Guidelines for rapid tests.

Table 2. Comparison of test results obtained by novel test and urine culture method.

Contingency Tables			
AIIMS ($n = 982$)	**Urine Culture Positive**	**Urine Culture Negative**	**Total**
Index test Positive	566 (92.9%)	72 (19.3%)	638
Index test Negative	43 (7.1%)	301 (80.7%)	344
Total	609	373	982
Gandhi ($n = 853$)	**Urine Culture Positive**	**Urine Culture Negative**	**Total**
Index test Positive	250 (91.6%)	100 (17.2%)	350
Index test Negative	23 (8.4%)	480 (82.8%)	503
Total	273	580	853
Combined ($n = 1835$)	**Urine Culture Positive**	**Urine Culture Negative**	**Total**
Index test Positive	816 (92.5%)	172 (18.0%)	988
Index test Negative	66 (7.5%)	781 (82.0%)	847
Total	882	953	1835
Diagnostic Accuracy			
Parameters	**AIIMS ($n = 982$)**	**Gandhi ($n = 853$)**	**Combined ($n = 1835$)**
Sensitivity	92.9% (95% CI: 90.6–94.8%)	91.6% (95% CI: 87.6–94.6%)	92.5% (95% CI: 90.6–94.2%)
Specificity	80.7% (95% CI: 76.3–84.6%)	82.8% (95% CI: 79.4–85.8%)	82.0% (95% CI: 79.4–84.3%)
Agreement Analysis			
Parameters	**AIIMS ($n = 982$)**	**Gandhi ($n = 853$)**	**Combined ($n = 1835$)**
Kappa value [1]	0.748	0.692	0.741
Standard error [1]	0.022	0.025	0.016
p value	<0.0005	<0.0005	<0.0005

[1] Kappa value and its standard error measures agreement between results of two dichotomous variables (here two diagnostic tests providing positive or negative results).

3.2.2. Agreement Analysis

Good agreement was observed at both validation sites, as seen by a Kappa = 0.741. The observed agreement is statistically significant as reflected by a p value of <0.0005.

3.3. Identification of Bacteria

The index test correctly reported the causative bacteria as reported positive by urine culture in 82% cases in AIIMS cohort and 80% cases in Gandhi Hospital cohort (Table 3). In Gandhi Hospital, four cases of *Streptococcus* were not reported by the index test as it is not designed to identify the same. Out of 17 mixed growth in Gandhi cohort, the index test identified seven as individual bacteria, while among 49 in AIIMS cohort, it identified 41 as individual bacteria.

Table 3. Identification of bacteria in the two cohorts.

Identification of Bacteria (Single Species Identification)							
AIIMS	*E. coli*	*Enterococcus*	*Klebsiella*	*Proteus*	*Staphylococcus*	*Pseudomonas*	**Total**
"n" (based on urine culture)	324	104	79	4	1	48	560
% correct identification by index test	93%	74%	68%	75%	100%	48%	82%
Gandhi	*E. coli*	*Enterococcus*	*Klebsiella*	*Proteus*	*Staphylococcus*	*Pseudomonas*	**Total**
"n" (based on urine culture)	92	22	100	8	22	8	252
% correct identification by index test	85%	82%	83%	63%	50%	88%	80%

3.4. Antibiotic Susceptibility

The index test used the same set of 14 antibiotics for every sample, while AIIMS and Gandhi Hospital laboratories used specific antibiotics based on identified bacteria. Hence, only a subset of antibiotics overlapped for both tests. Further, as the conventional method relied on the choice of antibiotics by the microbiologist in-charge, sets of antibiotics tested in both tests were also not used for all the samples tested. Antibiotics tested for at least 30 samples in both the tests were included in analysis presented in Table 4. The rapid index test correctly reported sensitivity and resistance to antibiotics in 91% and 96% cases, respectively, in AIIMS cohort, and these numbers were 87% in the case of sensitivity to tested antibiotics and 92% in the case of resistance to antibiotics reported for the Gandhi Hospital cohort.

Table 4. Comparison of antibiotic susceptibility report in the two cohorts using both tests.

		AIIMS		
	AIIMS Result	**Total Tests Done Together**	**Agreement in Results**	**Disagreement in Results**
Gentamycin	R	149	141 (95%) [a]	8 (5%) [b]
	S	259	237 (92%) [a]	22 (8%) [c]
	I	7	0	7 [d]
Amikacin	R	65	65 (100%) [a]	0 [b]
	S	29	26 (90%) [a]	3 (10%) [c]
	I	3	0	3 [d]
Ciprofloxacin	R	49	43 (88%) [a]	6 (12%) [b]
	S	1	1 (100%) [a]	0 [c]
	I	0	0	0 [d]
Ceftriaxone	R	269	263 (98%) [a]	6 (2%) [b]
	S	99	85 (86%) [a]	14 (14%) [c]
	I	4	0	4 [d]
Piperacillin-Tazobactum	R	121	118 (98%) [a]	3 (2%) [b]
	S	286	266 (93%) [a]	20 (7%) [c]
	I	22	0	22 [d]
Cefazolin	R	34	24 (71%) [a]	10 (29%) [b]
	S	12	10 (83%) [a]	2 (17%) [c]
	I	0	0	0 [d]
Imipenem	R	56	56 (100%) [a]	0 [b]
	S	21	19 (90%) [a]	2 (10%) [c]
	I	3	0	3 [d]
Overall	R	743	710 (96%) [a]	33 (4%) [b]
	S	707	644 (91%) [a]	63 (9%) [c]
		Gandhi		
	Gandhi Result	**Total Tests Done Together**	**Agreement in Results**	**Disagreement in Results**
Gentamycin	R	56	54 (96%) [a]	2 (4%) [b]
	S	120	103 (86%) [a]	17 (14%) [c]
	I	0	0	0 [d]
Amikacin	R	12	12 (100%) [a]	0 [b]
	S	27	23 (85%) [a]	4 (15%) [c]
	I	0	0	0 [d]
Cefepime	R	35	34 (97%) [a]	1 (3%) [b]
	S	10	8 (80%) [a]	2 (20%) [c]
	I	0	0	0 [d]
Piperacillin-Tazobactum	R	13	12 (92%) [a]	1 (8%) [b]
	S	21	20 (95%) [a]	1 (5%) [c]
	I	0	0	0 [d]
Cefotaxime	R	28	28 (100%) [a]	0 [b]
	S	14	14 (100%) [a]	0 [c]
	I	0	0	0 [d]
Levofloxacin	R	23	15 (65%) [a]	8 (35%) [b]
	S	8	6 (75%) [a]	2 (25%) [c]
	I	0	0	0 [d]
Cefazolin	R	56	50 (89%) [a]	6 (11%) [b]
	S	20	18 (90%) [a]	2 (10%) [c]
	I	0	0	0 [d]
Overall	R	223	205 (92%) [a]	18 (8%) [b]
	S	220	192 (87%) [a]	28 (13%) [c]

R = Resistant; S = Sensitive; and I= Intermediate; a—complete agreement, b—very major error, c—major error, and d—minor error. (Same test results either susceptible or resistant by both tests, were classified as "complete agreement" and result reported as resistant by culture and susceptible by novel test was labelled as "very major error"; susceptible by culture but resistant by novel test was labelled as "major error"; intermediate by culture and susceptible or resistant by novel test was labelled as "minor error"). Please note that no intermediate results were reported by novel test and by Gandhi Hospital culture reports.

4. Discussion

Treating patients, including UTIs caused by bacteria, is a challenging task, and development of rapid AST is very important to provide better healthcare services. Use of microbiological culture method and Kirby–Bauer disc diffusion tests are well established for diagnosis of UTIs in healthcare facilities worldwide. However, this entire method needs trained microbiologists and its major limitations are long turn-around time, resource intensiveness in the form of lab infrastructure, and requirement of cold chain for supply and storage of reagents [44]. In resource-constrained settings with poor or limited access to laboratory-based testing, performing urine culture and AST is not feasible. Therefore, initial antibiotic therapy in infectious diseases such as UTIs which accounts for ~40% cases of all infections as per World Health Organization (WHO), is mostly empirical. Hence, an alternative method, like the index test described herein, for reporting antibiotic sensitivity in a short period of 4 h, with no ancillary resource requirement, will not only be beneficial for patient care, but also curtail unnecessary antibiotic prescriptions. Additionally, availability of results in 4 h saves the repeat visit of patients to collect lab reports made available only after three days under best conditions and often even longer in remote and hard-to-reach geographical locations.

The high-cost, resource-intensive, non-portable, most commonly used automated systems Vitek 2 and MicroScan Walkaway provide AST and identification results in more than 28 h [6,7]. Reports evaluating the susceptibility of only Gram-negative bacilli to 11 antibacterial using these two systems showed the results in 92.7% of isolates and overall concurrence with the standard test being 94% with a 3.4% major error rate [45]. With reference to preventing emergence of resistance to antibiotics, they still pose a major limitation in terms of time taken to complete the identification and antibiogram profile of UTI causing pathogen. Most of the newer technologies tried for UTI [18] are facing limitations like the need for an overnight incubation, extensive initial sample preparation, need for an upstream screening test, and lack of integrated technology platform for clinical adoption. These technologies are expensive and not easy to use. Most of them do not give antimicrobial susceptibility. Previously tried strip-based tests also showed less sensitivity [46]. Even automated urine analyzers have resulted in low sensitivity [47]. In comparison, this index test is portable, can be used in all healthcare settings, costs less than 0.4 million INR (~5000 USD), needs no ancillary equipment or dedicated space, and provides ready-to-use antibiogram results and microbial identification within 4 h. The sensitivity and limitation of other tests are summarized in Table 5. The higher sensitivity, >90%, and specificity, >80%, of the index test, with kappa values indicating very good agreement with gold reference standard test, show that it has good diagnostic accuracy as a rapid test [48] for its role as a preliminary triage test and its intended use of diagnosing bacteriuria and preventing irrational prescription of antibiotics. Although the gold standard for diagnosing UTI remains as urine culture, the high cost, laboratory requirements, and long turnaround times (24–72 h) are its disadvantages. Further, in this type of testing, recognition and classification of bacteria is associated with the experience of laboratory technicians. The novel/index test developed is a simpler system and shows better agreement (Kappa = 0.741, significant substantial agreement) with the gold standard and is therefore best suited for routine use in clinical laboratories.

This novel test correctly identified sensitivity to multiple antibiotics in more than 75% instances (and in several cases with 100% accuracy), which then becomes the basis for evidence-based, rational use of antibiotics for specific therapy. The availability of results within 4 h will discourage unnecessary prescription of antibiotics in case of absence of bacterial disease and help the physician to prescribe antibiotics that are identified to be effective against the causative pathogen.

Table 5. Accuracy of different methods for estimating presence of bacteria.

Sl. No.	Method	Sensitivity	Specificity	Detection of Bacteriuria	Identification of Bacteria	Antibiotic Susceptibility	Limitations	Reference
1	MALDI-TOF	67% to 86%	Nearly 60%	Yes	Yes	No	Overnight incubation needed, expensive, extensive sample preparation	[18]
2	FISH	>96%	>96%	Yes	Yes	No	Requires multiple probes for all pathogens	[18]
3	PCR	82%	60%	Yes	Yes	No	Does not provide quantification, needs extensive initial processing and multiple probes	[18]
4	Integrated microfluidics-biosensor systems	91% to 95%	95% to 99%	Yes	Yes	Yes	Confounded results by urine variability and low bacterial count	[18]
5	Gram staining	85.1%	98.9%	Yes	No	No		[20]
6	Dipstick with nitrite & leucocyte esterase	53.1%	100%	Yes	No	No		[20]
7	Pus cell count	42.5%	95.5%	Yes	No	No		[20]
8	Urine analysis and microscopy	46.4%	89%	Yes	No	No		[21]
9	Chlorhexidine	100%	54%	Yes	No	No		[22]
10	Interleukin-8	70%	67%	Yes	No	No		[23]
11	Griess test	63.3%	99.5%	Yes	No	No		[24]
12	Serum procalcitonin level	30%	100%	Yes	No	No		[26]
13	Uriscreen Test	100%	68.6%	Yes	No	No		[27]
14	Antibody-based Lateral flow immunoassay	86%	94%	Yes	No	No		[28]
15	Chromogenic amoebocyte lysate assay	88.7%	98.7%	Yes	No	No		[29]
16	Flow cytometry-based systems	99%	58%	Yes	No	No		[30,31]
17	Genetic signature identification CAPTURE assay	100%	90%	Yes	Yes	No	Expensive, resource intensive, infrastructure, highly skilled manpower	[35]
18	Time-lapse microscopy	96% (agreement)	96% (agreement)	Yes	Yes	Yes	Imprecise phenotypic identification measures in direct urine, not easy-to-use	[36,37]
19	Kirby Bauer Method	51%	99%	No	No	Yes	Time-consuming, resource intense, and not user-friendly	[41,42]

Table 5. *Cont.*

Sl. No.	Method	Sensitivity	Specificity	Detection of Bacteriuria	Identification of Bacteria	Antibiotic Susceptibility	Limitations	Reference
20	Semiquantitative culture method	72.7%	95.7%	Yes	Yes	Yes	Time-consuming, resource intense, and not user-friendly	[44]
21	Quantitative culture method	59.3%	94.4%	Yes	Yes	Yes	Time-consuming, resource intense, and not user-friendly	[44]
22	Strip-based Urinalysis DongJiu	31.1%	91.8%	Yes	No	No		[46]
23	Automated Urinalysis system (URISED)	47%	91.1%	Yes	No	No		[47]
24	Detection of bacteriuria by a non-culture method	90% to 95%	90% to 95%	Not Applicable	Not Applicable	Not Applicable	European Guidelines for Urinalysis	[48]
25	Detection of bacteriuria by a rapid non-culture method	80% to 90%	80% to 90%	Not Applicable	Not Applicable	Not Applicable	European Guidelines for Urinalysis	[48]
26	Index Test	91.6 to 93.8%	80.7 to 96.7%	Yes	Yes	Yes	User-friendly, portable, affordable, rapid-fastest available, no special training required	Data from current study described above

The incidence of UTI from this hospital-based study may not be generalized over the entire population as the present study was conducted in tertiary hospitals to enroll enough participants in the shortest possible time and simultaneous comparison with reference gold standard test without any loss of time in processing or transport of collected samples. Due to the conventional practice in microbiology labs on the choice of antibiotics, which may also be governed by the availability of antibiotics discs, antibiotics could be compared for sensitivity in a subgroup of samples tested. In spite of this, the novel test reported resistance to antibiotics with an accuracy of 80% to 100%, except for two antibiotics, cefazolin (71%) and levofloxacin (65%). This was primarily seen in samples with more than one bacterial entity with a high probability of quorum sensing, impacting the sensitivity to the given antibiotic/s.

Rapid assay described herein determines the efficacy of an antibiotic not only in the shortest possible time, but also with literally no dependence on trained manpower and lab infrastructure. Although this novel test is suitable for use in all healthcare settings, it can prove to be of immense and unsurpassable value for healthcare facilities in low-resource settings due to features like portability, point-of-use testing, and no additional requirements. A consensus using Delphi technique, obtained from experts regarding criteria required for an acceptable point-of-care test for UTI detection, was reported by Weir et al. [49]. This novel test fulfils 25 out of 26 accepted criteria, except for just one, i.e., use of small sample volume. The novel test also fulfils six out of seven of the WHO's ASSURED criteria for ideal characteristics for a point-of-care test in resource-limited settings, the sole unfulfilled one being equipment free, and also matches all the revised criteria suggested by Paul et al. [50]. Effective diagnosis is a prerequisite for successful therapy, and early and accurate diagnosis results in timely and appropriate treatment.

5. Conclusions

In conclusion, it can be said that this novel test, with high sensitivity and specificity for detecting bacterial UTI and reporting antibiogram, can be used as a triage test for diagnosing UTIs and suggesting appropriate treatment for an evidence-based prescription for antibiotics in any kind of healthcare settings. In the wake of growing AMR, the prevalent "lack of priority for diagnostics over treatment" needs to be addressed urgently and this novel test enables physicians and labs to achieve this by adopting this affordable and portable IVD test before prescribing antibiotics for treatment of infectious diseases.

Author Contributions: Conceptualization, S.K., and S.S.; methodology, M.G.; software, S.K.; validation, M.G., S.K., N.K., P.B.,V.N., and S.M.D.; formal analysis, M.G.; investigation, M.G. and S.M.D.; resources, S.K., N.K., and V.N.; data curation, P.B. and M.G.; writing—original draft preparation, M.G., S.K., and S.S.; writing—review and editing, M.G., S.K., and S.S.; visualization, S.K. and S.S.; supervision, S.K., S.S., N.K., P.B., V.N., and S.M.D.; project administration, M.G., V.N., S.M.D., and S.K.; funding acquisition, S.K.

Acknowledgments: We gratefully acknowledge the support provided by the Government of Telangana supported Microbiology Department of Gandhi Medical College and All India Institute of Medical Sciences, Jodhpur for conducting the study and providing space and facilities for hosting the index test in their premises. We also acknowledge the support of Mr. M. Rajesh Bhatt, the lab technician for coordinating sample collection at Gandhi Hospital. Technical help from the technicians in Genomics Laboratory of BITS Pilani, Hyderabad Campus is also gratefully acknowledged.

References

1. World Health Organization. *The World Health Report 1996: Fighting DISEASE, Fostering Development*; Report of the Director-General; World Health Organization: Geneva, Switzerland, 1996.
2. Lal, P. *Report of the National Commission on Macroeconomics and Health*; Report of the National Commission on Health; Ministry of Health and Family Welfare: New Delhi, India, 2005.
3. Dixit, A.; Kumar, N.; Kumar, S.; Trigun, V. Antimicrobial Resistance: Progress in the Decade since Emergence of New Delhi Metallo-β-Lactamase in India. *Indian J. Community Med.* **2019**, *44*, 4–8. [PubMed]
4. Ganguly, N.K.; Arora, N.K.; Chandy, S.J.; Fairoze, M.N.; Gill, J.P.S.; Gupta, U.; Hossain, S.; Joglekar, S.; Joshi, P.C.; Kakkar, M.; et al. Rationalizing antibiotic use to limit antibiotic resistance in India. *Indian J. Med. Res.* **2011**, *134*, 281–294. [PubMed]
5. Baquero, F. Low-level antibacterial resistance: A gateway to clinical resistance. *Drug Resist. Updat.* **2001**, *4*, 93–105. [CrossRef] [PubMed]
6. Eigner, U.; Schmid, A.; Wild, U.; Bertsch, D.; Fahr, A.-M. Analysis of the comparative workflow and performance characteristics of the VITEK 2 and Phoenix systems. *J. Clin. Microbiol.* **2005**, *43*, 3829–3834. [CrossRef] [PubMed]
7. Thomson, K.S.; Cornish, N.E.; Hong, S.G.; Hemrick, K.; Herdt, C.; Moland, E.S. Comparison of Phoenix and VITEK 2 extended-spectrum-beta-lactamase detection tests for analysis of Escherichia coli and Klebsiella isolates with well-characterized beta-lactamases. *J. Clin. Microbiol.* **2007**, *45*, 2380–2384. [CrossRef]
8. Dolk, F.C.K.; Pouwels, K.B.; Smith, D.R.M.; Robotham, J.V.; Smieszek, T. Antibiotics in primary care in England: Which antibiotics are prescribed and for which conditions? *J. Antimicrob. Chemother.* **2018**, *73*, ii2–ii10. [CrossRef]
9. Chua, K.-P.; Fischer, M.A.; Linder, J.A. Appropriateness of outpatient antibiotic prescribing among privately insured US patients: ICD-10-CM based cross sectional study. *BMJ* **2019**, *364*, k5092. [CrossRef]
10. Schmiemann, G.; Kniehl, E.; Gebhardt, K.; Matejczyk, M.M.; Hummers-Pradier, E. The diagnosis of urinary tract infection: A systematic review. *Deutsches Ärzteblatt Int.* **2010**, *107*, 361–367.
11. Kim, H.Y.; Lee, S.-J.; Lee, D.S.; Yoo, J.M.; Choe, H.-S. Microbiological Characteristics of Unresolved Acute Uncomplicated Cystitis. *Microb. Drug Resist.* **2016**, *22*, 387–391. [CrossRef]
12. Seifu, W.D.; Gebissa, A.D. Prevalence and antibiotic susceptibility of Uropathogens from cases of urinary tract infections (UTI) in Shashemene referral hospital, Ethiopia. *BMC Infect. Dis.* **2018**, *18*, 30. [CrossRef]
13. Chang, P.-C.; Hsu, Y.-C.; Hsieh, M.-L.; Huang, S.-T.; Huang, H.-C.; Chen, Y. A pilot study on Trichomonas vaginalis in women with recurrent urinary tract infections. *Biomed. J.* **2016**, *39*, 289–294. [CrossRef] [PubMed]
14. Frej-Mądrzak, M.; Teryks-Wołyniec, D.; Jama-Kmiecik, A.; Sarowska, J.; Choroszy-Król, I. Diagnosing Chlamydia Trachomatis Urinary Tract Infections—Preliminary Report. *Adv. Clin. Exp. Med.* **2015**, *24*, 441–445. [CrossRef] [PubMed]
15. Lee, J.B.L.; Neild, G.H. Urinary tract infection. *Medicine* **2007**, *35*, 423–428. [CrossRef]
16. Mathai, E.; Thomas, R.J.; Chandy, S.; Mathai, M.; Bergstrom, S. Antimicrobials for the treatment of urinary tract infection in pregnancy: Practices in southern India. *Pharmacoepidemiol. Drug Saf.* **2004**, *13*, 645–652. [CrossRef] [PubMed]
17. U.S. Preventive Services Task Force. Screening for asymptomatic bacteriuria in adults: Reaffirmation recommendation statement. *Am. Fam. Phys.* **2010**, *81*, 505.
18. Davenport, M.; Mach, K.E.; Shortliffe, L.M.D.; Banaei, N.; Wang, T.-H.; Liao, J.C. New and developing diagnostic technologies for urinary tract infections. *Nat. Rev. Urol.* **2017**, *14*, 296–310. [CrossRef]
19. Gehani, M.; Kapur, S.; Bhardwaj, P.; Nag, V.; Balasubramaniam, S.; Kammili, N.; Madhuri, S. Unmet need of antenatal screening for asymptomatic bacteriuria: A risk factor for adverse outcomes of pregnancy. *Indian J. Community Med.* **2019**, *44*, 193. [CrossRef]
20. Jayalakshmi, J.; Jayaram, V.S. Evaluation of various screening tests to detect asymptomatic bacteriuria in pregnant women. *Indian J. Pathol. Microbiol.* **2008**, *51*, 379–381. [CrossRef]
21. Van Nostrand, J.D.; Junkins, A.D.; Bartholdi, R.K. Poor Predictive Ability of Urinalysis and Microscopic Examination to Detect Urinary Tract Infection. *Am. J. Clin. Pathol.* **2000**, *113*, 709–713. [CrossRef]
22. Okusanya, B.O.; Aigere, E.O.S.; Eigbefoh, J.O.; Okome, G.B.O.; Gigi, C.E. Is a chlorhexidine reaction test better than dipsticks to detect asymptomatic bacteriuria in pregnancy? *J. Obstet. Gynaecol.* **2014**, *34*, 21–24. [CrossRef]

23. Shelton, S.D.; Boggess, K.A.; Kirvan, K.; Sedor, F.; Herbert, W.N. Urinary interleukin-8 with asymptomatic bacteriuria in pregnancy. *Obstet. Gynecol.* **2001**, *97*, 583–586. [PubMed]
24. Mathews, J.E.; George, S.; Mathews, P.; Mathai, E.; Brahmadathan, K.N.; Seshadri, L. The Griess test: An inexpensive screening test for asymptomatic bacteriuria in pregnancy. *Aust. N. Z. J. Obstet. Gynaecol.* **1998**, *38*, 407–410. [CrossRef] [PubMed]
25. Archbald, F.J.; Verma, U.; Tejani, N.A. Screening for asymptomatic bacteriuria with Microstix. *J. Reprod. Med.* **1984**, *29*, 272–274. [PubMed]
26. Bilir, F.; Akdemir, N.; Ozden, S.; Cevrioglu, A.S.; Bilir, C. Increased serum procalcitonin levels in pregnant patients with asymptomatic bacteriuria. *Ann. Clin. Microbiol. Antimicrob.* **2013**, *12*, 25. [CrossRef] [PubMed]
27. Waisman, Y.; Zerem, E.; Amir, L.; Mimouni, M. The Validity of the Uriscreen Test for Early Detection of Urinary Tract Infection in Children. *Pediatrics* **1999**, *104*, e41. [CrossRef]
28. Stapleton, A.E.; Cox, M.E.; DiNello, R.K.; Geisberg, M.; Abbott, A.; Roberts, P.L.; Hooton, T.M. Performance of a New Rapid Immunoassay Test Kit for Point-of-Care Diagnosis of Significant Bacteriuria. *J. Clin. Microbiol.* **2015**, *53*, 2805–2809. [CrossRef]
29. Nachum, R.; Arce, J.J.; Berzofsky, R.N. Gram-negative bacteriuria of pregnancy: Rapid detection by a chromogenic Limulus amoebocyte lysate assay. *Obstet. Gynecol.* **1986**, *68*, 215–219.
30. Moshaver, B.; de Boer, F.; van Egmond-Kreileman, H.; Kramer, E.; Stegeman, C.; Groeneveld, P. Fast and accurate prediction of positive and negative urine cultures by flow cytometry. *BMC Infect. Dis.* **2016**, *16*, 211. [CrossRef]
31. Duong, H.P.; Wissing, K.M.; Tram, N.; Mascart, G.; Lepage, P.; Ismaili, K. Accuracy of Automated Flow Cytometry-Based Leukocyte Counts to Rule Out Urinary Tract Infection in Febrile Children: A Prospective Cross-Sectional Study. *J. Clin. Microbiol.* **2016**, *54*, 2975–2981. [CrossRef]
32. Hale, D.C.; Wright, D.N.; McKie, J.E.; Isenberg, H.D.; Jenkins, R.D.; Matsen, J.M. Rapid screening for bacteriuria by light scatter photometry (Autobac): A collaborative study. *J. Clin. Microbiol.* **1981**, *13*, 147–150.
33. Jenkins, R.D.; Hale, D.C.; Matsen, J.M. Rapid semiautomated screening and processing of urine specimens. *J. Clin. Microbiol.* **1980**, *11*, 220–225. [PubMed]
34. Tran, A.; Alby, K.; Kerr, A.; Jones, M.; Gilligan, P.H. Cost Savings Realized by Implementation of Routine Microbiological Identification by Matrix-Assisted Laser Desorption Ionization-Time of Flight Mass Spectrometry. *J. Clin. Microbiol.* **2015**, *53*, 2473–2479. [CrossRef] [PubMed]
35. O'Keefe, L.C.; Koelle, P.; McGee, Z.; Dewberry, L.S.; Wright, C.; Stallings, J.E.; Gates, E.; Chittur, K. Innovations in Worksite Diagnosis of Urinary Tract Infections and the Occupational Health Nurse. *Workplace Health Saf.* **2019**, *67*, 268–274. [CrossRef] [PubMed]
36. Fredborg, M.; Rosenvinge, F.S.; Spillum, E.; Kroghsbo, S.; Wang, M.; Sondergaard, T.E. Rapid antimicrobial susceptibility testing of clinical isolates by digital time-lapse microscopy. *Eur. J. Clin. Microbiol. Infect. Dis.* **2015**, *34*, 2385–2394. [CrossRef] [PubMed]
37. Price, C.S.; Kon, S.E.; Metzger, S. Rapid antibiotic susceptibility phenotypic characterization of Staphylococcus aureus using automated microscopy of small numbers of cells. *J. Microbiol. Methods* **2014**, *98*, 50–58. [CrossRef] [PubMed]
38. Bossuyt, P.M.; Irwig, L.; Craig, J.; Glasziou, P. Comparative accuracy: Assessing new tests against existing diagnostic pathways. *BMJ* **2006**, *332*, 1089–1092. [CrossRef]
39. Kapur, S.; Gupta, S. Indigenous rapid diagnostic technology for antibiotic susceptibility testing in urinary tract infection: From bench side to bedside. *BMJ Innov.* **2017**, *3*, 7–11. [CrossRef]
40. Kapur, S.; Gupta, S.; Dv, P.; Pal, A.; Pant, J.; Jain, R. Rapid Sensor Based Technology: A Novel Tool for Direct Antimicrobial Susceptibility Testing in Urinary Tract Infection. *Transl. Med. Biotecnol.* **2014**, *2*, 22–28.
41. Clinical and Laboratory Standards Institute (CLSI). *Performance Standards for Antimicrobial Susceptibility Testing*, 26th ed.; CLSI Supplement M100S; Clinical and Laboratory Standards Institute: Wayne, PA, USA, 2016; ISBN1 56238-923-8, ISBN2 56238-924-6.
42. Infectious Diseases Society of America; American Society of Nephrology; American Geriatric Society; Nicolle, L.E.; Bradley, S.; Colgan, R.; Rice, J.C.; Schaeffer, A.; Hooton, T.M. Infectious Diseases Society of America Guidelines for the Diagnosis and Treatment of Asymptomatic Bacteriuria in Adults. *Clin. Infect. Dis.* **2005**, *40*, 643–654. [CrossRef]
43. Gehani, M.; Kapur, S. Rapid Diagnostic Test for Antimicrobial Susceptibility. *Harv. Dataverse* **2019**, *V1*. [CrossRef]

44. Riboli, D.F.M.; Lyra, J.C.; Silva, E.P.; Valadão, L.L.; Bentlin, M.R.; Corrente, J.E.; de Souza Rugolo, L.M.S.; de Souza, M.D.L.R. Diagnostic accuracy of semi-quantitative and quantitative culture techniques for the diagnosis of catheter-related infections in newborns and molecular typing of isolated microorganisms. *BMC Infect. Dis.* **2014**, *14*, 283. [CrossRef] [PubMed]
45. Salmanzadeh-Ahrabi, S.; Kocagöz, T. Evaluation of a liquid-phase colorimetric method for rapid antibacterial susceptibility testing. *Iran. J. Microbiol.* **2013**, *5*, 259–262. [PubMed]
46. Kocer, D.; Sariguzel, F.M.; Ciraci, M.Z.; Karakukcu, C.; Oz, L. Diagnostic Accuracy of a New Urinalysis System, DongJiu, for Diagnosis of Urinary Tract Infection. *Ann. Clin. Lab. Sci.* **2015**, *45*, 686–691. [PubMed]
47. Huysal, K.; Budak, Y.U.; Ulusoy Karaca, A.; Aydos, M.; Kahvecioğlu, S.; Bulut, M.; Polat, M. Diagnostic accuracy of urised automated urine microscopic sediment analyzer and dipstick parameters in predicting urine culture test results. *Biochem. Medica* **2012**, *23*, 211–217. [CrossRef]
48. Kouri, T.; Fogazzi, G.; Gant, V.; Hallander, H.; Hofmann, W.; Guder, W.G. European Urinalysis Guidelines. *Scand. J. Clin. Lab. Investig. Suppl.* **2000**, *60*, 1–96. [CrossRef]
49. Weir, N.-J.M.; Pattison, S.H.; Kearney, P.; Stafford, B.; Gormley, G.J.; Crockard, M.A.; Gilpin, D.F.; Tunney, M.M.; Hughes, C.M. Criteria required for an acceptable point-of-care test for UTI detection: Obtaining consensus using the Delphi technique. *PLoS ONE* **2018**, *13*, e0198595. [CrossRef]
50. Drain, P.K.; Hyle, E.P.; Noubary, F.; Freedberg, K.A.; Wilson, D.; Bishai, W.R.; Rodriguez, W.; Bassett, I.V. Diagnostic point-of-care tests in resource-limited settings. *Lancet Infect. Dis.* **2014**, *14*, 239–249. [CrossRef]

Permissions

All chapters in this book were first published by MDPI; hereby published with permission under the Creative Commons Attribution License or equivalent. Every chapter published in this book has been scrutinized by our experts. Their significance has been extensively debated. The topics covered herein carry significant findings which will fuel the growth of the discipline. They may even be implemented as practical applications or may be referred to as a beginning point for another development.

The contributors of this book come from diverse backgrounds, making this book a truly international effort. This book will bring forth new frontiers with its revolutionizing research information and detailed analysis of the nascent developments around the world.

We would like to thank all the contributing authors for lending their expertise to make the book truly unique. They have played a crucial role in the development of this book. Without their invaluable contributions this book wouldn't have been possible. They have made vital efforts to compile up to date information on the varied aspects of this subject to make this book a valuable addition to the collection of many professionals and students.

This book was conceptualized with the vision of imparting up-to-date information and advanced data in this field. To ensure the same, a matchless editorial board was set up. Every individual on the board went through rigorous rounds of assessment to prove their worth. After which they invested a large part of their time researching and compiling the most relevant data for our readers.

The editorial board has been involved in producing this book since its inception. They have spent rigorous hours researching and exploring the diverse topics which have resulted in the successful publishing of this book. They have passed on their knowledge of decades through this book. To expedite this challenging task, the publisher supported the team at every step. A small team of assistant editors was also appointed to further simplify the editing procedure and attain best results for the readers.

Apart from the editorial board, the designing team has also invested a significant amount of their time in understanding the subject and creating the most relevant covers. They scrutinized every image to scout for the most suitable representation of the subject and create an appropriate cover for the book.

The publishing team has been an ardent support to the editorial, designing and production team. Their endless efforts to recruit the best for this project, has resulted in the accomplishment of this book. They are a veteran in the field of academics and their pool of knowledge is as vast as their experience in printing. Their expertise and guidance has proved useful at every step. Their uncompromising quality standards have made this book an exceptional effort. Their encouragement from time to time has been an inspiration for everyone.

The publisher and the editorial board hope that this book will prove to be a valuable piece of knowledge for researchers, students, practitioners and scholars across the globe.

List of Contributors

Hélène Gardeney, Arthur Bobin, Cécile Gruchet, Florence Sabirou, Anthony Lévy, Laly Nsiala, Laura Cailly, Cécile Tomowiak, Jose Torregrosa, Niels Moya and Stéphanie Guidez
Service d'Hematologie et Therapie Cellulaire, and Inserm CIC U1402, 86000 Poitiers, France

Cyrille Hulin
Service d'Hématologie et de Thérapie Cellulaire, CHU de Bordeaux, 33000 Bordeaux, France

Xavier Leleu
Service d'Hematologie et Therapie Cellulaire, and Inserm CIC U1402, 86000 Poitiers, France
Service d'Hématologie et Thérapie Cellulaire, Universite de Medecine et Pharmacie, 33000 Poitiers, France

Tina Wang, Sariah Liu, Thomas Joseph and Yung Lyou
Department of Medical Oncology & Experimental Therapeutics, City of Hope Comprehensive Cancer Center, Duarte, CA 91010, USA

Arturo Cuomo, Marco Cascella, Cira Antonietta Forte, Sabrina Bimonte and Gennaro Esposito
Division of Anesthesia and Pain Medicine, Istituto Nazionale Tumori, IRCCS. Fondazione G. Pascale, 80131 Napoli, Italy

Stefano De Santis
Palliative Care and Oncologic Pain Service, S. Camillo-Forlanini Hospital, 00149 Rome, Italy

Luigi Cavanna
Department of Oncology-Hematology, G. da Saliceto Hospital, 29121 Piacenza, Italy

Flavio Fusco
Palliative Home Care Unit, ASL 3, 16153 Genova, Italy

Mario Dauri and Silvia Natoli
Department of Anesthesiology and Resuscitation, II University of Rome, Tor Vergata, 00133 Roma, Italy

Marco Maltoni
Palliative Care Unit, Istituto Scientifico Romagnolo per lo Studio e la Cura dei Tumori (IRST) IRCCS, 47014 Meldola, Italy

Alessandro Morabito
Medical Oncology Unit, Istituto Nazionale Tumori, IRCCS. Fondazione G. Pascale, 80131 Napoli, Italy

Rocco Domenico Mediati
Palliative Care and Pain Therapy Unit, University Hospital Careggi, 50134 Firenze, Italy

Vito Lorusso
UO Oncologia Medica, Istituto Tumori "G Paolo II", 70124 Bari, Italy

Sandro Barni
Oncology Unit, ASST Bergamo Ovest, 24047 Treviglio, Italy

Giampiero Porzio
Medical Oncology Unit, San Salvatore Hospital, University of L'Aquila, 67100 L'Aquila, Italy

Sebastiano Mercadante
Main regional center for Pain Relief & Supportive Care, La Maddalena Cancer Center, 90146 Palermo, Italy

Anna Crispo
Epidemiology and Biostatistics Unit, Istituto Nazionale Tumori, IRCCS. Fondazione G. Pascale, 80131 Napoli, Italy

Ricardo Jorge Dinis-Oliveira
IINFACTS—Institute of Research and Advanced Training in Health Sciences and Technologies, Department of Sciences, University Institute of Health Sciences (IUCS), CESPU, CRL, 4585-116 Gandra, Portugal
Department of Public Health and Forensic Sciences, and Medical Education, Faculty of Medicine, University of Porto, 4200-319 Porto, Portugal
UCIBIO-REQUIMTE, Laboratory of Toxicology, Department of Biological Sciences, Faculty of Pharmacy, University of Porto, 4050-313 Porto, Portugal

Teresa Magalhães
IINFACTS—Institute of Research and Advanced Training in Health Sciences and Technologies, Department of Sciences, University Institute of Health Sciences (IUCS), CESPU, CRL, 4585-116 Gandra, Portugal
Department of Public Health and Forensic Sciences, and Medical Education, Faculty of Medicine, University of Porto, 4200-319 Porto, Portugal
Fidelidade—Companhia de Seguros, SA, R. Direita de Campinas 324, 4100-207 Porto, Portugal

Jing Guo
School of Public Health, Peking University, Beijing 100191, China

Se Hee Lee, Chae-Man Lim, Younsuck Koh, Sang-Bum Hong and Jin Won Huh
Department of Pulmonary and Critical Care Medicine, Asan Medical Center, University of Ulsan College of Medicine, 88, Olympic-ro 43-gil, Songpa-gu, Seoul 05505, Korea

Roman Jurik and Petr Stastny
Department of Sport, Faculty of Physical Education and Sport, Charles University, 162 52 Prague, Czech Republic

Shangyuan Ye
Department of Population Medicine, Harvard Pilgrim Health Care Institute and Harvard Medical School, Boston, MA 02115, USA

Hui Zhang
Division of Biostatistics, Department of Prevention Medicine, Northwestern University Feinberg School of Medicine, Chicago, IL 60611, USA

Fuyan Shi and Suzhen Wang
School of Public Health and Management,Weifang Medical University, Weifang, Shandong 261053, China

Bo Zhang
Department of Neurology and ICCTR Biostatistics and Research Design Center, Boston Children's Hospital and Harvard Medical School, Boston, MA 02115, USA

Hao-Hsien Lee
Department of General Surgery, Chi Mei Medical Center, Liouying 73657, Taiwan

Chong-Chi Chiu
Department of General Surgery, Chi Mei Medical Center, Liouying 73657, Taiwan
Department of General Surgery, Chi Mei Medical Center, Tainan 71004, Taiwan
Department of Electrical Engineering, Southern Taiwan University of Science and Technology, Tainan 71005, Taiwan

Ding-Ping Sun
Department of General Surgery, Chi Mei Medical Center, Tainan 71004, Taiwan

King-Teh Lee
Division of Hepatobiliary Surgery, Department of Surgery, Kaohsiung Medical University Hospital, Kaohsiung 80708, Taiwan
Department of Healthcare Administration and Medical Informatics, Kaohsiung Medical University, Kaohsiung 80708, Taiwan

Jhi-Joung Wang
Department of Medical Research, Chi Mei Medical Center, Tainan 71004, Taiwan

Chien-Cheng Huang
Department of Emergency Medicine, Chi Mei Medical Center, Tainan 71004, Taiwan
Department of Senior Services, Southern Taiwan University of Science and Technology, Tainan 71005, Taiwan

Hon-Yi Shi
Department of Healthcare Administration and Medical Informatics, Kaohsiung Medical University, Kaohsiung 80708, Taiwan
Department of Business Management, National Sun Yat-sen University, Kaohsiung 80424, Taiwan
Department of Medical Research, Kaohsiung Medical University Hospital, Kaohsiung 80708, Taiwan

Aelee Jang
Department of Nursing, University of Ulsan, 93, Daehak-ro, Nam-gu, Ulsan 44610, Korea

Yang Cao
Clinical Epidemiology and Biostatistics, School of Medical Sciences, Orebro University, 70182 Orebro, Sweden

Mustafa Raoof, Johan Ottosson and Ingmar Näslund
Department of Surgery, Faculty of Medicine and Health, Orebro University, 70182 Orebro, Sweden

Scott Montgomery
Clinical Epidemiology and Biostatistics, School of Medical Sciences, Orebro University, 70182 Orebro, Sweden
Clinical Epidemiology Division, Department of Medicine, Karolinska Institutet, 17177 Stockholm, Sweden
Department of Epidemiology and Public Health, University College London, London WC1E 6BT, UK

Jong-Han Lee and Juwon Kim
Department of Laboratory Medicine, Yonsei University Wonju College of Medicine, Wonju 26426, Korea

Tae Hwa Go and Dae Ryong Kang
Center of Biomedical Data Science, Institute of Genomic Cohort, Yonsei University Wonju College of Medicine, Wonju 26426, Korea

San-Hui Lee
Department of Obstetrics and Gynecology, Yonsei University Wonju College of Medicine, Wonju 26426, Korea

Ji Hye Huh and Jang Young Kim
Department of Internal Medicine, Yonsei University Wonju College of Medicine, Wonju 26426, Korea

Seongmun Jeong
Genome Editing Research Center, Korea Research Institute of Bioscience and Biotechnology, Daejeon 34141, Korea

Sang-Baek Koh
Department of Preventive Medicine and Institute of Occupational and Environmental Medicine, Wonju College of Medicine, Yonsei University, Wonju 26426, Korea

Jung Ran Choi
Institute of Genomic Cohort, Yonsei University Wonju College of Medicine, Wonju 26426, Korea

Sunga Kong
Department of Clinical Research Design and Evaluation, SAIHST, Sungkyunkwan University, Seoul 06351, Korea
Patient-Centered Outcomes Research Institute, Samsung Medical Center, Seoul 06351, Korea

Jae Kyung Lee and Genehee Lee
Patient-Centered Outcomes Research Institute, Samsung Medical Center, Seoul 06351, Korea

Hye Yun Park and O Jung Kwon
Division of Pulmonary and Critical Care Medicine, Department of Medicine, Samsung Medical Center, Sungkyunkwan University School of Medicine, Seoul 06351, Korea

Danbee Kang
Department of Clinical Research Design and Evaluation, SAIHST, Sungkyunkwan University, Seoul 06351, Korea
Center for Clinical Epidemiology, Samsung Medical Center, Sungkyunkwan University School of Medicine, Seoul 06351, Korea

Young Mog Shim and Jae Ill Zo
Department of Thoracic and Cardiovascular Surgery, Samsung Medical Center, Sungkyunkwan University School of Medicine, Seoul 06351, Korea

Juhee Cho
Department of Clinical Research Design and Evaluation, SAIHST, Sungkyunkwan University, Seoul 06351, Korea
Center for Clinical Epidemiology, Samsung Medical Center, Sungkyunkwan University School of Medicine, Seoul 06351, Korea
Departments of Epidemiology and Health, Behavior and Society, Johns Hopkins Bloomberg School of Public Health, Baltimore, MD 21205, USA

Eric Chiwei Shiao
Graduate Institute of Biomedical Electronics and Bioinformatics, National Taiwan University, Taipei 10617, Taiwan

Po-Ling Kuo
Graduate Institute of Biomedical Electronics and Bioinformatics, National Taiwan University, Taipei 10617, Taiwan
Department of Electrical Engineering, Department of Physical Medicine and Rehabilitation, College of Medicine, Health Science and Wellness Center, National Taiwan University, Taipei 10617, Taiwan

Fuu-Cheng Jiang and Chao-Tung Yang
Department of Computer Science, Tunghai University, No. 1727, Section 4, Taiwan Boulevard, Taichung 40704, Taiwan

Yun-Ming Wang
Department of Biological Science and Technology, National Chiao Tung University, No. 1001, Daxue Rd, Hsinchu 30010, Taiwan

Yi-Ju Chiang
Information and Communication Research Division, National Chung-Shan Institute of Science & Technology, Taoyuan 32546, Taiwan

Cheng-Min Shih
Department of Biological Science and Technology, National Chiao Tung University, No. 1001, Daxue Rd, Hsinchu 30010, Taiwan
Department of Orthopedics, Taichung Veterans General Hospital, No. 1650, Section 4, Taiwan Boulevard, Taichung 40705, Taiwan

Cheng-Hung Lee
Department of Orthopedics, Taichung Veterans General Hospital, No. 1650, Section 4, Taiwan Boulevard, Taichung 40705, Taiwan
Department of Food Science and Technology, Hung Kuang University, No. 1018, Section 6, Taiwan Boulevard, Taichung 43302, Taiwan

Kaechang Park
Research Organization for Regional Alliance, Kochi University of Technology, Kochi 782-0003, Japan

Kiyotaka Nemoto, Keitaro Yoshida, Masashi Tamura and Tetsuaki Arai
Department of Psychiatry, Faculty of Medicine, University of Tsukuba, Tsukuba 305-8575, Japan

Yoshinori Yamakawa
ImPACT Program of Council for Science, Technology and Innovation (Cabinet Office, Government of Japan), Tokyo 100-8974, Japan

Fumio Yamashita and Makoto Sasaki
Division of Ultrahigh Field MRI, Institute for Biomedical Sciences, Iwate Medical University, Morioka 028-3694, Japan

Atsushi Kawaguchi
Center for Comprehensive Community Medicine, Faculty of Medicine, Saga University, Saga 849-8501, Japan

Yu Kume
Department of Occupational Therapy, Graduate School of Medicine, Akita University, Akita 010-8543, Japan

Tomoko Takahashi
Integrated Community Support Center, Public Health and Welfare Department, City Hall of Yokote, Akita 013- 0525, Japan

Yuki Itakura and Hidetaka Ota
Advanced Research Center for Geriatric and Gerontology, Akita University, Akita 010-8543, Japan

Sangyoon Lee and Hiroyuki Shimada
Center for Gerontology and Social Science, National Center for Geriatrics and Gerontology, Obu, Aichi 474-8511, Japan

Tsuyosi Ono
Omori Municipal Hospital, Akita 013-0525, Japan

Hyuma Makizako
Department of Physical Therapy, School of Health Sciences, Faculty of Medicine, Kagoshima University, Kagoshima 890-8544, Japan

Youn Huh and Jun Hyung Lee
Department of Family Medicine, Inje University Ilsan Paik Hospital, College of Medicine, Inje University, 170, Juhwa-ro, Ilsanseo-gu, Goyang-si, Gyeonggi-do, Seoul 10380, Korea

Ga Eun Nam and Yang-Hyun Kim
Department of Family Medicine, Korea University Anam Hospital, Korea University College of Medicine, 73, Goryeodae-ro, Seongbuk-gu, Seoul 02841, Korea

Suman Kapur and Manish Gehani
Department of Biological Sciences, Birla Institute of Technology and Science, Pilani, Hyderabad Campus, Hyderabad, Telangana 500078, India

Sudha M. Devara and Nagamani Kammili
Department of Microbiology, Gandhi Medical College and Hospital, Hyderabad, Telangana 500003, India

Pankaj Bhardwaj and Vijayalakshmi Nag
All India Institute of Medical Sciences, Jodhpur, Rajasthan 342005, India

Shashwat Sharad
Center for Prostate Disease Research, Department of Surgery, Uniformed Services University of the Health Sciences and the Walter Reed National Military Medical Center, Bethesda, MD 20817, USA

Index